Allergic Diseases: Clinical Advances

Allergic Diseases: Clinical Advances

Edited by **Kevin Parker**

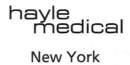

New York

Published by Hayle Medical,
30 West, 37th Street, Suite 612,
New York, NY 10018, USA
www.haylemedical.com

Allergic Diseases: Clinical Advances
Edited by Kevin Parker

International Standard Book Number: 978-1-63241-036-8 (Hardback)

Contents

Preface

This book presents some latest perspectives connected to one of the most common clinical expression disease. The attempts of a group of excellent experts from several countries present a set of very promising scientific studies on clinical allergy, inflammation and basic mechanisms linked to the immune system response. The inflammatory reaction understanding in allergic disease has been clearly explained, along with new strategies for further researches.

Significant researches are present in this book. Intensive efforts have been employed by authors to make this book an outstanding discourse. This book contains the enlightening chapters which have been written on the basis of significant researches done by the experts.

Finally, I would also like to thank all the members involved in this book for being a team and meeting all the deadlines for the submission of their respective works. I would also like to thank my friends and family for being supportive in my efforts.

Editor

Part 1

Specific Aspects of Allergic Diseases

Obesity, Diet, Exercise and Asthma in Children

Luis Garcia-Marcos and Manuel Sanchez-Solis
University of Murcia,
Spain

1. Introduction

During the past decades, an increase in several pediatric morbid conditions has been well documented. Two of the most important of these conditions are obesity and asthma. While the increase of asthma prevalence has been explained in part by the so-called hygiene hypothesis, which claims for a shift from a Th1 to a Th2 environment (if the immunological system does not have to deal with infections –Th1- due to a much more aseptic environment, it will turn to an allergic predisposition –Th2) (von Mutius, 2007). However, this hypothesis does not explain the high prevalences among inner city populations (Platts-Mills et al., 2005) or developing countries as found in the International Study of Asthma and Allergies in Childhood (ISAAC) (Asher et al., 2006). On the other hand, the increased prevalence of obesity is most probably due to an imbalance between the energy intake (both in quantity as well as quality) and the expenditure, in which the lack of exercise is a key point. In this chapter we will explore the complex relationship between asthma, obesity diet and exercise in children.

2. Obesity and asthma are linked together

2.1 The epidemiological link

In this section some of the epidemiological evidence regarding the link between asthma and obesity is reviewed.

2.1.1 Obesity/overweight is associated and precedes asthma

Numerous studies support the epidemiological association between asthma and obesity. Though many of them are cross-sectional, thus making it difficult to establish a casual relationship, some have been specifically aimed at disentangling the first question of which is first in those two apparently connected diseases. The meta-analysis by Sutherland and Beuther (Beuther & Sutherland, 2007) included seven studies which fulfilled their criteria of including adult individuals followed for at least one year in which the main outcome variable was incident asthma and whose obesity was measured using body mass index (BMI). The aforementioned studies included more than 300,000 individuals and the result clearly demonstrated that BMI was associated to incident asthma in a dose-response manner: the association was higher with obesity than it was with overweight.

There are also a number of epidemiological clues which suggest that obesity in childhood precedes asthma later in life. For instance, in a Tasmanian cohort study (Burgess et al., 2007) of children recruited at the age of seven years, adiposity (defined as overweight at 7 years, or as highest quartile BMI) was associated with incident asthma between the ages of 21 and 32 years in girls, but not in boys. Although the number of subjects was low, the association was considerably high. Similarly, females who became overweight or obese between 6 and 11 years of age were seven times more likely to develop new asthma symptoms at ages 11 or 13, according to the Tucson Children Respiratory Study (Castro-Rodriguez et al., 2001). However, not all studies have found a higher association in girls. In fact, in the Children's Health Study (Southern California) the risk of new-onset asthma was higher in boys than in girls, although it was significant in both genders.

Not only do overweight or obesity seem to precede asthma but birth weight has also been shown to be related to later asthma. Although not all the reports coincide it does seem quite consistent that extreme high birth weights are strongly associated to asthma symptoms in school years (To et al., 2010). Furthermore, children with a predisposition for asthma may have a higher risk of developing asthma during childhood when their mothers are overweight before pregnancy, irrespective of the child's BMI (Scholtens et al., 2010). It is also of interest that infants breast fed for at least six moths have a better lung function, and this seems to be related to a lower weight gain. This was shown by Turner at al. (Turner et al., 2008) who followed 154 infants from birth. Maximal flow at functional residual capacity (V'maxFRC) was measured at 1 and 12 months of life: the change in V'maxFRC was inversely associated with change in weight. The group with lower V'maxFRC at 1 month and reduced change in V'maxFRC over infancy had the greatest weight gain and increased risk for asthma symptoms by the age of three years but not afterwards. Those authors concluded that postnatal weight gain may be indirectly associated with early transient asthma symptoms which might be the result of impaired lung growth during infancy, a situation which could be modifiable by breast feeding. A Danish cohort study in which lung function was measured at 6 weeks of age showed that infants in the upper quartile of BMI had lower $FEV_{0.5}$ (Bisgaard et al., 2009). To what extent this circumstance of the early years can be translated to older ages and established asthma is difficult to say, although a connection between obesity and architectural changes in the lung is suggestive, especially if the action of adipokines (which will be reviewed later in this chapter) is taken into account.

Taken together, epidemiological data indicate that body weight and asthma are related in some way, and that excess weight seems to precede asthma or asthma-related symptoms. This fact does not necessarily rule out that the two conditions develop in parallel with the former being apparent before. Furthermore, there are factors which modify the relationship between obesity and asthma. This has been shown in a cross-sectional study (Garcia-Marcos et al., 2008) including a very high number of children: although the association was highly significant for the whole group, it changed dramatically when the group was stratified between those asthmatics also suffering or not from rhinoconjunctivitis. Obesity was not a risk factor for those children with significant asthma who also suffered rhinoconjunctivitis. Although the study has limitations and rhinoconjunctivitis is not a perfect marker of atopy, it raises the question as to whether obesity may be related only to specific asthma phenotypes.

2.1.2 Obesity and asthma develop in parallel, especially in periods of fast growth and maturation

Rather than obesity being the cause of asthma, some findings support the hypothesis of parallel processes which may be related to a change of the environment in which children develop. It is probably when development is more intense (immediately after birth and during puberty) when those processes may be more obvious. Some facts support this view:

- Perinatal events (Jaakkola et al., 2006; Sukalich et al., 2006) or mother food consumption during pregnancy have an influence on later obesity and asthma (Chatzi et al., 2008; Castro-Rodriguez et al., 2010).
- Breast feeding and dietary habits during infancy and later on, are related to obesity and asthma (Matheson et al., 2007); (Moreno & Rodriguez, 2007).
- It is among pre-puberal girls where the association between obesity and asthma is most apparent (Castro-Rodriguez et al., 2001); (Garcia-Marcos et al., 2007), and obesity favours early menarche.
- Epidemiological studies show that females who became overweight or obese between 6 and 11 years of age were seven times more likely to develop new asthma symptoms at age 11 or 13 (Castro-Rodriguez et al., 2001). Moreover, the early onset of puberty has been associated with the persistence of asthma after puberty (Guerra et al., 2004).
- Obesity and asthma are linked conditions during puberty. Although both obesity and asthma can start early in the child life, it is probably around puberty when the connections between those conditions may be better revealed, as some epidemiological studies have shown (Castro-Rodriguez et al., 2001); (Herrera-Trujillo et al., 2005). Some mechanisms might explain this process. For instance, leptin is a key permissive factor (Navarro et al., 2007) –probably through the activation of kisspeptin neurons (Kauffman et al., 2007)- for the onset of puberty. Furthermore, the increase in body weight which occurs during the pubertal spurt induces a corresponding increase of circulating leptin, but also of interleukin (IL)-6 and tumour necrosis factor alpha (TNF-α).
- Several areas in the genome are common to mediators related both to asthma and obesity.

2.1.3 The association between obesity/overweight and bronchial hyperresponsiveness is conflicting

A recent review by Shore (Shore, 2010) lists eight studies dealing with the association of obesity and bronchial hyperresponsiveness (BHR) in adults and a further eight in children. Except for one, all the studies in adults were carried out using metacholine in the challenge test. In children, there were studies using metacholine (n=3), histamine (n=1) and exercise (n=3). The results do not point in the same direction even in the two longitudinal studies (one in adults and one in children). The study in adults reported that high initial BMI was un-linearly associated to later BHR; and weight gain was also associated linearly with the risk of later BHR. On the contrary, the study performed in children (Hancox et al., 2005) did not find any association. Interestingly, however, a high BMI was associated to asthma only in women. This might indicate that the link between obesity and asthma might not necessarily be mediated through airway inflammation revealed by metacholine challenge testing. The cross-sectional studies in children which used metacholine in the challenge test showed all types of results: no association; association only in males; or association only in females. On the contrary, all three cross-sectional studies using exercise as the challenge test found a positive association. The cross-sectional studies in adults (none of them using exercise) also found mixed results, including one study which observed that BMI increased BHR in non-asthmatics but not in asthmatics.

Although a number of factors such as gender, type of challenge test, non-linear association between BMI and BHR (which might counteract the effect of BMI if both low and high BMI are associated to BHR), age groups, asthma control, lack of control for diet, etc. may explain the discrepancy between studies, it seems quite clear that the evidence of an association (if any) between BMI and BHR is not as strong as it is for asthma diagnosis or asthma symptoms. It is interesting that the results are concordant only for the exercise challenge test which does not produce smooth muscle reactivity (as metacholine does) but provokes mast cell activation. It might be hypothesized that obese individuals either create a different osmolality of the airways (the mechanism thought to be responsible for BHR with exercise) while exercising, which in turn causes a higher mast cell activation; or have more mast cells in their airways; or they are more sensitive to osmolality. Although findings in animal models are difficult to translate to humans, it is of great interest that obese mice sensitized and challenged with ovoalbumin have increased numbers of mast cells in their lungs as compared to lean controls (Mito et al., 2002).

2.2 The clinical link

Further evidence that obesity and asthma are related to each other is the fact that BMI predicts asthma control as an independent factor. For instance, in a very recent study, Farah et al. (Farah et al., 2011) reported on asthma control in 49 asthmatic subjects before and after three months of treatment with high doses of inhaled corticosteroids. The effects of treatment were stratified according to BMI (normal, overweight and obese) and the degree of control was assessed by means of the asthma control questionnaire (ACQ-5) although other variables, such as forced expiratory volume during the first second (FEV1), airways resistance (Rrs) and reactance (Xrs) as measured by the forced oscillation technique, BHR to metacholine, and exhaled nitric oxide (FeNO), were also measured before and after treatment. After the treatment period neither FeNO (as a surrogate of bronchial eosinophilic inflammation) nor FEV1 predicted asthma control according to ACQ-5. The two independent predictors of ACQ-5 were Rrs and BMI. The authors conclude that BMI is a factor which determines asthma control and is independent of airway inflammation, lung function and BHR. Furthermore, after ICS treatment, BMI again predicts ACQ-5, and this seems independent of obesity-related changes in lung mechanics.

From a different angle, but adding some evidence to the argument, one study (Maniscalco et al., 2008) has shown that weight loss helps to control asthma in asthmatic individuals. In a series of 12 consecutive asthmatic females who had laparoscopic adjustable gastric banding and consecutively a significant weight loss, asthma control was significantly improved as compared to a control group. Interestingly, no changes in FeNO were found before and after the surgical procedure. Previously, another study showed that a small group of asthmatics (mainly women) significantly improved their asthma control after a very-low-calorie-diet period of 8 weeks (Hakala et al., 2000). In this case, spirometric variables significantly improved leading the authors to think that improvement may be due to better lung mechanics. To the best of our knowledge there are no controlled studies evaluating the effect of weight loss in obese children.

2.3 A genetic link?

There are some regions of the genome that are linked with both asthma and obesity, as occurs with chromosome 5q, 6, 11q13 and 12q (Tantisira & Weiss, 2001). Chromosome 5q contains genes coding the β_2-adrenergic receptor, which has been related to different asthma phenotypes, asthma severity and differential response to β_2-agonists (Hall et al., 1995). A change of Gln for Glu in this receptor has been also associated to obesity (Ishiyama-Shigemoto et al., 1999). Additionally, chromosome 5q contains the glucocorticoid receptor gene which has been involved in inflammatory responses associated to obesity and asthma. Chromosome 6 contains the gene for TNF-α, an interleukin which is important for both obesity and asthma. Another genome region which is linked with asthma and with obesity independently is that of chromosome 11q13 which contains genes for the uncoupling proteins UCP2-UCP3 (related to baseline metabolism) and for the low affinity receptor for IgE. To end, chromosome 12 contains the genes for inflammatory cytokines both related to asthma (such as IFN-γ, or nitric oxide synthase-1) and to obesity (such as signal transducer and activator of transcription protein 6 -STAT6-, or type 1 insulinoid growth factor) (Delgado et al., 2008). To what extent specific but very large areas of the genome are involved in the genesis of the parallel development of asthma and obesity is questionable. How epigenetic changes taking place under certain environments might influence genome areas related to both diseases is even more questionable.

2.4 The inflammation link

The hypothesis that the increase in the prevalence of asthma and obesity, being parallel, could be related to one another (Chinn & Rona, 2001) seems quite plausible. However, a definite link between the two conditions has yet to be definitely established, as it seems to be related to the age and gender of the studied population (Castro-Rodriguez et al., 2001; Chen et al., 2002; Garcia-Marcos et al., 2007), and also to the asthma phenotype (Garcia-Marcos et al., 2008; Gilliland et al., 2003). However, some of the epidemiological and experimental information reviewed in former sections seems to indicate that obesity may precede asthma. To explain this, several inflammatory mechanisms have been evoked:

2.4.1 Adipokines

Adipokines are cytokines produced by the adipose tissue. Some of them are associated both to obesity and to asthma.

2.4.1.1 Leptin

Leptin is mainly produced by white adipose tissue proportionally to the amount of such tissue. Leptin production is regulated by food intake: food consumption up regulates the *ob* gene, thus increasing leptin synthesis; conversely, fasting reduces leptin levels. Infection and sepsis and various pro-inflammatory cytokines including TNF-α and IL-1 increase leptin. Conversely to this acute response, chronic inflammation causes a reduction in leptin levels. Leptin is also moderated by sex hormones: while testosterone inhibits leptin production, ovarian sex steroids increase it, a fact which keeps up with gender-related dimorphism of this adipokine: leptin levels are higher in females than BMI and age-matched males. The main target organ for leptin is the hypothalamus in which it triggers efector pathways to suppress appetite and increase energy expenditure. Apart from the metabolic processes, leptin is also involved in other functions, including the immune response both innate and adaptative: it increases several pro-inflammatory cytokines, such as TNF-α, IL-6 and IL-12, and increases chemotaxis and the functioning of natural killer cells. Overall, leptin increases Th1 and suppresses Th2 response by acting on T regulatory cells (Treg). The leptin receptor gene (*db* gene) is expressed in the lung tissue of several animals and also in humans (Tsuchiya et al., 1999). Although the role of those receptors is not yet clear their presence indicates that the lung is a target organ for leptin. There is also some evidence that leptin can stimulate surfactant protein synthesis (Malli et al., 2010). However, the evidence that leptin influences lung growth and maturation comes from animal models, thus extrapolation to humans remains a major limitation. There also appears to be some role of leptin in respiratory function control, at least in mice (Groeben et al., 2004; Tankersley et al., 1996).

Asthmatic 12-year-old children who are overweight have higher levels of leptin than overweight children who are not asthmatics, despite there being no difference of BMI between the two groups (Mai et al., 2004). This has been also shown in preschool children with normal weight, although reduced to male gender (Guler et al., 2004). Very interestingly, however, is that leptin and BMI are both associated to asthma in adults in an independent way, so when adjusting for leptin levels there is still an association of BMI with asthma (Sood et al., 2006). Furthermore, in asthmatic children leptin and IgE serum levels are highly correlated to each other (Guler et al., 2004). Atopic asthmatic boys have higher leptin levels than non-atopic asthmatic boys. The extent to which leptin has the ability to recruit eosinophils into the lungs and to augment leukotriene synthesis by macrophages may actually be the explanation of its association with atopy still remains controversial (Mancuso et al., 2004; Wong et al., 2007). Further than allergic inflammation as a possible pathway to asthma mediated by leptin, this hormone seems to also have some up-regulatory effect on the sympathetic nervous system, although it does not seem to be important in regulating airway smooth muscle tone (Nair et al., 2008), a fact which might be in connection to the non-consistent findings related to the association between obesity and BHR. However, its is interesting that leptin and leptin receptor are significantly reduced in bronchial epithelial cells in patients with mild asthma which is uncontrolled and in severe treated asthmatics as compared to mild asthmatics under good control, and healthy controls. Additionally, leptin and leptin receptor expression correlated inversely with the thickness of the basement membrane, which is a salient feature of lung remodeling (Bruno et al., 2009).

2.4.1.2 Adiponectin

Adiponectin has an anti-inflammatory role, and decreases with increasing obesity. Contrary to this apparent anti-inflammatory role favoured by obesity, adiponectin is increased in other chronic inflammatory conditions such as rheumatoid arthritis, systemic lupus erythematosus or inflammatory bowel disease. Moreover, elevated levels of adiponectin in cord blood have been associated with an increased risk of asthma in children born from atopic mothers (Rothenbacher et al., 2007). More importantly, adiponectin decreases during puberty only in boys, and remains unchanged in girls (Andersen et al., 2007), a situation that would make gender a modifying factor in the association between obesity and asthma during puberty. Adiponectin and all its currently known receptors are expressed in multiple cell types in the lung (Hug et al., 2004; Miller et al., 2009; Takemura et al., 2007) which makes it a suitable candidate for an additional link between obesity and asthma. In ovoalbumin sensitized mice, administration of exogenous adiponectin protects against cell infiltration and cytokine levels. Serum adiponectin reduces allergic airway inflammation and BHR in mice (Shore et al., 2006). On the other hand and also in mice, adiponectin inhibits the proliferation of vessels associated to smooth muscles although it does not affect muscle itself (Medoff et al., 2009). These findings suggest that adiponectin is involved in allergic inflammation and pulmonary vascular remodeling in a mouse model of chronic asthma.

The number of studies in humans is scarce and the study by Rothenbacher et al. (Rothenbacher et al., 2007) seems to be contradictory to the animal model. Among children with a maternal history of atopy, lower level of adiponectin was associated to lower incidence of asthma or obstructive bronchitis during the first two years of life. Conversely, higher levels of cord serum adiponectin were associated to higher incidence of those respiratory conditions. Among those children without a maternal history of atopy, there was no association of the adipokine and the incidence of asthma or obstructive bronchitis. Other epidemiological studies in humans have rendered inconclusive results. In two cross-sectional studies with a relatively low number of school children, serum adiponectin was not associated to an ever diagnosis of asthma (Nagel et al., 2009) or to current asthma confirmed by metacholine challenge test (Kim et al., 2008). In two very large epidemiological studies in adults, although a clear association between higher BMI and asthma was found in both of them, adiponectin was only inversely associated with current asthma in premenopausal women in one. In a more recent study, 368 adolescent asthmatics were followed for one year: adiponectin was inversely associated to asthma symptoms and exacerbations and positively to FEV1/FVC but only in male subjects (Kattan et al., 2010). FeNO was not associated to serum adiponectin. Conversely, a study in adults did find that adiponectin was associated to lower values of FeNO in men but not in women. No further association of the adipokine and different asthma markers was found in any gender. (Sutherland et al., 2009).

2.4.1.3 Resistin

Resistin is also known as adipocyte-secreted factor or "found in inflammatory zone 3" (FIZZ3). It has recently been discovered and has been proposed as a link between obesity and diabetes. In contrast to mice, resistin is expressed in human adipocytes in low amounts; in fact it is in bone marrow where this adipokine is most expressed in humans (Filkova et al., 2009). Resistin has recently been shown to initiate a pro-inflammmatory state "in vitro" and "in vivo". Pro-inflammatory mediators such as TNF-α, IL-1β or IL-6 can strongly increase the expression of resistin in peripheral mononuclear cells. As stated above, resistin is minimally expressed in human adipose tissue, but adipocytes may be targets for it. Nagaev et al. have demonstrated that resistin, similarly to its action on peripheral blood mononuclear cells, can induce adipocytes to express IL-6 and TNF-α (Nagaev et al., 2006). Resistin has been shown to be increased in the murine models of genetic as well as in diet-induced obesity. This has also been shown in humans. In an asthma cohort study on adult asthma, levels of resistin were higher in asthmatic patients as compared to controls, and resistin levels increased with increased severity of the disease (Larochelle et al., 2007). Conversely, atopic asthmatic children have lower resistin levels as compared to the non-atopic asthma and control groups (Kim et al., 2008). However, in a recent study (Arshi et al., 2010) in children of a similar age to those in the previous study (11 years) resistin levels were not different between a group of atopic asthmatics and a control group. In fact, its levels in the former study were about double than in the latter both in the control and in the atopic asthmatic groups. More recently, a study has shown that in a group of non-obese corticosteroid naïve adult female recently diagnosed asthmatics resistin predicted favourable anti-inflammatory effects of inhaled corticosteroids as assessed by levels of eosinophil cationic protein, eosinophil protein X and myeloperoxidase. Furthermore, an "in vitro" assay found that fluticasone significantly reduced resistin-induced IL-6 and TNF-α production in cultured monocytes/macrophages (Leivo-Korpela et al., 2011).

2.4.1.4 Adipsin

This adipokine is the rate-limiting enzyme in the alternate pathway of complement activation and is primarily expressed by adipocytes and monocytes/macrophages in humans. Adipsin has however been barely studied in asthma or allergic diseases. In a group of non-obese corticosteroid naïve adult female recently diagnosed asthmatics and with a positive bronchodilator tests, levels of adipsin were similar to the control group (Leivo-Korpela et al., 2011); however this adipokine has been reported to be significantly increased in individuals with seasonal allergic rhinitis, but only in males. Sublingual immunotherapy did not seem to affect adipsin levels (Ciprandi et al., 2009). Information regarding whether adipsin might have a role in asthma (if any) is still very scarce and we will have to wait until new studies publish their results.

2.4.1.5 Visfatin

Visfatin is identical to pre-B cell colony enhancing factor, a cytokine which is increased in the bronchoalveolar lavage fluid in animal models of acute lung injury and in neutrophils of septic patients. Exercise training with weight loss induced a significant reduction of plasma visfatin in non-diabetic women (Choi et al., 2007). Although this protein represents an additional link between obesity and inflammation, its role in asthma (if any) is still to be elucidated.

2.4.2 Immunologic properties of adipose tissue

The view of adipose tissue as a sole storage system has radically changed in the last decade. Further than being able to synthesize adipokines, adipocytes share some similarities with macrophages. In fact, preadipocytes can differentiate into macrophages, but the two cell types are distinct. On the other hand, about 10% of cells in the adipose tissue are macrophages. The number of macrophages in the adipose tissue is directly related to adiposity and to the size of adipocytes both in humans and in mice (Curat et al., 2004). Apart from secreting adipokines, adipocytes also secrete chemokines and cytokines, such as TNF-α, IL-6, Il-10, IL-1β and other factors such as monocyte chemoattractant protein-1 (MCP-1). It is thought that those mediators are secreted by the adipocyte itself since when adipose tissue is increased there is an up-regulation of genes related to inflammation. Indeed macrophages of the adipose tissue are an additional source of inflammatory mediators.

-    TNF-α is the most important of cytokines produced by adipose tissue. It increases formation of Th2 cytokines such as IL-4 and Il-5, IL-6 and Il-1β by the bronchial epithelial cells. On the other hand, TNF-α increases the expression of leptin and adiponectin in cultured adipocytes (Kirchgessner et al., 1997). TNF-α is an important cytokine in the innate immune response and has been involved in the pathophysiology of several chronic inflammation diseases, including asthma (Thomas et al., 1995; Thomas & Heywood, 2002). This cytokine has an array of effects on the immunological system which have direct implications for the asthmatic response, such as recruitment of neutrophils, macrophages and mast cells; recruitment and activation of eosinophils; up-regulation of adhesion molecules both in the respiratory epithelium and on the vascular endothelium, which in turn can further increase inflammatory cell recruitment; proliferation and differentiation of fibroblasts (related to asthma remodeling and potentially to a more severe type of asthma); activation and increased release of cytokines by T cells of the Th2 arm; and induction of corticoisosteroid resistance (Brightling et al., 2008).

- IL-6 is a proinflammatory cytokine which has a central role in host defence against infection and tissue injury. This interleukin derived from antigen presenting cells can induce production of IL-4 in naïve CD4+ cells, thus polarizing them into Th2 cells; i.e. to the allergic type of inflammation. This interleukin also modulates the intensity of the immune response by inhibiting Treg cell development. Additionally IL-6 promotes generation of Th17 cells (cells involved in autoimmune diseases) in mice, though its ability to do so in humans is subject to debate (Wilson et al., 2007). It has been recently shown that IL-6 levels are elevated in sputum of asthmatic patients as compared to healthy volunteers (Neveu et al., 2010).
- IL-10 is a cytokine with important regulatory function, having multiple biological effects in different cell-types. IL-10 modulates allergic disease in humans: the expression of IL-10 by antigen presenting cells in the airway of healthy subjects is important for inducing and maintaining tolerance to allergens (Commins et al., 2008).
- IL-1β is a potent mediator in response to infection and injury, and is increased in asthmatic airways as it is in other chronic inflammatory diseases. Apart from its pro-inflammatory effects, IL-1β has been shown to induce migration of vascular smooth muscle cells in culture and to provoke migration of endothelial cells. Its potential effects on the airway epithelial cell have been recently shown in cell cultures (White et al., 2008).

It should not be forgotten that apart from adipocytes, adipose tissue contains a considerable number of macrophages. Those cells are located in the white adipose tissue, which –as compared to brown adipose tissue which has as main role non-shivering thermogenesis- is the majority of adipose tissue and serves as energy storage. The number of macrophages in this tissue is proportional to adiposity and adipocyte size, both in mice and humans, and no difference exists between visceral and subcutaneous white fat (Weisberg et al., 2003).

2.4.3 Other endogenous molecules relating obesity with asthma

There are other hormones which may be related to obesity and asthma since they can be associated with processes related to food intake/body weight and inflammation.

2.4.3.1 Alpha-melanocyte stimulating hormone

Alpha-melanocyte stimulating hormone (α-MSH) belongs to a group of hormones called melanocortins, which include ACTH among others, with a common precursor (proopiomelanocortin). This hormone produces a significant down-regulation of pro-inflammatory cytokines such as IL-1β, IL-6 and TNF-α, as well as chemokines such as IL-8 and interferon gamma (IFN-γ). Furthermore, chemotaxis induced by IL-8 in human neutrophils and monocytes is blunted by α-MSH. Additionally, this hormone has been shown to induce IL-10 production (Brzoska et al., 2010). In a murine model, α-MSH was able to inhibit airway inflammation induced by aerosol sensitization and subsequent challenges with OVA. Additionally, the levels of two important interleukins related to the allergic response, IL-4 and IL-13, were highly decreased in the broncho-alveolar lavage fluid of mice treated with α-MSH. In agreement with the important role of IL-10 as an anti-inflammatory mediator, the action of α-MSH was dependent on the presence of IL-10, as IL-10 knock-out mice were resistant to treatment with α-MSH (Raap et al., 2003). In the context of an association between asthma and obesity, what is on interest of α-MSH is the fact that the hormone is included in one of the main mechanisms of energy balance. There are melanocortin receptors in the CNS and effects on food intake and on energy expenditure have been observed with treatments containing ligands of those receptors (Williams et al., 2000). Those receptors are hypothesized to be downstream mediators of the effects of leptin signaling: leptin increases the expression of the proopiomelanocortin gene in neurons of the nucleus tractus solitarius (Schwartz et al., 1997). Thus, α-MSH may play a role both in allergic inflammation and in food-intake control. In fact, the melanocortin system appears to be a common pathway for mediation of both leptin and ghrelin (Lebrethon et al., 2007).

2.4.3.2 Ghrelin

Ghrelin is not only a mere growth-hormone releasing factor but also an important appetite regulator, energy conservator and suppressor of the sympathetic nervous system. Ghrelin, secreted from the peripheral organ, has its regulatory region in the hypothalamic arcuate nucleus, where the regulatory region of appetite is located. Circulating ghrelin excites this region and stimulates food intake after passing through the blood-brain barrier. Additionally, this hormone can exert its action through receptors in the vagus nerve (Kojima & Kangawa, 2010). Apart from being an orexigenic hormone, ghrelin has an interesting association with IgE in humans. In a case-control study of obese school children, Matsuda et al. (Matsuda et al., 2006) found that ghrelin was inversely and significantly correlated with BMI but also with IgE both in allergic and non-allergic subjects as defined from a combination of asthma and skin symptoms. This correlation with IgE is higher among overweight patients as compared to normal weight ones, in which the correlation is still significant (Okamatsu et al., 2009). The strong inverse correlation between plasma ghrelin and serum IgE levels suggests that ghrelin may inhibit IgE production in some manner. In this context, it is of interest that in splenic murine T lymphocytes, mRNA levels of IL-4 and IL-10, which both increase IgE synthesis, are suppressed by ghrelin (Xia et al., 2004).

2.4.3.3 Eotaxin

Eotaxin is a key chemotactic agent responsible for the eosinophil-mediated bronchial inflammation. In their pivotal study, Vasudevan et al. (Vasudevan et al., 2006) showed that eotaxin circulating levels are increased in diet-induced obese mice. They also showed that after weight loss in humans eotaxin was significantly reduced. In a group of obese and non-obese Korean women it was shown that circulating eotaxin was similar in both groups, although women with central obesity had significantly higher levels of eotaxin than those without it. This study also showed that weight reduction after following an exercise program for 12 weeks was associated to a significant decrease in circulating eotaxin levels in the whole group (Choi et al., 2007).

Not only has eotaxin been studied in relation to obesity but also as to how this chemokine interacts with allergy inflammation in the context of obesity. In a murine allergy model (Calixto et al., 2010), diet-induced obesity enhanced eosinophil trafficking from bone marrow to lung tissues, and delayed their transit through the airway epithelium into the airway lumen. Consequently, eosinophils remain longer in lung peribronchiolar segments. Furthermore, Kim et al. (Kim et al., 2011) cultivated and differentiated pre-adypocites and investigated eotaxin expression during differentiation and found that levels of this chemokine increased as adipocytes differentiated. Eotaxin was further expressed when cultured cells were challenged with TNF-α and IL-4.

2.4.3.4 Plasminogen activator inhibitor 1

Remodeling of the airway is a key feature of asthma and is associated to a more severe type of disease. Plasminogen activator inhibitor 1 (PAI-1) is a potent inhibitor of both tissue-type plasminogen activator (t-PA) and urokinase-type plasminogen activator (u-PA). Both t-PA and u-PA are involved in the dissolution of fibrin and in the degradation of the extracellular matrix. Activated mast cells are a major source of PAI-1, and mast cell-derived PAI-1 is highly expressed in patients with fatal asthma (Cho et al., 2000). Furthermore, a gene polymorphism associated with PAI-1 levels is preferably transmitted to asthmatic patients; and deletion of PAI-1 prevents extracellular matrix deposition in a murine model of asthma (Cho et al., 2001); (Oh et al., 2002). In a very recent study (Cho et al., 2011), it was found that plasma levels of PAI-1 were significantly higher in obese subjects as compared to controls after adjusting for race and smoking status; furthermore, PAI-1 plasma levels were significantly and inversely correlated to forced vital capacity. Thus, it could be hypothesized that the reduction of FVC in obese patients may be in part mediated by PAI-1. Although research on the association of PAI-1 as a link between obesity and asthma is still very scarce, this is a field which warrants further investigation.

2.5 The mechanical link

The mechanical load of obesity might affect lung growth, leading to reduced pulmonary function. For instance, leptin-deficient mice which are obese very early in their development have substantially smaller lungs than normal ones (Shore et al., 2003). Maternal obesity in pregnancy increases the risk of pregnancy complications, caesarean sections and adverse birth outcomes, which have in turn been associated with respiratory illness in children. However, little is known of the effect of obesity in the mother during pregnancy with regard to respiratory diseases in the offspring. A recent Norwegian study (Haberg et al., 2009) (Norwegian and Child Study) which includes 100,000 pregnant mothers was able to analyse data from more than 33,000 mother-children pairs up to the age of 18 months of the infants and demonstrated that after adjustment for many factors including birth weight, preterm birth and pregnancy complications, infants born from obese mothers had a modest but significant increased risk (3.3%) of suffering from at least one episode of wheezing during the follow-up period. To what extent this finding is related to the low-grade inflammation status of mothers during pregnancy or to mechanical factors "in utero" and how they might affect lung development in the foetus is still to be determined. Furthermore, it is not known if this effect is maintained in later years.

Independently of its effects on lung development either in the fetal period or later on, obese subjects have a low functional residual capacity due to changes in the elastic properties of the chest wall (Shore & Johnston, 2006). At low volumes, the retractile forces of the lung parenchyma are reduced, thus airway smooth muscle has a lower load when functional residual capacity is reduced. Consequently it might shorten still further when activated (either by parasympathetic tone or broncho-constricting agents such as metacholine) (Naimark & Cherniack, 1960). However, some studies have noted that there is bronchial constriction in obese subjects after correcting for lung volume, which suggests that other mechanisms are involved. Apparently low tidal volume (which is common in obese individuals) may be one such mechanism: stretching of the airways smooth muscles causes cross-bridging of actin-myosin to detach, and the bigger the tidal volume (stretch) the easier it is for bronchodilation to occur. Low tidal volume facilitates more cross-bridging between actin and myosin, thus making airway smooth muscle stiffer and harder to stretch. Hence reduction of tidal volume in obese subjects could lead to a vicious circle in which small airway muscle strain leads to greater stiffness, and this leads to even less muscle strain in every breath (Shore, 2008). This paradigm is supported by the fact that both obese and asthmatic subjects have lower bronchodilation after deep breaths (Hakala et al., 1995; Skloot & Togias, 2003).

There could be additional mechanical explanations as to the reasons why airways in obese subjects are more easily constricted than in normal ones. Closure of small peripheral airways is common in obese individuals, especially in the supine posture (Hakala et al., 1995). Some authors have postulated that the frequent opening and closure of those airways may lead to the rupture of alveolar attachment to bronchioles, thus disconnecting airways from the attached parenchyma and exacerbating constriction (Milic-Emili et al., 2007). To what extent those less oxygenated areas could lead to higher artery pressures and pulmonary edema, further complicating the situation, is still very speculative although there is some evidence of edema in obese subjects and pulmonary hypertension in obese women (Bergeron et al., 2005); (Taraseviciute & Voelkel, 2006). Hypoxemia might exacerbate local hypoxia occurring in obese adipose tissue, a situation which contributes to the general inflammation of obesity (Hosogai et al., 2007; Ye et al., 2007). Situations related to obesity such as obesity hypoventilation syndrome or sleep disordered breathing could further aggravate this situation and although extreme and far from asthma, could add some clues to the mechanical associations between asthma and obesity.

2.6 The experimental link (animal models)

Three are several models in which the lung features of obese mice have been characterized. According to Shore (Shore, 2007), those are:

-   *ob/ob* Mice: This is a type of mice which is not capable of synthesizing leptin, which is a satiety hormone formed in the adipose tissue. These mice eat in excess and are already obese at four weeks of age. These mice have smaller lungs than the wild type.
-   *db/db* Mice: In this type of mice there is an altered leptin receptor in the hypothalamus (Ob-R$_b$) so the effect of leptin on satiety is lost. Thus, *db/db* mice are similar to *ob/ob* mice. As in the case of *ob/ob* mice, *db/db* mice have smaller lungs than the wild type.
-   *Cpe^{fat}* Mice: These mice have a missense mutation of the enzyme carboxipeptidase E (Cpe) which makes it inactive. Cpe cleaves neuropeptides such as corticotrophin-releasing factor and neuropeptide Y which control eating behaviours and energy consumption. In the absence of Cpe mice become obese but not as fast as *ob/ob* or *db/db* mice. These mice have lung size comparable to that of the wild type.
-   Diet-induced obese mice: feeding recently weaned mice with a diet in which 45-60% of calories are derived from fat produces obesity. Obesity is milder than in the three prior models and lung size is again similar to that of the wild type.

Taken together, the results from the studies from animal models in obese mice suggest that obesity might be related to asthma in several ways. In the first place very early obese mice have smaller lungs and this might have implications both at the mechanical and at the ultra-structural level, in particular in the way lungs are alveolarized. Secondly, obesity either acquired very early or later on in the mice's lives increases BHR and this neither seems to be directly mediated by leptin nor is secondary to a prior inflammation. Lastly, obesity might have some effect on asthma through allergic sensitization as that hormone seems to increase sensitization, and thus BHR to allergen challenge (Shore et al., 2005), this being dependent on when obesity and sensitization develop.

2.7 A distinct asthma phenotype in the obese?

There seems to be enough epidemiological, clinical and mechanistic evidence that obesity and asthma "live" together in some individuals. Whether this comorbidity is a distinct phenotype as suggested by some authors; or obesity is a risk factor for asthma incidence and worse control, is difficult to say (Castro-Rodriguez & Garcia-Marcos, 2008; Lessard et al., 2008; Lugogo et al., 2010). However, both the mechanical, hormonal and immunological links between the two conditions suggest that obesity probably leads to asthma in many cases and could be in part responsible for the "asthma epidemic". Moreover, there are two other important factors –diet and exercise- which can favour both asthma and obesity in parallel. An official American Thoracic Society workshop report recently published concludes that obesity is a risk factor for asthma in all age groups and that asthma in the obese might represent a distinct phenotype with a more severe disease with a worse response to treatment (Dixon et al., 2010). The report states the urgent need to further investigate the mechanisms of asthma in this risk group and to develop new therapies directed to this specific population.

3. Diet as an independent factor in the development of asthma and obesity

Diet and exercise are probable common pathways for asthma and obesity irrespective of which of the two conditions starts first. This is quite well documented during the first months after birth. Infants who are breastfed have a different bacterial colonization of their intestine than those who are fed with artificial formulas (Harmsen et al., 2000). Similarly, children fed with the latter formulas gain weight more rapidly, although this does not seem to be translated into later obesity (Burdette et al., 2006). Although the information is still sparse, it is quite probable that the so-called microflora fingerprinting –which remains very stable throughout the years- is related to diet. Either by this mechanism which might be included into de hygiene hypothesis or by others, such as the antioxidant or pro-oxidant properties of some foods (Roberts et al., 2006), or the modulating properties of prebiotics - like fibers- to adjust intestinal microflora (Schley & Field, 2002), may have an effect on asthma and obesity.

There are currently enough studies to conclude that there is an association between consumption of some types of nutrients or foods and asthma. An ecological analysis of the European Community Respiratory Health Survey (ECRHS) showed a trend towards decreasing sensitization (specific IgE) prevalence with higher intakes of fruit and vitamins A and C (Farchi et al., 2003). Furthermore, other studies have found an association between consuming citrus/kiwi fruit and a lower last year prevalence of several asthma symptoms (Forastiere et al., 2000; Wickens et al., 2005); and also of rhinitis. The frequent intake of vegetables showed an inverse relationship with prevalence rates of asthma, allergic rhinoconjunctivitis and atopic eczema (Weiland et al., 1999). The intake of cereals has also been shown to be associated to a lower prevalence of asthma (Garcia-Marcos et al., 2007; To et al., 2004). A recent meta-analysis on food intake and asthma arrived at interesting conclusions (Nurmatov et al., 2011) in spite of the limitations of applying the meta-analysis technique to epidemiological studies which cannot be –by definition- perfectly controlled. With respect to individual nutrients, vitamins A, D, E and zinc seem to be protective, while vitamin C and selenium do seem to be neither a protective nor a risk factor. Higher consumption of fruit and vegetables are associated to a lower prevalence of asthma, with fruit having a higher impact. However the associations were not adjusted for obesity or exercise.

Two different groups, including ours, have very recently associated Mediterranean diet to a lower prevalence of asthma at different ages (Castro-Rodriguez et al., 2008; Chatzi et al., 2007; Garcia-Marcos et al., 2007) independently of exercise. Furthermore, Mediterranean diet also showed this protective effect in the offspring when the mother consumed it during pregnancy (Chatzi et al., 2008), although the effect might be restricted just to olive oil intake (Castro-Rodriguez et al., 2010). The reasons why this type of diet is associated with a lower prevalence of asthma could be explained in several ways. Considering that Mediterranean diet is rich in both antioxidants and *cis* monounsaturated fatty acids this is not an unexpected finding. Individually, a more frequent intake of seafood and also of cereals is associated with a lower prevalence of significant asthma. At 8-10 years of age atopy is a risk factor for a more severe asthma (Ponsonby et al., 2002), so it could be speculated that at least in part the protection offered by this diet is mediated through allergy modulation. The protection from asthma that Mediterranean diet seems to offer is probably due to a mixed effect of taking "protective" foods and avoiding "risky" foods. Protective foods may be those with antioxidant properties and rich in prebiotics, such as fibers (as in the Mediterranean diet); and risky foods may be those rich in *trans* fatty acids and unsaturated fat (as in fast foods) (Garcia-Marcos et al., 2007; Innis & King, 1999; von Kries et al., 2001). In fact, Mediterranean diet has been shown to increase the total antioxidant capacity in healthy adults (Pitsavos et al., 2005). Mediterranean diet has additionally been associated to a reduced prevalence of obesity. Due to its content in fibre and unsaturated fat (olive oil, fish) this diet is associated to better weight control (Schroder, 2007). On the contrary, fast food is related to an increase of calorie intake (Schmidt et al., 2005) and is greatly related to the school and family environment, especially during the transition to adulthood (Nelson et al., 2006)

3.1 Oxidant-antioxidant imbalance in asthma

Reactive oxygen species (ROS), formed in every cell during metabolic processes, are increased in asthma and can mediate pathophysiologic changes which are characteristic of this condition, such as initiating lipid peroxidation and favouring the release of arachidonic acid from cell membranes; contracting smooth muscle; increasing airway reactivity and vascular permeability; augmenting the synthesis and release of cytokines and chemokines; impairing the response to β_2 adrenergic drugs; and decreasing cholinesterase and neutral endopeptidase activities (Nadeem et al., 2008). Lungs have several antioxidant mechanisms including enzymatic (catalase, glutathione peroxidase ans superoxide dismutase) and non-enzymatic ones (vitamin C, E, albumin, uric acid, cerulopasmin and glutathione). Increased ROS generation is found when the activity of neutrophils, eosinophils, monocytes and macrophages is increased, as occurs in asthma (Kelly et al., 1988). Oxidative stress (a situation of imbalance between the production of ROS and the ability to detoxify the reactive intermediates or to repair the resulting damage) is an important consequence of asthma inflammation; is associated with an altered activity in anti-oxidation in lungs and blood; and also with airway reactivity (Katsumata et al., 1990; Nadeem et al., 2005; Sackesen et al., 2008).

There are numerous reports showing deficiencies of antioxidants in asthma: low levels of vitamin C in airway lining fluid, serum, plasma, whole blood and brochoalveolar lavage fluid; vitamin E in brochio-alveolar lavage fluid, red cells and plasma; or beta-carotene in serum (Kalayci et al., 2000; Kelly et al., 1999; Sackesen et al., 2008; Shanmugasundaram et al., 2001; Vural & Uzun, 2000; Wood et al., 2008). The cooperation of several antioxidants provides a better defense against ROS, so the total antioxidant capacity of serum is probably a better index than the measurement of a specific antioxidant. Again, antioxidant capacity in serum is reduced in asthmatics during exacerbations as compared with healthy individuals and is less reduced in subjects with stable asthma (Katsoulis et al., 2003). Very recently, oxidative stress has been shown to be increased in children with previous bronchilitis obliterans (Mallol et al., 2011) and although in this study the authors did not find correlation with lung function tests, several studies have indeed shown an inverse relationship between oxidative stress and lung function in asthmatics (Nadeem et al., 2005; Ochs-Balcom et al., 2006; Picado et al., 2001; Wood et al., 2000).

Taken together these results indicate that an oxidant-antioxidant imbalance could play a crucial role in the development of asthma symptoms and in the severity of the disease. Accordingly, certain diets may favor or protect from asthma depending upon their ability to maintain a better oxidant-antioxidant balance.

4. Exercise is an independent protective factor for asthma and obesity

Although it would be expected that asthmatics perform less exercise and severe asthmatic perform even less, it is not so straightforward that the lack of exercise favours obesity, which in turn favours asthma. Although this causal pathway may be present in some asthmatics, more exercise –independently of BMI- has been associated to a lower prevalence of mild asthma, although it does not influence severe asthma. If the association of asthma with exercise was a reverse causation effect it should be expected that at least in severe asthmatics, there was an inverse association, which does not seem the case when diet and BMI are controlled: in their study Garcia-Marcos et al. showed that after adjusting for BMI and Mediterranean diet exercise was not associated with severe asthma; and mild asthma was less prevalent among children who exercise more (Garcia-Marcos et al., 2007). Therefore, it might be hypothesized that at least in mild cases, the lack of exercise is associated to asthma. In this context, a very interesting and challenging hypothesis was proposed by Alexander in 2005 who maintains that the increase of asthma prevalence might be due in part to a "disuse contracture" which reminds of the mechanical link between obesity and asthma (Alexander, 2005). The following paragraphs are a brief explanation of that hypothesis.

Bronchial constriction and BHR are crucial features of asthma and are both driven by bronchial smooth muscle. When lumen is narrower than normal in a permanent way, there is also a reduction in the length of the annular components of the bronchii, namely smooth muscle fibres and collagen. Under-extension causes contracture: elastic components (smooth muscle and collagen) need a certain tension to operate correctly and when this is not provided by intermittent stretching they either fail to extend during growth (infants and schoolchildren) or reduce in length (adults) to a point in which habitual usage is enough to provoke a peak tension needed for effective functioning. This situation maybe reversible in its first stages but becomes permanent with time due to fixed cross-linking (Akeson et al., 1977). While this is typical of the joint tissues, it is most probably applicable to muscles and elastic tissues of the airways, which in continued growing (as in infancy and childhood) without stretching to their potential length the result would result in an increased thickness of the wall and narrowing of the lumen, which, in turn, will start a vicious cycle: thicker wall, less ability to stretch and more difficult distension to inspiration, less distension, less lumen and thicker wall again. If lumen is reduced to a critical point and according to Laplace's law, the product of atmospheric pressure times radius will not be able to counteract wall tension and bronchii would collapse. In this situation a very small increase of muscle tone will be enough to cause bronchial closure. Moreover, exercise increases respiratory rate and speed of airflow, thus reducing transmural pressure and further favouring collapse.

In summary, this hypothesis contemplates asthma as a lack of lung expansion by exercise during growth. While just a hypothesis, the idea of a lack of "sufficient" inspiration has been contemplated as a feasible explanation for the influence in asthma prevalence of TV watching. The ALSPAC study, after following a large sample of more than 5,000 children, found that new asthma cases, as diagnosed by a doctor, between the ages of 3.5 and 11.5 years were associated to the number of hours of TV watching after controlling for other risk factors including BMI: those watching more than 2h/day had double odds of having new onset asthma a compared to those watching 1-2h/day, while those watching less than 1h/day had just half the odds (Sherriff et al., 2009). While previous studies showed that new cases of asthma during adolescence are associated to lower fitness (Rasmussen et al., 2000; Vogelberg et al., 2007), sometimes confused by smoking, children in the ALSPAC study were too young to consider smoking-related TV watching as a plausible explanation. Sedentary lifestyle ("disuse contracture") is a more plausible explanation. Additionally, the ALSPAC group suggested as an additional explanation of their results that respiratory patterns associated to TV watching may also play a role: prolonged periods of watching a videotape are associated with lower sigh rates than while reading (Hark et al., 2005). Thus, "modern" as opposed to "classical" sedentary lifestyle maybe and additional factor favouring the "disuse contracture".

5. Conclusion

Obesity and asthma are linked together, a link which has been shown at different levels and has plausible pathways. However, it is still to be established if obesity causes asthma (or a specific asthma phenotype) or if the two conditions are part of a parallel development in the context of the western lifestyle in which sedentary habits and unhealthy diets (together with lower contact with germs and/or with "non-traditional" germs) may interact to favour an internal environment in which not only obesity and asthma, but other diseases such as type II diabetes or rheumatoid arthritis develop more easily.

The epidemiological and animal studies carried out to date have probably rendered all possible information and it is the time of more controlled trials. New pregnancy/birth cohort studies specifically designed to disentangle the interrelationship between asthma, obesity, exercise and diet are needed. Creative clinical trials will also have an important role here, although designing and performing them is a great challenge. The implications of the results of such studies on public health policies are crucial.

6. References

Akeson WH, Amiel D, Mechanic GL, Woo SL, Harwood FL, Hamer ML. (1977) Collagen cross-linking alterations in joint contractures: changes in the reducible cross-links in periarticular connective tissue collagen after nine weeks of immobilization, *Connect Tissue Res* 5(1): 15-19

Alexander CJ. (2005) Asthma: a disuse contracture?, *Med Hypotheses* 64(6): 1102-1104

Andersen KK, Frystyk J, Wolthers OD, Heuck C, Flyvbjerg A. (2007) Gender differences of oligomers and total adiponectin during puberty: a cross-sectional study of 859 Danish school children, *J Clin Endocrinol Metab* 92(5): 1857-1862

Arshi M, Cardinal J, Hill RJ, Davies PS, Wainwright C. (2010) Asthma and insulin resistance in children, *Respirology* 15(5): 779-784

Asher MI, Montefort S, Bjorksten B, Lai CK, Strachan DP, Weiland SK, Williams H. (2006) Worldwide time trends in the prevalence of symptoms of asthma, allergic rhinoconjunctivitis, and eczema in childhood: ISAAC Phases One and Three repeat multicountry cross-sectional surveys, *Lancet* 368(9537): 733-743

Bergeron C, Boulet LP, Hamid Q. (2005) Obesity, allergy and immunology, *J Allergy Clin Immunol* 115(5): 1102-1104

Beuther DA, Sutherland ER. (2007) Overweight, obesity, and incident asthma: a meta-analysis of prospective epidemiologic studies, *Am J Respir Crit Care Med* 175(7): 661-666

Bisgaard H, Loland L, Holst KK, Pipper CB. (2009) Prenatal determinants of neonatal lung function in high-risk newborns, *J Allergy Clin Immunol* 123(3): 651-657

Brightling C, Berry M, Amrani Y. (2008) Targeting TNF-alpha: a novel therapeutic approach for asthma, *J Allergy Clin Immunol* 121(1): 5-10

Bruno A, Pace E, Chanez P, Gras D, Vachier I, Chiappara G, La Guardia M, Gerbino S, Profita M, Gjomarkaj M. (2009) Leptin and leptin receptor expression in asthma, *J Allergy Clin Immunol* 124(2): 230-7, 237

Burdette HL, Whitaker RC, Hall WC, Daniels SR. (2006) Breastfeeding, introduction of complementary foods, and adiposity at 5 y of age, *Am J Clin Nutr* 83(3): 550-558

Burgess JA, Walters EH, Byrnes GB, Giles GG, Jenkins MA, Abramson MJ, Hopper JL, Dharmage SC. (2007) Childhood adiposity predicts adult-onset current asthma in females: a 25-yr prospective study, *Eur Respir J* 29(4): 668-675

Calixto MC, Lintomen L, Schenka A, Saad MJ, Zanesco A, Antunes E. (2010) Obesity enhances eosinophilic inflammation in a murine model of allergic asthma, *Br J Pharmacol* 159(3): 617-625

Castro-Rodriguez JA, Garcia-Marcos L. (2008) Wheezing and Asthma in childhood: an epidemiology approach, *Allergol Immunopathol (Madr)* 36(5): 280-290

Castro-Rodriguez JA, Garcia-Marcos L, Alfonseda Rojas JD, Valverde-Molina J, Sanchez-Solis M. (2008) Mediterranean diet as a protective factor for wheezing in preschool children, *J Pediatr* 152(6): 823-8, 828

Castro-Rodriguez JA, Garcia-Marcos L, Sanchez-Solis M, Perez-Fernandez V, Martinez-Torres A, Mallol J. (2010) Olive oil during pregnancy is associated with reduced wheezing during the first year of life of the offspring, *Pediatr Pulmonol* 45(4): 395-402

Castro-Rodriguez JA, Holberg CJ, Morgan WJ, Wright AL, Martinez FD. (2001) Increased incidence of asthmalike symptoms in girls who become overweight or obese during the school years, *Am J Respir Crit Care Med* 163(6): 1344-1349

Chatzi L, Apostolaki G, Bibakis I, Skypala I, Bibaki-Liakou V, Tzanakis N, Kogevinas M, Cullinan P. (2007) Protective effect of fruits, vegetables and the Mediterranean diet on asthma and allergies among children in Crete, *Thorax* 62(8): 677-683

Chatzi L, Torrent M, Romieu I, Garcia-Esteban R, Ferrer C, Vioque J, Kogevinas M, Sunyer J. (2008) Mediterranean diet in pregnancy is protective for wheeze and atopy in childhood, *Thorax* 63(6): 507-513

Chen Y, Dales R, Tang M, Krewski D. (2002) Obesity may increase the incidence of asthma in women but not in men: longitudinal observations from the Canadian National Population Health Surveys, *Am J Epidemiol* 155(3): 191-197

Chinn S, Rona RJ. (2001) Can the increase in body mass index explain the rising trend in asthma in children?, *Thorax* 56(11): 845-850

Cho S, Kang J, Lyttle C, Harris K, Daley B, Grammer L, Avila P, Kumar R, Schleimer R. (2011) Association of elevated plasminogen activator inhibitor 1 levels with diminished lung function in patients with asthma, *Ann Allergy Asthma Immunol* 106(5): 371-377

Cho SH, Hall IP, Wheatley A, Dewar J, Abraha D, Del Mundo J, Lee H, Oh CK. (2001) Possible role of the 4G/5G polymorphism of the plasminogen activator inhibitor 1 gene in the development of asthma, *J Allergy Clin Immunol* 108(2): 212-214

Cho SH, Tam SW, Demissie-Sanders S, Filler SA, Oh CK. (2000) Production of plasminogen activator inhibitor-1 by human mast cells and its possible role in asthma, *J Immunol* 165(6): 3154-3161

Choi KM, Kim JH, Cho GJ, Baik SH, Park HS, Kim SM. (2007) Effect of exercise training on plasma visfatin and eotaxin levels, *Eur J Endocrinol* 157(4): 437-442

Ciprandi G, De Amici M, Marseglia G. (2009) Serum adipsin levels in patients with seasonal allergic rhinitis: preliminary data, *Int Immunopharmacol* 9(12): 1460-1463

Commins S, Steinke JW, Borish L. (2008) The extended IL-10 superfamily: IL-10, IL-19, IL-20, IL-22, IL-24, IL-26, IL-28, and IL-29, *J Allergy Clin Immunol* 121(5): 1108-1111

Curat CA, Miranville A, Sengenes C, Diehl M, Tonus C, Busse R, Bouloumie A. (2004) From blood monocytes to adipose tissue-resident macrophages: induction of diapedesis by human mature adipocytes, *Diabetes* 53(5): 1285-1292

Delgado J, Barranco P, Quirce S. (2008) Obesity and asthma, *J Investig Allergol Clin Immunol* 18(6): 420-425

Dixon AE, Holguin F, Sood A, Salome CM, Pratley RE, Beuther DA, Celedon JC, Shore SA. (2010) An official American Thoracic Society Workshop report: obesity and asthma, *Proc Am Thorac Soc* 7(5): 325-335

Farah CS, Kermode JA, Downie SR, Brown NJ, Hardaker KM, Berend N, King GG, Salome CM. (2011) Obesity is a determinant of asthma control, independent of inflammation and lung mechanics, *Chest*

Farchi S, Forastiere F, Agabiti N, Corbo G, Pistelli R, Fortes C, Dell'Orco V, Perucci CA. (2003) Dietary factors associated with wheezing and allergic rhinitis in children, *Eur Respir J* 22(5): 772-780

Filkova M, Haluzik M, Gay S, Senolt L. (2009) The role of resistin as a regulator of inflammation: Implications for various human pathologies, *Clin Immunol* 133(2): 157-170

Forastiere F, Pistelli R, Sestini P, Fortes C, Renzoni E, Rusconi F, Dell'Orco V, Ciccone G, Bisanti L. (2000) Consumption of fresh fruit rich in vitamin C and wheezing symptoms in children. SIDRIA Collaborative Group, Italy (Italian Studies on Respiratory Disorders in Children and the Environment), *Thorax* 55(4): 283-288

Garcia-Marcos L, Arnedo PA, Busquets-Monge R, Morales Suarez-Varela M, Garcia dA, Batlles-Garrido J, Blanco-Quiros A, Lopez-Silvarrey VA, Garcia-Hernandez G, Aguinaga-Ontoso I et al . (2008) How the presence of rhinoconjunctivitis and the severity of asthma modify the relationship between obesity and asthma in children 6-7 years old, *Clin Exp Allergy* 38(7): 1174-1178

Garcia-Marcos L, Canflanca IM, Garrido JB, Varela AL, Garcia-Hernandez G, Guillen GF, Gonzalez-Diaz C, Carvajal-Uruena I, Arnedo-Pena A, Busquets-Monge RM et al . (2007) Relationship of asthma and rhinoconjunctivitis with obesity, exercise and Mediterranean diet in Spanish schoolchildren, *Thorax* 62(6): 503-508

Gilliland FD, Berhane K, Islam T, McConnell R, Gauderman WJ, Gilliland SS, Avol E, Peters JM. (2003) Obesity and the risk of newly diagnosed asthma in school-age children, *Am J Epidemiol* 158(5): 406-415

Groeben H, Meier S, Brown RH, O'Donnell CP, Mitzner W, Tankersley CG. (2004) The effect of leptin on the ventilatory responseto hyperoxia, *Exp Lung Res* 30(7): 559-570

Guerra S, Wright AL, Morgan WJ, Sherrill DL, Holberg CJ, Martinez FD. (2004) Persistence of asthma symptoms during adolescence: role of obesity and age at the onset of puberty, *Am J Respir Crit Care Med* 170(1): 78-85

Guler N, Kirerleri E, Ones U, Tamay Z, Salmayenli N, Darendeliler F. (2004) Leptin: does it have any role in childhood asthma?, *J Allergy Clin Immunol* 114(2): 254-259

Haberg SE, Stigum H, London SJ, Nystad W, Nafstad P. (2009) Maternal obesity in pregnancy and respiratory health in early childhood, *Paediatr Perinat Epidemiol* 23(4): 352-362

Hakala K, Mustajoki P, Aittomaki J, Sovijarvi AR. (1995) Effect of weight loss and body position on pulmonary function and gas exchange abnormalities in morbid obesity, *Int J Obes Relat Metab Disord* 19(5): 343-346

Hakala K, Stenius-Aarniala B, Sovijarvi A. (2000) Effects of weight loss on peak flow variability, airways obstruction, and lung volumes in obese patients with asthma, *Chest* 118(5): 1315-1321

Hall IP, Wheatley A, Wilding P, Liggett SB. (1995) Association of Glu 27 beta 2-adrenoceptor polymorphism with lower airway reactivity in asthmatic subjects, *Lancet* 345(8959): 1213-1214

Hancox RJ, Milne BJ, Poulton R, Taylor DR, Greene JM, McLachlan CR, Cowan JO, Flannery EM, Herbison GP, Sears MR. (2005) Sex differences in the relation between body mass index and asthma and atopy in a birth cohort, *Am J Respir Crit Care Med* 171(5): 440-445

Hark WT, Thompson WM, McLaughlin TE, Wheatley LM, Platts-Mills TA. (2005) Spontaneous sigh rates during sedentary activity: watching television vs reading, *Ann Allergy Asthma Immunol* 94(2): 247-250

Harmsen HJ, Wildeboer-Veloo AC, Raangs GC, Wagendorp AA, Klijn N, Bindels JG, Welling GW. (2000) Analysis of intestinal flora development in breast-fed and formula-fed infants by using molecular identification and detection methods, *J Pediatr Gastroenterol Nutr* 30(1): 61-67

Herrera-Trujillo M, Barraza-Villarreal A, Lazcano-Ponce E, Hernandez B, Sanin LH, Romieu I. (2005) Current wheezing, puberty, and obesity among mexican adolescent females and young women, *J Asthma* 42(8): 705-709

Hosogai N, Fukuhara A, Oshima K, Miyata Y, Tanaka S, Segawa K, Furukawa S, Tochino Y, Komuro R, Matsuda M et al . (2007) Adipose tissue hypoxia in obesity and its impact on adipocytokine dysregulation, *Diabetes* 56(4): 901-911

Hug C, Wang J, Ahmad NS, Bogan JS, Tsao TS, Lodish HF. (2004) T-cadherin is a receptor for hexameric and high-molecular-weight forms of Acrp30/adiponectin, *Proc Natl Acad Sci U S A* 101(28): 10308-10313

Innis SM, King DJ. (1999) trans Fatty acids in human milk are inversely associated with concentrations of essential all-cis n-6 and n-3 fatty acids and determine trans, but not n-6 and n-3, fatty acids in plasma lipids of breast-fed infants, *Am J Clin Nutr* 70(3): 383-390

Ishiyama-Shigemoto S, Yamada K, Yuan X, Ichikawa F, Nonaka K. (1999) Association of polymorphisms in the beta2-adrenergic receptor gene with obesity, hypertriglyceridaemia, and diabetes mellitus, *Diabetologia* 42(1): 98-101

Jaakkola JJ, Ahmed P, Ieromnimon A, Goepfert P, Laiou E, Quansah R, Jaakkola MS. (2006) Preterm delivery and asthma: a systematic review and meta-analysis, *J Allergy Clin Immunol* 118(4): 823-830

Kalayci O, Besler T, Kilinc K, Sekerel BE, Saraclar Y. (2000) Serum levels of antioxidant vitamins (alpha tocopherol, beta carotene, and ascorbic acid) in children with bronchial asthma, *Turk J Pediatr* 42(1): 17-21

Katsoulis K, Kontakiotis T, Leonardopoulos I, Kotsovili A, Legakis IN, Patakas D. (2003) Serum total antioxidant status in severe exacerbation of asthma: correlation with the severity of the disease, *J Asthma* 40(8): 847-854

Katsumata U, Miura M, Ichinose M, Kimura K, Takahashi T, Inoue H, Takishima T. (1990) Oxygen radicals produce airway constriction and hyperresponsiveness in anesthetized cats, *Am Rev Respir Dis* 141(5 Pt 1): 1158-1161

Kattan M, Kumar R, Bloomberg GR, Mitchell HE, Calatroni A, Gergen PJ, Kercsmar CM, Visness CM, Matsui EC, Steinbach SF et al . (2010) Asthma control, adiposity, and adipokines among inner-city adolescents, *J Allergy Clin Immunol* 125(3): 584-592

Kauffman AS, Clifton DK, Steiner RA. (2007) Emerging ideas about kisspeptin- GPR54 signaling in the neuroendocrine regulation of reproduction, *Trends Neurosci* 30(10): 504-511

Kelly C, Ward C, Stenton CS, Bird G, Hendrick DJ, Walters EH. (1988) Number and activity of inflammatory cells in bronchoalveolar lavage fluid in asthma and their relation to airway responsiveness, *Thorax* 43(9): 684-692

Kelly FJ, Mudway I, Blomberg A, Frew A, Sandstrom T. (1999) Altered lung antioxidant status in patients with mild asthma, *Lancet* 354(9177): 482-483

Kim HJ, Kim CH, Lee DH, Han MW, Kim MY, Ju JH, Do MS. (2011) Expression of eotaxin in 3T3-L1 adipocytes and the effects of weight loss in high-fat diet induced obese mice, *Nutr Res Pract* 5(1): 11-19

Kim KW, Shin YH, Lee KE, Kim ES, Sohn MH, Kim KE. (2008) Relationship between adipokines and manifestations of childhood asthma, *Pediatr Allergy Immunol* 19(6): 535-540

Kirchgessner TG, Uysal KT, Wiesbrock SM, Marino MW, Hotamisligil GS. (1997) Tumor necrosis factor-alpha contributes to obesity-related hyperleptinemia by regulating leptin release from adipocytes, *J Clin Invest* 100(11): 2777-2782

Kojima M, Kangawa K. (2010) Ghrelin: more than endogenous growth hormone secretagogue, *Ann N Y Acad Sci* 1200140-148

Larochelle J, Freiler J, Dice J, Hagan L. (2007) Plasma resistin levels in asthmatics as a marker of disease state, *J Asthma* 44(7): 509-513

Lebrethon MC, Aganina A, Fournier M, Gerard A, Parent AS, Bourguignon JP. (2007) Effects of in vivo and in vitro administration of ghrelin, leptin and neuropeptide mediators on pulsatile gonadotrophin-releasing hormone secretion from male rat hypothalamus before and after puberty, *J Neuroendocrinol* 19(3): 181-188

Leivo-Korpela S, Lehtimaki L, Vuolteenaho K, Nieminen R, Kankaanranta H, Saarelainen S, Moilanen E. (2011) Adipokine resistin predicts anti-inflammatory effect of glucocorticoids in asthma, *J Inflamm (Lond)* 8(1): 12-

Lessard A, Turcotte H, Cormier Y, Boulet LP. (2008) Obesity and asthma: a specific phenotype?, *Chest* 134(2): 317-323

Lugogo NL, Kraft M, Dixon AE. (2010) Does obesity produce a distinct asthma phenotype?, *J Appl Physiol* 108(3): 729-734

Mai XM, Bottcher MF, Leijon I. (2004) Leptin and asthma in overweight children at 12 years of age, *Pediatr Allergy Immunol* 15(6): 523-530

Malli F, Papaioannou AI, Gourgoulianis KI, Daniil Z. (2010) The role of leptin in the respiratory system: an overview, *Respir Res* 11152-

Mallol J, Aguirre V, Espinosa V. (2011) Increased oxidative stress in children with post infectious Bronchiolitis Obliterans, *Allergol Immunopathol (Madr)*

Mancuso P, Canetti C, Gottschalk A, Tithof PK, Peters-Golden M. (2004) Leptin augments alveolar macrophage leukotriene synthesis by increasing phospholipase activity and enhancing group IVC iPLA2 (cPLA2gamma) protein expression, *Am J Physiol Lung Cell Mol Physiol* 287(3): L497-L502

Maniscalco M, Zedda A, Faraone S, Cerbone MR, Cristiano S, Giardiello C, Sofia M. (2008) Weight loss and asthma control in severely obese asthmatic females, *Respir Med* 102(1): 102-108

Matheson MC, Erbas B, Balasuriya A, Jenkins MA, Wharton CL, Tang ML, Abramson MJ, Walters EH, Hopper JL, Dharmage SC. (2007) Breast-feeding and atopic disease: a cohort study from childhood to middle age, *J Allergy Clin Immunol* 120(5): 1051-1057

Matsuda K, Nishi Y, Okamatsu Y, Kojima M, Matsuishi T. (2006) Ghrelin and leptin: a link between obesity and allergy?, *J Allergy Clin Immunol* 117(3): 705-706

Medoff BD, Okamoto Y, Leyton P, Weng M, Sandall BP, Raher MJ, Kihara S, Bloch KD, Libby P, Luster AD. (2009) Adiponectin deficiency increases allergic airway inflammation and pulmonary vascular remodeling, *Am J Respir Cell Mol Biol* 41(4): 397-406

Milic-Emili J, Torchio R, D'Angelo E. (2007) Closing volume: a reappraisal (1967-2007), *Eur J Appl Physiol* 99(6): 567-583

Miller M, Cho JY, Pham A, Ramsdell J, Broide DH. (2009) Adiponectin and functional adiponectin receptor 1 are expressed by airway epithelial cells in chronic obstructive pulmonary disease, *J Immunol* 182(1): 684-691

Mito N, Kitada C, Hosoda T, Sato K. (2002) Effect of diet-induced obesity on ovalbumin-specific immune response in a murine asthma model, *Metabolism* 51(10): 1241-1246

Moreno LA, Rodriguez G. (2007) Dietary risk factors for development of childhood obesity, *Curr Opin Clin Nutr Metab Care* 10(3): 336-341

Nadeem A, Masood A, Siddiqui N. (2008) Oxidant--antioxidant imbalance in asthma: scientific evidence, epidemiological data and possible therapeutic options, *Ther Adv Respir Dis* 2(4): 215-235

Nadeem A, Raj HG, Chhabra SK. (2005) Increased oxidative stress in acute exacerbations of asthma, *J Asthma* 42(1): 45-50

Nagaev I, Bokarewa M, Tarkowski A, Smith U. (2006) Human resistin is a systemic immune-derived proinflammatory cytokine targeting both leukocytes and adipocytes, *PLoS One* 1e31-

Nagel G, Koenig W, Rapp K, Wabitsch M, Zoellner I, Weiland SK. (2009) Associations of adipokines with asthma, rhinoconjunctivitis, and eczema in German schoolchildren, *Pediatr Allergy Immunol* 20(1): 81-88

Naimark A, Cherniack RM. (1960) Compliance of the respiratory system and its components in health and obesity, *J Appl Physiol* 15377-382

Nair P, Radford K, Fanat A, Janssen LJ, Peters-Golden M, Cox PG. (2008) The effects of leptin on airway smooth muscle responses, *Am J Respir Cell Mol Biol* 39(4): 475-481

Navarro VM, Castellano JM, Garcia-Galiano D, Tena-Sempere M. (2007) Neuroendocrine factors in the initiation of puberty: the emergent role of kisspeptin, *Rev Endocr Metab Disord* 8(1): 11-20

Nelson MC, Gordon-Larsen P, North KE, Adair LS. (2006) Body mass index gain, fast food, and physical activity: effects of shared environments over time, *Obesity (Silver Spring)* 14(4): 701-709

Neveu WA, Allard JL, Raymond DM, Bourassa LM, Burns SM, Bunn JY, Irvin CG, Kaminsky DA, Rincon M. (2010) Elevation of IL-6 in the allergic asthmatic airway is independent of inflammation but associates with loss of central airway function, *Respir Res* 1128-

Nurmatov U, Devereux G, Sheikh A. (2011) Nutrients and foods for the primary prevention of asthma and allergy: systematic review and meta-analysis, *J Allergy Clin Immunol* 127(3): 724-733

Ochs-Balcom HM, Grant BJ, Muti P, Sempos CT, Freudenheim JL, Browne RW, McCann SE, Trevisan M, Cassano PA, Iacoviello L et al . (2006) Antioxidants, oxidative stress, and pulmonary function in individuals diagnosed with asthma or COPD, *Eur J Clin Nutr* 60(8): 991-999

Oh CK, Ariue B, Alban RF, Shaw B, Cho SH. (2002) PAI-1 promotes extracellular matrix deposition in the airways of a murine asthma model, *Biochem Biophys Res Commun* 294(5): 1155-1160

Okamatsu Y, Matsuda K, Hiramoto I, Tani H, Kimura K, Yada Y, Kakuma T, Higuchi S, Kojima M, Matsuishi T. (2009) Ghrelin and leptin modulate immunity and liver function in overweight children, *Pediatr Int* 51(1): 9-13

Picado C, Deulofeu R, Lleonart R, Agusti M, Mullol J, Quinto L, Torra M. (2001) Dietary micronutrients/antioxidants and their relationship with bronchial asthma severity, *Allergy* 56(1): 43-49

Pitsavos C, Panagiotakos DB, Tzima N, Chrysohoou C, Economou M, Zampelas A, Stefanadis C. (2005) Adherence to the Mediterranean diet is associated with total antioxidant capacity in healthy adults: the ATTICA study, *Am J Clin Nutr* 82(3): 694-699

Platts-Mills TA, Erwin E, Heymann P, Woodfolk J. (2005) Is the hygiene hypothesis still a viable explanation for the increased prevalence of asthma?, *Allergy* 60(Suppl 79): 25-31

Ponsonby AL, Gatenby P, Glasgow N, Mullins R, McDonald T, Hurwitz M. (2002) Which clinical subgroups within the spectrum of child asthma are attributable to atopy?, *Chest* 121(1): 135-142

Raap U, Brzoska T, Sohl S, Path G, Emmel J, Herz U, Braun A, Luger T, Renz H. (2003) Alpha-melanocyte-stimulating hormone inhibits allergic airway inflammation, *J Immunol* 171(1): 353-359

Rasmussen F, Lambrechtsen J, Siersted HC, Hansen HS, Hansen NC. (2000) Low physical fitness in childhood is associated with the development of asthma in young adulthood: the Odense schoolchild study, *Eur Respir J* 16(5): 866-870

Roberts CK, Barnard RJ, Sindhu RK, Jurczak M, Ehdaie A, Vaziri ND. (2006) Oxidative stress and dysregulation of NAD(P)H oxidase and antioxidant enzymes in diet-induced metabolic syndrome, *Metabolism* 55(7): 928-934

Rothenbacher D, Weyermann M, Fantuzzi G, Brenner H. (2007) Adipokines in cord blood and risk of wheezing disorders within the first two years of life, *Clin Exp Allergy* 37(8): 1143-1149

Sackesen C, Ercan H, Dizdar E, Soyer O, Gumus P, Tosun BN, Buyuktuncer Z, Karabulut E, Besler T, Kalayci O. (2008) A comprehensive evaluation of the enzymatic and nonenzymatic antioxidant systems in childhood asthma, *J Allergy Clin Immunol* 122(1): 78-85

Schley PD, Field CJ. (2002) The immune-enhancing effects of dietary fibres and prebiotics, *Br J Nutr* 87(Suppl 2): S221-S230

Schmidt M, Affenito SG, Striegel-Moore R, Khoury PR, Barton B, Crawford P, Kronsberg S, Schreiber G, Obarzanek E, Daniels S. (2005) Fast-food intake and diet quality in black and white girls: the National Heart, Lung, and Blood Institute Growth and Health Study, *Arch Pediatr Adolesc Med* 159(7): 626-631

Scholtens S, Wijga AH, Brunekreef B, Kerkhof M, Postma DS, Oldenwening M, de Jongste JC, Smit HA. (2010) Maternal overweight before pregnancy and asthma in offspring followed for 8 years, *Int J Obes (Lond)* 34(4): 606-613

Schroder H. (2007) Protective mechanisms of the Mediterranean diet in obesity and type 2 diabetes, *J Nutr Biochem* 18(3): 149-160

Schwartz MW, Seeley RJ, Woods SC, Weigle DS, Campfield LA, Burn P, Baskin DG. (1997) Leptin increases hypothalamic pro-opiomelanocortin mRNA expression in the rostral arcuate nucleus, *Diabetes* 46(12): 2119-2123

Shanmugasundaram KR, Kumar SS, Rajajee S. (2001) Excessive free radical generation in the blood of children suffering from asthma, *Clin Chim Acta* 305(1-2): 107-114

Sherriff A, Maitra A, Ness AR, Mattocks C, Riddoch C, Reilly JJ, Paton JY, Henderson AJ. (2009) Association of duration of television viewing in early childhood with the subsequent development of asthma, *Thorax* 64(4): 321-325

Shore SA. (2007) Obesity and asthma: lessons from animal models, *J Appl Physiol* 102(2): 516-528

Shore SA. (2008) Obesity and asthma: possible mechanisms, *J Allergy Clin Immunol* 121(5): 1087-1093

Shore SA. (2010) Obesity, airway hyperresponsiveness, and inflammation, *J Appl Physiol* 108(3): 735-743

Shore SA, Johnston RA. (2006) Obesity and asthma, *Pharmacol Ther* 110(1): 83-102

Shore SA, Rivera-Sanchez YM, Schwartzman IN, Johnston RA. (2003) Responses to ozone are increased in obese mice, *J Appl Physiol* 95(3): 938-945

Shore SA, Schwartzman IN, Mellema MS, Flynt L, Imrich A, Johnston RA. (2005) Effect of leptin on allergic airway responses in mice, *J Allergy Clin Immunol* 115(1): 103-109

Shore SA, Terry RD, Flynt L, Xu A, Hug C. (2006) Adiponectin attenuates allergen-induced airway inflammation and hyperresponsiveness in mice, *J Allergy Clin Immunol* 118(2): 389-395

Skloot G, Togias A. (2003) Bronchodilation and bronchoprotection by deep inspiration and their relationship to bronchial hyperresponsiveness, *Clin Rev Allergy Immunol* 24(1): 55-72

Sood A, Ford ES, Camargo CA, Jr. (2006) Association between leptin and asthma in adults, *Thorax* 61(4): 300-305

Sukalich S, Mingione MJ, Glantz JC. (2006) Obstetric outcomes in overweight and obese adolescents, *Am J Obstet Gynecol* 195(3): 851-855

Sutherland TJ, Sears MR, McLachlan CR, Poulton R, Hancox RJ. (2009) Leptin, adiponectin, and asthma: findings from a population-based cohort study, *Ann Allergy Asthma Immunol* 103(2): 101-107

Takemura Y, Ouchi N, Shibata R, Aprahamian T, Kirber MT, Summer RS, Kihara S, Walsh K. (2007) Adiponectin modulates inflammatory reactions via calreticulin receptor-dependent clearance of early apoptotic bodies, *J Clin Invest* 117(2): 375-386

Tankersley C, Kleeberger S, Russ B, Schwartz A, Smith P. (1996) Modified control of breathing in genetically obese (ob/ob) mice, *J Appl Physiol* 81(2): 716-723

Tantisira KG, Weiss ST. (2001) Complex interactions in complex traits: obesity and asthma, *Thorax* 56(Suppl 2): ii64-ii73

Taraseviciute A, Voelkel NF. (2006) Severe pulmonary hypertension in postmenopausal obese women, *Eur J Med Res* 11(5): 198-202

Thomas PS, Agrawal S, Gore M, Geddes DM. (1995) Recall lung pneumonitis due to carmustine after radiotherapy, *Thorax* 50(10): 1116-1118

Thomas PS, Heywood G. (2002) Effects of inhaled tumour necrosis factor alpha in subjects with mild asthma, *Thorax* 57(9): 774-778

To T, Guan J, Wang C, Radhakrishnan D, McLimont S, Latycheva O, Gershon AS. (2010) Is large birth weight associated with asthma risk in early childhood?, *Arch Dis Child*

To T, Vydykhan TN, Dell S, Tassoudji M, Harris JK. (2004) Is obesity associated with asthma in young children?, *J Pediatr* 144(2): 162-168

Tsuchiya T, Shimizu H, Horie T, Mori M. (1999) Expression of leptin receptor in lung: leptin as a growth factor, *Eur J Pharmacol* 365(2-3): 273-279

Turner S, Zhang G, Young S, Cox M, Goldblatt J, Landau L, Le Souef P. (2008) Associations between postnatal weight gain, change in postnatal pulmonary function, formula feeding and early asthma, *Thorax* 63(3): 234-239

Vasudevan AR, Wu H, Xydakis AM, Jones PH, Smith EO, Sweeney JF, Corry DB, Ballantyne CM. (2006) Eotaxin and obesity, *J Clin Endocrinol Metab* 91(1): 256-261

Vogelberg C, Hirsch T, Radon K, Dressel H, Windstetter D, Weinmayr G, Weiland SK, von Mutius E, Nowak D, Leupold W. (2007) Leisure time activity and new onset of wheezing during adolescence, *Eur Respir J* 30(4): 672-676

von Kries R, Hermann M, Grunert VP, von Mutius E. (2001) Is obesity a risk factor for childhood asthma?, *Allergy* 56(4): 318-322

von Mutius E. (2007) Allergies, infections and the hygiene hypothesis--the epidemiological evidence, *Immunobiology* 212(6): 433-439

Vural H, Uzun K. (2000) Serum and red blood cell antioxidant status in patients with bronchial asthma, *Can Respir J* 7(6): 476-480

Weiland SK, von Mutius E, Husing A, Asher MI. (1999) Intake of trans fatty acids and prevalence of childhood asthma and allergies in Europe. ISAAC Steering Committee, *Lancet* 353(9169): 2040-2041

Weisberg SP, McCann D, Desai M, Rosenbaum M, Leibel RL, Ferrante AW, Jr. (2003) Obesity is associated with macrophage accumulation in adipose tissue, *J Clin Invest* 112(12): 1796-1808

White SR, Fischer BM, Marroquin BA, Stern R. (2008) Interleukin-1beta mediates human airway epithelial cell migration via NF-kappaB, *Am J Physiol Lung Cell Mol Physiol* 295(6): L1018-L1027

Wickens K, Barry D, Friezema A, Rhodius R, Bone N, Purdie G, Crane J. (2005) Fast foods - are they a risk factor for asthma?, *Allergy* 60(12): 1537-1541

Williams DL, Kaplan JM, Grill HJ. (2000) The role of the dorsal vagal complex and the vagus nerve in feeding effects of melanocortin-3/4 receptor stimulation, *Endocrinology* 141(4): 1332-1337

Wilson NJ, Boniface K, Chan JR, McKenzie BS, Blumenschein WM, Mattson JD, Basham B, Smith K, Chen T, Morel F et al . (2007) Development, cytokine profile and function of human interleukin 17-producing helper T cells, *Nat Immunol* 8(9): 950-957

Wong CK, Cheung PF, Lam CW. (2007) Leptin-mediated cytokine release and migration of eosinophils: implications for immunopathophysiology of allergic inflammation, *Eur J Immunol* 37(8): 2337-2348

Wood LG, Fitzgerald DA, Gibson PG, Cooper DM, Garg ML. (2000) Lipid peroxidation as determined by plasma isoprostanes is related to disease severity in mild asthma, *Lipids* 35(9): 967-974

Wood LG, Garg ML, Blake RJ, Simpson JL, Gibson PG. (2008) Oxidized vitamin E and glutathione as markers of clinical status in asthma, *Clin Nutr* 27(4): 579-586

Xia Q, Pang W, Pan H, Zheng Y, Kang JS, Zhu SG. (2004) Effects of ghrelin on the proliferation and secretion of splenic T lymphocytes in mice, *Regul Pept* 122(3): 173-178

Ye J, Gao Z, Yin J, He Q. (2007) Hypoxia is a potential risk factor for chronic inflammation and adiponectin reduction in adipose tissue of ob/ob and dietary obese mice, *Am J Physiol Endocrinol Metab* 293(4): E1118-E1128

2

Psychological Factors in Asthma and Psychoeducational Interventions

Lia Fernandes
Department of Psychiatry and Mental Health,
Faculty of Medicine, University of Oporto,
Psychiatry Service of S. João Hospital, Oporto,
Portugal

1. Introduction

This subject is of interest as asthma has increased over the last two decades. Despite therapeutic advances, morbidity and mortality are increasing (Global Initiative for Asthma [GINA], 2010), particularly due to the development of western standards of living, where psychological factors have regained notability (Busse et al., 2000). This brings about a worsening in psychological factors and quality of life which entails high socioeconomic costs (direct and indirect) (Sulivan 1996; Suissa 2000).

Since the most remote times of medical history (Maimonides 1990, Alexander 1940, Dunbar 1948), it has been possible to determine a connection between asthma and emotional factors. In this study, besides the epidemiological aspects and the determinant psychopathological issues of this illness, some of the main psychological factors that influence and are influenced by this complex illness are reviewed in a multidimensional systemic vision (Gregerson, 2000; Jasnoski et al., 1994; Dirks et al., 1978).

Parallel to the importance given to biological factors, social and physical variables have also been enhanced, as have conditionings brought about by stress, which intervene and condition psychoneuroimmunohormonal mechanisms in the evolution of the illness (Goodwin & Eaton, 2003).

In the most severe cases of asthma, psychological factors such as depression, anxiety, stress, psychopathology, psychiatric expression of asthma and side effects of medication will be implicated. In this context, the coping mechanisms involved, as well as different life events and other psychosocial conditions are of the utmost importance. The transformation of these people's lives inevitably involves their families, making problem solving difficult, and determining the outcome and the treatment of this pathology (Scott et al., 2007; Fernandes et al., 2010; Thomas et al., 2011; Di Marco et al., 2011).

On the other hand, less adapted behaviours become related to minor compliance in the care of asthma, which leads to the worsening of the symptoms of asthma, causing self-perpetuation mechanisms, with chronically inflammatory processes, pulmonary remodelling and irreversibility in the size of the airways (Rietveld, 2000; Fonseca et al., 2004).

Therapeutically, in people with moderate to severe asthma, besides the usual, preventive and pharmacological approaches, it is essential to turn to psychoeducational and multifamily programmes, in order to increase the control of the illness, and allow more efficient treatment (Yorke et al., 2007; Smith et al., 2007).

It is in this multisystemic context only by deepening the reciprocal relationships among psychological and biological, family and social factors can one find answers for the enormous complexity of the asthmatic illness. As a corollary of this, the confirmation that only a sufficiently widespread intervention that simultaneously combines the premises previously formulated, will allow an increased therapeutic effectiveness (Fernandes, 2009).

This conceptual transformation into a multifactorial model influences also methodologically the psychosomatic research (Gregerson, 1995). The focus of this approach is based not so much on the causes (as in the linear model) but above all, in intervention and treatment (Mathison, 1993; Stout & Creer, 1997).

Illustrating this, two studies will be presented. The first one, Psychological and Psychosocial Factors in Asthma, will study the influence of the psychological (anxiety, depression, psychopathology) and psychosocial variables of asthmatics with the clinical variables (symptoms, spirometry, inflammatory marker, severity and duration) and morbidity (quality of life, control of asthma, medication, use of health care and absenteeism). In the second study, Psychoeducational and Multifamily Interventions in asthma will presented the effectiveness of these interventions in this illness.

2. Clinical review

Asthma is a chronic inflammatory disease of the airways, which has a great impact on the quality of life of these patients.

In Portugal, as in the majority of western countries, asthma is increasing, which brings about high socioeconomic costs and an increase in mortality and morbidity (GINA, 2010).

For a long time the involvement of psychosocial factors in this disease has been known. Among different respiratory illnesses asthma presents the most profound links between psychological, social, biological and physiological factors. This is why it is considered the prototype of psychosomatic diseases (Isenberg et al., 1992; Lehrer et al., 1993; Mackenzie, 1886).

Much has been achieved since the 1960s, with the psychoanalytic approach to asthma in children, viewed as crying repression (French & Alexander, 1941).

Great progress has been made in the field of medical knowledge namely concerning the neuroimunohormonal mechanisms involved in the etiopathogenesis of this disease. There is increasing evidence that the immune system is not working autonomously. In spite of this it will be connected with many psychophysiological processes under the regulatory modulation of the brain (Ader & Cohen, 1985). This branch of study we call psychoneuroimmunology. In this way it makes sense that we speak in the long term about changes that can stabilize resistance to the disease. This individual stability could be organized in each patient's personality structure, which could confront the different challenges and stress events of daily life (Goldstein & Dekker, 2001).

However the precise physiological mechanisms involved are very complex, needing more profound research. The psychological disorders seem to produce systemic effects in the immune system function, in metabolic and hormonal processes and in the peripheral and central nervous system, in interactional and reciprocal mechanisms instead of being focused on one organ, as was commonly thought for a long time (Kang et al., 1997; Cohen et al., 1991; Rietveld & Everaerd, 2000; Di Marco et al., 2011).

Nowadays in a more realistic perspective, it is considered that negative emotions (fear, panic, anger, anxiety and depression) are linked in a fluctuating process of bronchoconstriction of the airways, based on a mechanism of worsening crises of asthma (Hollaender & Florin, 1983; Silverglade et al., 1994; Lehrer, 1998; ten Brinke et al., 2001).

In an indispensable holistic vision of this disease the psychological aspects become inseparable from the remaining symptoms when it is a question of making a diagnosis or prognosis or treating asthma (Lehrer et al., 2002).

It is well known that these patients' behaviour strongly influences the course of the illness and the treatment, determining the exposure to allergic factors, in the perception and assessment of the symptoms, in the search for adequate medical care and compliance with the therapeutic plan, being strongly predictive for the frequency and severity of the worsening of the disease (Levy, 1994; van der Berg et al., 1997; Miller & Hotses, 1995; Devriese et al., 2000).

Determinants of this behaviour are indubitable the psychopathology and familiar disorganization which is reflected in the worsening of the disease, in a decrease in quality of life as well as in the increasing health care costs involved. In some more extreme conditions these factors increase risk to life (Nouwen et al., 1999).

Near-fatal asthma deserves scrutiny due to the severity of these events and because of its impact on subsequent asthma morbidity and healthcare costs. The first studies emphasized the role of psychological variables (Campbell et al., 1994; Strunk et al., 1999; Innes et al., 1998; Di Marco et al., 2011).

Furthermore, special attention has to be devoted to the subgroup of severe asthma which is difficult and complex - implying avoidance of multiple environmental stimuli, with a variety of medications for controlling chronic inflammation or acute broncho-dilatation, with complex planning and high costs (Boulet et al., 1991; Woller et al., 1993; Kelloway et al., 2000).

Besides that, knowing that asthma is not a behavioural disease, there is evidence that some changes in some asthmatic groups can condition the evolution of the disease. On the other hand there is also evidence that asthma has a role in the development of some psychiatric diseases (Lehrer et al., 2002; Scott et al., 2007).

Some negative emotions, particularly panic and depression, even not severe enough to be classified as psychiatric disorders, can produce respiratory effects and lead to worsening of asthma, directly by psychophysiological effects or indirectly by neglecting self-management of the illness. Conversely, these emotional disorders can also be worsened by asthma itself (Nouwen et al., 1999; ten Brinke et al., 2001; Lehrer et al., 2004).

A prospective Swiss community-based longitudinal cohort study (Hasler et al., 2005) reported that having a diagnosis of asthma may result in the subsequent development of panic in some patients with an odds ratio of 4.5. On the other hand, the same study also reported that the presence of panic disorder predicted subsequent asthma with an odds ratio of 6.3, suggesting that psychological dysfunction may precede the development of asthma.

A UK primary care survey published in 2007 (Cooper et al., 2007), reported higher anxiety and depression scores in adults with asthma than the general community, and a prevalence of panic disorder of 16% in those with asthma.

There are other psychological factors with a similar relationship to asthma worsening, which deserve a deeper study, particularly personality characteristics and their relation to the perception of asthma symptoms. The state of the art test pinpoints for endorphin activity on the basis of this respiratory sensitivity (Rietveld et al., 2000).

In a recent study (Fernandes et al., 2005) the predominance of neurotic characteristics in asthmatic patients was confirmed. They also presented lower extroversion, openness to experience, agreeableness and conscientiousness when compared to the general population. These characteristics were linked to the severity and duration of the disease.

On the other hand, an increasing consensus is becoming established concerning the emotional triggers of asthma, focusing on psychophysiological mechanisms. This is demonstrated in recent studies where in response to emotional states there is a bronchoconstriction as well as registered cardiovascular and electrodermal modifications. Particularly in asthma the respiratory reaction in the airways is well known, when psychologically induced, including the variations in airways narrowing, which characterize the typical fluctuations of the disease (Lehrer et al., 2003, 2004).

Nowadays bronchoconstriction in asthma is defined by direct sympathetic nervous system action or indirect parasympathetic nervous system action by a rebound effect (Manto, 1969; Isenberg et al., 1992; Lehrer et al., 1997), under some specific psychological states (sadness, stress, etc.), or by an inflammatory reaction. Although it remains less well-investigated, it is the last characteristic component in the pathology of asthma, i.e., blood vessel proliferations with increased airways wall thickness, as well as mucus hypersecrection (Lehrer et al., 1998). In some patients, stress in particular is the essential trigger for asthma attacks. Anxiety symptoms in asthmatics have been revealed as strong predictors of respiratory illness in those patients. Besides that, anxiety and depression seem to be much more prevalent in the asthmatic population than in the normal one (Rietveld et al., 2000; Thomas et al., 2011).

Different surveys using different methodologies and instruments indicate that anxiety and depression disorders are up to six times more common in people with asthma than in the general population (Goodwin & Eaton, 2003; Lavoie et al., 2006).

In a recent study (Fernandes et al., 2010) the high prevalence of anxiety in asthmatic patients as well as its associations with worse subjective asthma outcomes and increased used of medications/healthcare services was confirmed.

Anxiety and depression are also particularly reported with severe and difficult to control asthma (Heaney et al., 2005) and impaired emotional coping mechanisms (Lavoie et al., 2010).

Both psychological manifestations inherent in the asthmatic process itself and other clinical situations that can be asthma like, or present some aspects of this illness, have in core genesis a common mechanism: psychosomatic structure (Horton et al., 1978).

Some of that asthma like illnesses have present in their origin above all a psychological mechanism. These kinds of clinical expressions can vary from somatoform disorder to factitious or conversion disorder. In any case it is mainly a functional disturbance, with a physiological minor component (Luparello et al., 1968).

From an investigational perspective there has been a huge change in the techniques used. In the majority of the research, scientists look for physical data when trying to understand this complex system, where psychological factors and emotions are involved.

In this context, some respiratory changes are measured and studied, in some experiments with emotional content in films (Levenson, 1979), in contrast with saline solution inhalation, both by the action of suggestion (Luparello, 1968; McFadden et al., 1969; Neild & Cameron, 1985).

In spite of this, all researchers are using a model, which follows a linear mechanism of thinking. According to some authors (Ford, 1987; Ford & Urban, 1998), who mostly reflected on psychosomatic methodology research, this paradigm is considered completely inappropriate since we involve the behavioural component. In none of these studies, for example, was the individual and unique experience of each patient taken into account, neither were their past nor their future hopes, considered as a part of the study context.

In fact, any biological, physical or chemical system works like a complex system in which the inherent proprieties are not totally explained, by each constituent part (Gallagher & Appenzeller, 1999). This kind of approach has given rise to some findings in the chemical field (Whitesides & Ismagilov, 1999) in biological signal systems (Weng et al., 1999) and the nervous system (Koch & Laurent, 1999).

Alternatively a new model was suggested, with particular relevance to human being studies. In this, as underlined by Borkovec (1997), the involved processes are linked in a nonlinear dynamic, just as with attention, thinking, images, memory, emotion, physiology and behaviour, all in a permanent interaction, and answering to interpersonal and environmental changes, with a background of biological and developmental history.

In an attempt to adapt this model to the investigation of emotional phenomena in asthma, it will probably be as difficult as to adapt it to the chemical field (Whitesides & Ismagilov, 1999). This becomes even more difficult if we take into consideration that asthma is particularly sensitive to the initial conditions with small variations, having a great number of independent components, which interact in multiple pathways, through which all of these mechanisms could be involved. These conditions raise a multiplicity of potential respiratory patterns.

Through this kind of alternative approach, we will be able to allow a draw study project based above all on the reality of the phenomena investigated. This will bring us close to the necessary conditions to finally get solid evidence in the clarification of the complexity of all of these mechanisms involved with stress and emotions in the present disease. Not only will we get solutions for centuries of old mysteries but it will be possible to have new approaches in the treatment of asthma (Gallagher & Appenzeller, 1999; Koch & Laurent, 1999).

It is in this new contextualization that the importance of psychoeducational programs in asthma is growing. The preliminary data about this intervention gives emphasis to educational, communicational and self-efficacy aspects (Yorke et al., 2007; Fernandes, 2009).

There are already some series of randomized multicenter educational programmes for asthma (Taitel et al., 1995; Kotses et al., 1995; Wilson et al., 1996; Bruzzese et al., 2001). The focus of these programmes is in the clarification of the importance of specific components of the illness. In spite of this, feedback to patients with an assessment of these educational programmes is lacking, as well as an adaptation into short interventions that can work in clinical practice or even in a multifamily context (McFarlane et al., 1995; Devine, 1996; Fernandes, 2009).

Furthermore, it will be important to establish this kind of intervention in more specific groups, such as children with more vulnerability in asthmatic crises, people in high risk groups where stress clearly triggers the worsening of the disease (Bernard-Bonnin et al., 1995; Smith et al., 2005).

There is also some relevance of specific programmes for tobacco reduction, with use of psychotherapy, particularly in the cognitive and family therapy fields. These studies took a privileged focus on the control and treatment in daily life, of this complex chronic disease (Irvine et al., 1999; Silagy, 1999; Gustafsson & Cederblad, 1986; Lask & Matthew, 1979; Sun et al., 2010).

Another important aspect is the identification of some specific characteristics of these patients (in terms of severity, personality and even psychological aspects) in subpopulations that most benefit from these education programmes. Eventually the longitudinal assessment in different contexts will be fundamental.

In conclusion, from a research perspective, a distinct kind of approach will be necessary, based on a reality of these phenomena studied, that allows association mechanisms to be established among multiple factors involved, leading to a more modern methodology in a systemic framework, that puts emphasis on the multifactorial model (Fernandes, 2009).

3. Study 1: Psychological and psychosocial factors

3.1 Objectives

The present study aims to study the influence of psychological factors (state and trait anxiety, anger, depression, psychopathology) and psychosocial variables of asthma with clinical characteristics (spirometry, inflammatory marker, severity and duration) and morbidity criteria (quality of life, control of asthma, medication, use of health care services and absenteeism).

The second aim is to study the integration of these data into the cultural diversity of the present population, from a demographic perspective.

3.2 Methods

In this transversal study, 299 outpatients of the Immunoallergology department of the S. João Hospital, of both sexes, were recruited with asthma diagnosis, between the ages of 17 and 75 years.

With the 217 patients that participated, a psychiatric clinical interview was carried out, and psychiatric clinical cases were excluded, by the General Health Questionnaire – GHQ-28 (Goldberg & Hillier, 1979), as well as alcohol and drug abuse cases. Inclusion criteria were previous medical diagnosis of asthma and specific criteria (anti-asthmatic therapy, tests of unspecified bronchial hyper-reactivity and bronchodilation, inflammatory marker, spirometry).

Thus, 195 patients were studied according to the duration of the illness, symptoms, morbidity criteria (use of health care, medication and absenteeism), spirometry (FEV1, PEF), test of bronchial hyper-reactivity (PD20 metacolina), inflammatory markers (FENO), severity of asthma (GINA, 2010) and atopy and rhinitis.

They were evaluated according to the following scales: Self Anxiety Scale – SAS (Zung, 1971), State-Trait Anxiety Inventory – STAIY (Spielberger, 1983), State-Trait Anger Expression Inventory – STAXI (Spielberger, 1988), Beck Depression Inventory – BDI (Beck et al., 1961), Hopkins Symptom Distress Checklist 90-Revised – SCL90R (Derogatis & Savitz, 1999), Ways of Coping with Asthma in Everyday Life – WCAEL (Aalto et al., 2002), Mini Asthma Quality of Life Questionnaire – MiniAQLQ (Juniper et al., 1999a) and Asthma Control Questionnaire – ACQ (Juniper et al., 1999b).

Patient informed consent was obtained and the study was approved by the hospital Ethics Committee.

3.3 Results

In this sample (n=195), most of the patients were female (76.4%), with ages ranging from 17 to 75 years. The mean (sd) age was 38(14.5) years. Most of the patients have low education (70.2%). There was a predominance of low and very low classes (72.4%), according to the Graffar social classification (Graffar, 1956).

The mean duration of the disease was 19.8(14.0) years. The severity of the illness was distributed in the following way: Intermittent (8.2%), Mild persistent (12.8%), Moderate persistent (12.8%) and Severe persistent (66.2%).

The respiratory values found were: spirometry FEV1 83.5(22.4) (min.19%, max.120%), inflammatory marker FENO P50 28 (min.4, max.222). Most of these patients concomitantly have atopy (80.9%) and rhinitis (60.3%).

Total = 195		
Age (years) mean (sd)	38.0	(14.6)
Gender n(%)		
Male	46	(23.6)
Female	149	(76.4)
Education n(%)		
≤ 9	137	(70.2)
10-11	37	(19.0)
> 12	21	(10.8)
Socio-economic classification n(%)		
High and very high	16	(8.2)
Median	38	(19.5)
Low	59	(30.3)
Very low	82	(42.1)
Asthma duration (years) mean (sd)	19.8	(14.0)
Asthma severity n (%)		
Intermittent	16	(8.2)
Mild persistent	25	(12.8)
Moderate persistent	25	(12.8)
Severe persistent	129	(66.2)

Table 1. Demographic and clinical characteristics of sample

From a psychological point of view, the asthmatics of the sample were individuals with a high level of anxiety state (70%): 13.3% had scores suggesting anxiety and 56.4% suffered from high-anxiety (Ponciano et al., 1982).
Considering the anxiety trait, assessed by STAIY, there was a mean (sd) value of 40.82 (12.18). On this scale, state-anxiety had a mean (sd) of 44.8 (13.16).
In this sample, the mean values of contained and manifested anger (mean 15.94, sd 4.05; mean 13.31, sd 12.0) were much higher than the mean standard results found in the normative Portuguese population (Martins, 1995).
Additionally the analysis of the degree of depression, assessed by BDI, allowed us to conclude that in the majority of the sample (72%) depression was absent. Only 6.2% of these patients revealed symptoms of severe and 22% mild/moderate depression.
Psychopathology assessed in the different list of symptoms of Hopkins-Review SCL-90-R, had in general normal values, with the exception for somatization (mean 1.4, dp 0.8) and anxiety (mean 1.06, dp 0.68), higher than the mean values standardized for the Portuguese population.
In the present sample, the most important coping mechanism found was hiding asthma, with a mean (dp) value of 13.08 (2.21), followed by worry with the disease, with a mean (dp) value of 9 (2.12), corroborated by the global score (mean 82, dp 7.63).
The mean (sd) values for quality of life, according to the MiniAQLQ were 4.9 (1.3), with a minimum of 2 and a maximum of 7.

For asthma control, assessed by ACQ (with 0 FEV1), P50 (min.0 /max. 5.2), the mean (sd) was 1.5 (1.2).

In the present study we verified a correlation between sex (higher in women) and anxiety (p<0.001), as well as depression (p=0.000) and psychopathology (p=0.001).

There was a positive correlation between age and anxiety state (p=0.006) and trait (p=0.037), depression (p=0.001), psychopathology (p=0.025), as well as coping mechanism (p<0.001).

A worsening in breathing was noted (spirometry values) only with psychopathology – obsession (p=0.05).

On the other hand, these psychological variables (anxiety p≤0.001, psychopathology - somatization p=0.001) were related to the decrease in the inflammatory marker, indicating higher health care use and an increase in medication intake (mainly preventative).

Above all anxiety state was related to more hospitalization (p=0.007) as well as non-scheduled consultations (p=0.008) and routine ones (p=0.001).

Anxiety and depression also increased absenteeism (p=0.011; p=0.017).

These psychological variables also increased with the severity (p≤0.001; p≤0.001) and with the duration of the disease (p=0.002; p=0.023). However, psychopathology only increased with severity (p=0.002).

Another result found, was that anxiety (r=0.638; p≤0.001), anger (r=-0.343; ≤0.001) and depression (r=-0.527; p≤0.001) worsened the quality of life (Figure 1 and 2).

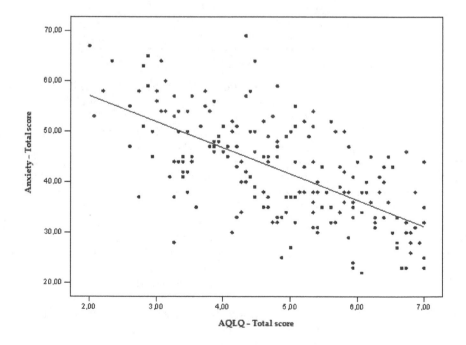

Fig. 1. Correlation between anxiety and quality of life

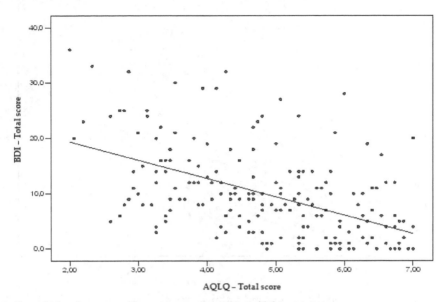

Fig. 2. Correlation between depression and quality of life

The control of asthma was correlated with anxiety state (r=0.554; p≤0.001) and trait (r=0.357; p=0.000), as well as anger (r=0.221; p=0.016) (Figure 3). Another clinical variable was also associated with control of asthma, which is depression (r=0.656; p≤0.001) (Figure 4).

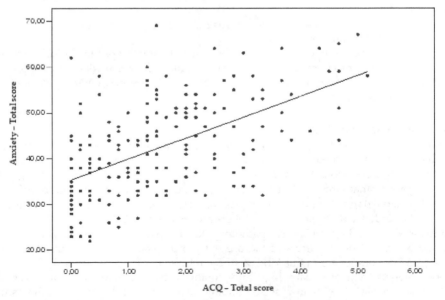

Fig. 3. Correlation between anxiety and asthma control

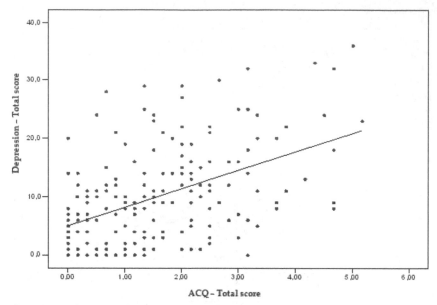

Fig. 4. Correlation between depression and asthma control

Increase in age implied better disease adaptation (p≤0.001). The severity of asthma sustained lower total coping mechanisms (p=0.021), as well as positive reappraisal (p=0.009), assessed by WCAEL.

Of special note, the coping mechanism restricted lifestyle (p=0.021) increased with duration of the disease. The positive reappraisal had a negative correlation with the duration of the disease (p=0.028).

Absenteeism was also directly related to restricted lifestyle and reverse with seeking information, the two coping mechanisms.

The coping mechanism worry with asthma decreased the quality of life (r=-0.239; p=0.044). The most mobilizing mechanism for looking for medical care: consultation (p=0.014) was restricted lifestyle. An opposite implication for denial (p=0.015) mechanism was found, and leading to less intake of corticosteroids.

3.4 Discussion and conclusion

According to the standard values for the Portuguese population (Ponciano et al., 1982), this group has a clear predominance of anxiety in 70% of the sample, as defined in the literature (Vila et al., 2000; Goodwin & Eaton, 2003). This is reinforced by the high levels of anger-in as well as anger-out, that almost all duplicated in this sample (when compared to the normal values of general population), which may be related to more physiological activation, as found for the studies with hypertension (Spielberger & London, 1990).

In contrast we found lower psychopathology levels, particularly depression, probably explained by the selection criteria of the present sample and because the influence of the well-known low compliance in this kind of study of these particular patients.

Anxiety, depression, psychopathology and coping increased with age. However, only anxiety was correlated with low socioeconomic level, as corroborated in other studies (Rumbak et al., 1993).

In the present sample a high correlation with sex, especially for women was found with anxiety, depression and psychopathology, which is in accordance in the previous studies (Eysenck, 1969; Dalton et al., 1975; Mayer-Cross et al., 1969; Thomas et al., 2011).

Anxiety, anger and depression correlated with the duration of asthma episodes and their acuteness (in the GINA classification), which is in agreement with former studies (Mrazeck et al., 1998; Sandberg et al., 2000; ten Brinke et al., 2001; Barton et al., 2005; Wainwright et al., 2007; Dahlem et al., 2009), associating the early onset of asthma with a negative impact on psychological adaptation to the disease, which implies the development of more clinical anxiety and depression.

The use of healthcare services by asthmatic patients as well medication (especially relief and preventive ones) was also directly linked with anxiety. Particularly, anxiety is predicted due to hospitalizations (Dirks et al., 1978, 1981; Kinsman et al., 1982) and their duration (Put et al., 1999).

These results agree with others, who argue that high anxiety leads to poor discrimination between anxiety symptoms and breathing symptoms, thus leading to an overuse of medical care (Spinhoven et al., 1997; Cluley & Cochrane, 2001). There was also a significant relationship between a great number of hospital admissions and higher scores of anxiety, which strengthens the conclusions of previous studies, where anxiety is predictive of more hospital admissions (Bender et al., 2006; Prueter & Norra, 2005) and longer duration.

There was a relationship between exhaled nitric oxide (FENO) and anxiety and somatization. This marker for airway inflammation had a negative correlation with anxiety. In other words, as the levels of anxiety increase, there is evidence of a decrease in inflammation. A possible interpretation of this inverse association may be found in the characteristics of high anxiety of this sample, calling for the use of greater medical care (ten Brinke et al., 2001b). In turn physicians may be influenced by the increased expression of symptoms by the patients. As a consequence more anti-inflammatory treatment is prescribed as patients are identified as more acutely ill (Hibbert & Pilsbury, 1988; Hornsveld & Garssen, 1996). The inflammatory marker decreases because it is particularly sensitive to changes in medication, specifically corticosteroids (Chetta et al., 1998). However, the changes are not reflected in other, less sensitive markers of this disease, namely, lung-function (FEV and PEF), for which no significant relationship with anxiety was found. This lack of association between lung function and anxiety has been previously reported (Thomas et al., 2001).

This tendency toward increasing anxiety was seen for the greater degrees of asthma severity. This agrees with studies in which anxiety in asthmatics is seen as a risk factor for increase in asthma morbidity and mortality (Wright et al., 1998; Forsythe et al., 2004). A similar correlation was found for psychopathology which is corroborated by other studies (Chetta et al., 1998), namely when this is linked with near-fatal asthma attacks (Yellowees et al., 1988; Boulet et al., 1991; Garden et al., 1993; Campbell et al., 1995a; McQuaid et al., 2001). This severity was also correlated positively with depression, in accordance with other studies (Strunk et al., 195; Picado et al., 1989; Campbell et al., 1995a; Martin et al., 1995). This relation between depression and severity asthma is particularly relevant in the case of recent bereavement (Levitan, 1985), as well as death by asthma with hopelessness and despair in the days before the relative's death (Miller et al., 1989).

By using STAI-Y, the average values for the anxiety trait (i.e., a measure for an individual's tendency for anxiety) were higher than those found in other studies for the Portuguese population (Santos & Silva, 1997; Silva & Campos, 1998) and that have been used as standard references. These characteristics agree with some other previous studies (Boulet et al., 1991; Chetta et al., 1998) which argue that there is a strong link between anxiety trait and asthma, as well as a greater manifestation of the symptoms of this ailment (Kinsman et al., 1973; Dirks et al., 1978; Friedman & Booth-Kewley, 1987; Yellowlees & Kalucy, 1990). More recently Rimington et al (2001) further supports this notion and states that as anxiety increases (state and trait) a poorer quality of life is evidenced, and Baumeister et al (2005) makes similar observations between higher anxiety and less asthma control (Thomas et al., 2011).

The present study also recognized worse control of the disease with anger and depression, as found in other studies (Cluley & Cochrane, 2001; Thomas et al., 2011). Is well known that patients classified as non-adherent (those taking less 70% of the prescription) presented high anxiety and depression levels (Zigmond et al., 1983; Thomas et al., 2011).

Corroborating former studies (Dirks et al., 1978; Staudenmayer et al., 1979; Dirks & Kinsman, 1981; Baron et al., 1986; Put et al., 1999), the data from this study suggest that the most anxious patients are more vigilant over their symptoms, use more medication and more often turn to healthcare services for help. With this behaviour they would suffer from great psychological stress with their disease in the short term (higher values of anxiety, with less quality of life associated with asthma), but in the long run it may result in better control over the illness. Thus, this anxiety which is specifically related to asthma can be beneficial, by making the individual aware of the bodily symptoms related to asthma, through a process of focusing attention. However, excessively high levels of anxiety may lead to super-perception of asthma symptoms, with the patient thus becoming more disorganized in behavioural terms, with negative consequences upon the development of the ailment. In this way we may understand the association observed: as the state of anxiety increases, asthma control becomes worse.

The most important coping mechanism in this study was hiding asthma, considered as a passive one. This mechanism as well as avoidance and denial were linked with less mobilized strategies in chronic diseases (Felton et al., 1984; Santavirta, 1997; Osowiecki & Compas, 1999). In other studies, asthma denial has been recognized as an important risk factor for asthma attacks, and more emergency treatment (Dirks et al., 1978; Miller, 1987; Steiner et al., 1987; Yellowlees & Ruffin, 1989; Lavoie et al., 2010). The coping mechanism in general (total scores) and particularly the positive reappraisal were also correlated with greater severity of asthma.

Another important mechanism found in this sample was worry about the disease, which is considered as the most emotionally involving, correlated with poor quality of life. This is in accordance with the worst adjustment to the disease, related to emotional involvement (Bombardier et al., 1990; Landreville & Veniza, 1994; Scharloo et al., 1998).

Related also with poor quality of life are depressive symptoms (Goethe et al., 2001), which seem to measure negative feelings as well as neuroticism (Koivumaa-Honkanen et al., 2000), and this is corroborated in the present study.

With these results we are witnessing a multiple confluence of biological, environmental, psychological and social factors in asthma, as well as in its evolution, treatment and prognosis, understandable in the complexity of systemic and multiple interaction of all these factors, which influence and are simultaneously influenced by the disease.

The behavioral disorders found are translated by clinical and morbidity criteria, leading to higher use of healthcare and medication, and absenteeism, with poorer disease control and quality of life.

In this way, the need for better and more accurate assessment emerge, not at a symptomatic level but also discriminating different types of anxiety, depression, associated psychopathology that determine the diagnosis and development of this disease.

In future studies a cluster selection of individuals will be required who combine physical and psychological characteristics, above all with severe or unstable asthma, with more adequate clinical interventions. This is taking into account that even if we cannot change personalities, we can at least modify behaviour, with efficacy in healthy habits and attitudes, namely concerning compliance to treatment.

4. Study 2: Psychoeducational and multifamily interventions in asthma

4.1 Objectives

This study aims to analyse the effects of psychoeducational and multifamily interventions in asthma, in biological variables (spirometry and inflammatory marker), morbidity criteria (health care use, absenteeism, medication, quality of life and control of disease) and psychological outcomes (anxiety, depression and coping mechanisms).

4.2 Methods

We conducted a five-month prospective study, randomized with simple occultation, with two intervention groups and a control group, according to the criteria defined and presented in the previous study, where 195 patients were studied. Of these, the ones with moderate or severe persistent asthma were selected.

This Random Control Trial was carried out in the Allergy & Immunology outpatients' department of the University Hospital S. João in Oporto.

The randomization resulted in the balanced inclusion of 141 patients, divided into three groups (according to levels of anxiety and depression). The studied sample, in two observations, was the following: Psychoeducational Group (PG) intervention and usual pharmacological treatment (n=38), Multifamily Group (MG) intervention and usual pharmacological treatment (n=29), Control group (CG) with only usual pharmacological treatment (n=44) (Figure 5).

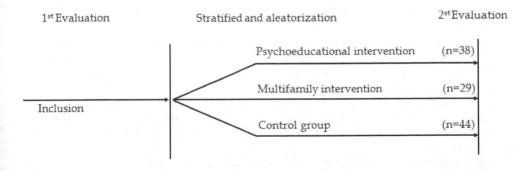

Fig. 5. Clinical study design

For comparison with the evaluation made in the second study, the following scales of evaluation were used: Self Anxiety Scale – SAS (Zung, 1971), State-Trait Anxiety Inventory – STAIY (Spielberger, 1983), Beck Depression Inventory – BDI (Beck et al., 1961), Ways of Coping with Asthma in Everyday Life – WCAEL (Aalto et al., 2002), Mini Asthma Quality of Life Questionnaire – MiniAQLQ (Juniper et al., 1999a) and Asthma Control Questionnaire – ACQ (Juniper et al., 1999b).

They were still compared according to their asthma symptoms, spirometry, inflammatory marker and morbidity criteria.

All psychological and clinical measures were assessed twice, before and after interventions.

Only adding information and knowledge became incomplete (Costa & MacCrane, 1987; Clark et al., 2002). With these interventions the aim is not to modify personalities, but change behaviour and attitudes (Costa & MacCrane, 1986).

In this context, the general principles of two interventions included both transmission of information, promoting behaviour change and improvement of self-efficacy. This implies a bidirectional process with interactions between health professionals and asthmatic patients and families. There are some objectives in this communication, mainly in answer to different issues, erasing false constructs, reduction of anxiety due to illness and promoting healthy habits and attitudes

Specifically for the **Psychoeducational programme**, the present intervention was focused on results in three levels of learning: knowledge transmission, education for instrumental attitudes and finally integration of the former. This empowered the patients by increasing self-efficacy and improvement in problem-solving of asthma. These sessions were not only didactic but also interactive.

The **Multifamily programme** was based on three distinct components: educational (sharing of experiences between families and patients, mediation by psychotherapists), social network (cross over difficult situations) and problem-solving (extending solutions, training strategies to deal with illness). This intervention was structured as a "group within a group", based on the Multifamily Discussion Group of Gonzalez and Steinglass (Gonzalez et al., 1986, Gonzalez & Steinglass, 2002; Steinglass, 1998).

4.3 Results

The intervention groups and control group had balanced demographic, psychological and clinical characteristics (Table 2).

Considering the total sample of asthmatics (n=141), the majority was female (78.7%), with a mean age (sd) of 39.3 (14.2). There was also a predominance of lower socio-economic classes (75.1%). The mean duration of the disease was 21.5 (14.8) years and most of the patients had severe persistent asthma (76.6%).

There was an improvement in both intervention programmes, in psychological variables. Depression only achieved statistical significance in the PG ($p \leq 0.05$), but anxiety state was significant in all groups (MG $p<0.01$; PG $p<0.01$), as well as anxiety trait (MG $p<0.001$; PG $p<0.01$) (Table 3).

In the MG, there was a relevant decrease in the coping mechanism of worry with asthma (p=0.000).

In both programs there was an improvement in the quality of life (MG $p<0.05$; PG $p<0.01$), increasing in 0.8U in PG and 0.5U in MG, taking into consideration effective results since 0.5U, according Juniper´s references (Juniper et al., 1999a).

	Multifamily (n=46)	Psychoeducacional (n=47)	Control (n=48)
Age (years) mean (sd)	40.2(16.3)	37.8(14.1)	40.0(12.3)
Gender n(%)			
Male	7(15.2)	8(17.0)	15(31.3)
Female	39(84.8)	39(83.0)	33(68.8)
Socio-economic classification n(%)			
High and very high	3(6.5)	3(6.4)	5(10.4)
Median	6(13.0)	11(23.4)	7(14.6)
Low	12(26.1)	10(21.3)	14(29.2)
Very low	25(54.3)	23(48.9)	22(45.8)
Disease duration (years) mean (sd)	24.4(15.0)	20.4(14.6)	19.7(14.8)
Asthma severity n(%)			
Moderate persistent	9(19.6)	8(17.0)	16(33.4)
Severe persistent	37(80.4)	39(83.0)	32(66.7)

Table 2. Demographic and clinical characteristics of sample

	MULTIFAMILY (n=29)			PSYCOEDUCACIONAL (n=38)		
	1° Av.	*2ª Av.*		*1° Av.*	*2ª Av.*	
Anxiety state[1]	11.2 (3.3)	9.8 (3.7)	Imp **	11.4 (3.0)	9.4 (2.6)	Imp **
Anxiety trait[2]	49.5 (12.4)	38.8 (11.4)	Imp ***	45.8 (11.8)	41.2 (10.7)	Imp **
Depression[3]	12.3 (9.1)	11.9 (10.2)	Imp. NS	10.7 (6.9)	8.0 (8.3)	Imp *
Quality of life[4]	4.5 (1.3)	5.0 (1.4)	Imp. *	4.3 (1.2)	5.1 (1.3)	Imp **
Asthma control[5]	2.0 (1.1)	1.5 (1.4)	Imp *	1.9 (1.1)	1.5 (1.3)	Imp *

Note: p<0.001 ***; p<0.01**; p<0.05*; NS – non-significant, imp. – improved; [1]SAS; [2]STAI-Y; [3]BDI; [4]MiniAQLQ; [5]ACQ

Table 3. Psychological and clinical outcomes in experimental groups

There was also an increase in the control of asthma in both groups (MG p<0.05; PG p<0.05). In morbidity criteria, there was a reduction in the use of corticotherapy (p=0.01) in the MG, and in hospitalization (p=0.000) in the PG. There was an improvement in spirometry: FEV1 (MG p<0.05, PG p<0.05) and PEF (MG p<0.05, PG p<0.01).

4.4 Discussion and conclusion

The intention of this pioneer study in Portugal was to contribute to the characterization of the clinical situation of asthmatic patients in a hospital context, as well as the importance of group interventions (mainly educational and communicational) carried out in the context of a multidisciplinary programme (Fernandes, 2009).

Rejecting the linear model of etiological causality, the multisystemic model is strengthened with this psychoeducational intervention, in which all factors influence and are influenced by the illness.

In moderate/severe asthma, besides the usual preventive and pharmacological approaches, it is essential to turn to a widespread intervention: psychoeducational and multifamily programmes, with a multidisciplinary team, to increase the control of the illness and allow therapeutic effectiveness (Wamboldt et al., 1995; Devine, 1996; Steinglass et al., 2002; Yorke et al., 2007)

The innovative therapeutic interventions (Psychoeducational and Multifamily) revealed promising results, as demonstrated in the present study. Namely in both interventional groups, there were good results, with statistically significant improvement in quality of life, asthma control, psychological variables (anxiety state and trait, depression and coping mechanisms) and clinical parameters (spirometry).

With the present intervention we try to demonstrate that behavioural changes brought about, improvement in the psychological parameters, as well as in the clinical parameters.

The present results encourage further studies, with larger samples and longitudinal interventions, in order to evaluate the stability of the positive effects found.

An accurate selection for a therapeutic approach is also necessary to cater for specific characteristics of these patients, more orientated for control and self-efficacy in psychoeducational or solution focused/emotional confrontation for more psychotherapeutic intervention.

Only in this way, can we pursue a holistic comprehension of the complexity of these physiopathological processes involved in asthma, with a more integrated and efficient treatment.

5. Acknowledgements

The author wish to thank J. Fonseca, S. Martins, M. Ribeiro, L. Delgado, A. Costa Pereira and M. Vaz.

6. References

Aalto, A.M.; Härkäpää, K.; Aro, A.R. & Rissanen, P. (2002). Ways of coping with asthma in everyday life validation of the asthma specific coping scale. *Journal of Psychosomatic Research*, Vol. 53, pp. 1061-1069.

Ader, R. & Cohen, N. (1985). CNS-immune system interaction conditioning phenomena. *Behavioral and Brain Sciences*, Vol. 8, pp- 379-394.

Baron, C., Lamarre, A., Veilleux, P., Ducharme, G., Spiet, S. & Lapierre, J.G. (1986). Psycho maintenance of childhood asthma: a study of 34 children. Journal of Asthma, Vol. 23, pp. 69-79.

Barton, C.A., McKenzie, D.P., Walters, E.H. & Abramson, M. (2005). Interactions between psychosocial problems and management of asthma: who is at risk of dying? *J Asthma*, Vol. 42, pp. 249-56.

Baumeister, H. (2005). [Bronchial asthma and mental disorders -- a systematic review of empirical studies]. *Psychother Psychosom Med Psychol*, May, Vol. 55, No. 5, pp. 247-55.

Beck, A.T., Ward, C.H., Mendelson, M., Mock, J. & Erbaugh, J. (1961). An Inventory for Measuring Depression. *Arch Gen Psychiat*, Vol. 4, pp. 561-571.

Bender, B.G. (2006). Risk taking, depression, adherence, and symptom control in adolescents and young adults with asthma. *Am J Respir Crit Care Med*, Vol. 173, No. 9, pp. 953-7

Bernard-Bonnin, A.C., Stachenko, S., Bonin, D., Charette, C. & Rousseau, E. (1995). Self-management teaching programs and morbidity of pediatric asthma: a meta-analysis. *Journal of Allergy and Clinical Immunology*, Vol. 95, pp. 34-41.

Bombardier, C.H., D'Amico, C. & Jordan, J.S. (1990). The relationship of appraisal and coping to chronic illness adjustment. *Behav Res Ther*, Vol. 28, pp. 297-304.

Borkovec, T.D. On the need for a basic science approach to psychotherapy research. *Psych Sci*, Vol. 8, pp. 145-147.

Boulet, L.P., Deschesnes, F., Turcotte, H. & Gignac, F. (1991). Near-fatal asthma: Clinical and physiologic features, perception of bronchoconstriction, and psychologic profile. *J Allergy Clin Immunol*, Vol. 88, No. 6, pp. 838-846.

Bruzzese, J.M., Markman, L.B., Appel, D. & Webber, M. (2001). An evaluation of Open Airways for Schools: using college students as intructors. *Journal of Asthma*, Vol. 38, pp. 337-342.

Busse, W.B. (2000). A 47-year-old woman with severe asthma. Clinical crossroads. *JAMA*, Vol. 284, pp. 2225-2233.

Campbell, D.A., McLennan, G., Coates, J.R., Frith, P.A., Gluyas, P.A., Latimer, K.M., Luke, C.G., Martin, A.J., Roder, D.M. & Ruffin, R.E. (1994). A comparison of asthma deaths and near-fatal asthma attacks in South Australia. *Eur Respir J*, Vol. 7, pp. 490–497.

Campbell, D.A., Yellowlees, P., McLennan, G., Coates, J.R., Frith, P.A., Gluyas, P.A., Latimer, K.M., Luke, C.G., Martin, A.J. & Ruffin, R.E. (1995a). Psychiatric and medical features of near fatal asthma. *Thorax*, Vol. 50, pp. 254-259.

Chetta, A., Gerra, G., Foresi, A., Zaimovic, A., Del Donno, M., Chittolini, B., Malorgio, R., Castagnaro, A. & Olivieri, D. (1998). Personality profiles and breathlessness perception in outpatients with different grading of asthma. *Am J Respir Crit Care Med*, Vol. 157, pp. 116-22.

Clark, N.M. & Partridge, M.R. (2002). Strengthening asthma education to enhance disease control. *Chest*, Vol. 121, pp. 1661-1669.

Cluley, S. & Cochrane, G.M. (2001). Psychological disorder in asthma is associated with poor control and poor adherence to inhaled steroids. *Respir Med*, Vol. 95, pp. 37- 9.

Cohen, S., Tyreli, D.A. & Smith, A.P. (1991). Psychological stress in humans and susceptibility to the common cold. *New England Journal of Medicine*, Vol. 325, pp. 606-612.

Cooper, C.L., Parry, D.G., Saul, C., Morice, A.H., Hutchcroft, B.J., Moore, J. & Esmonde, L. (2007). Anxiety and panic fear in adults with asthma: prevalence in primary care. BMC Fam Prat, Vol. 8, pp. 62.

Costa, P.T. & McCrae, R. (1986). Personality stability and its implications for clinical psychology. *Clinical Psychology Review*, Vol. 6, pp. 407-423.

Costa, P.T. & McCrae, R. (1987). Neuroticism, somatic complaints and disease: Is the bark worse than the bite? *Journal of Personality*, Vol. 55, No. 2, pp. 299-316.

Dahlem, N.K., Kinsman, R.A. & Horton, D.J. (2009). Panic-fear in asthma: requests for asneeded medication in relation to pulmonary function measurements. *J Allergy Clin Immunol*, Vol. 60, pp. 295-300.

Derogatis, L.R. & Savitz, K.L. (1999). The SCL-90-R, brief symptom inventory, and matching clinical rating scales. In: Maruish (Ed), *The use of psychological testing for treatment planning and outcomes assessment*. Mahwah, NJ. Erlbaum, pp. 679-724.

Devine, E.C. (1996). Meta-analysis of the effects of psychoeducational care in adults with asthma. *Research in Nursing and Health*, Vol. 19, pp. 367-376.

Devriese, S., Winters, W., Stegen, K., van Diest, I., Veulemans, H., Nemery, B., Eelen, P., Van de Woestijne, K. & Van den Bergh, O. (2000). Generalization of acquired somatic symptoms in response to odors: A Pavlovian perspective on multiple chemical sensitivity. *Psychosomatic Medicine*, Vol. 62, pp. 751-759.

Di Marco, F., Santus, P. & Centanni, S. (2011). Anxiety and depression in asthma. *Curr Opin Pulm Med*, Vol. 17, No. 1, pp. 39-44.

Dirks, J.F. & Kinsman, R.A. (1981). Clinical prediction of medical rehospitalization: psychological assessment with the battery of asthma illness behavior. *J Pers Assessment*, Vol. 45, pp. 608-613.

Dirks, J.F., Kinsman, R.A., Horton, D.J., Fross, K.H. & Jones, N.F. (1978). Panic-fear in asthma: rehospitalization following intensive long-term treatment. *Psychosom Med*, Vol. 40, pp. 5-13

Eysenck, H.J. (1969). Research findings with the MPI. In: Eysenck, H.J. & Eysenck, S.B.C., Personality Structure and Measurement. London: Routledge & Kegan Paul.

Felton, B.J., Revenson, T.A. & Hinrichsen, G.A. (1984). Stress and coping in explenation of psychosocial adjustment among chronically ill adults. *Soc Sci Med*, Vol. 18, pp. 889-98.

Fernandes, L. (2009). Dos Factores Biopsicológicos às Intervenções Multifamiliares e Psicoeducacionais na Asma. Edição Bial.

Fernandes, L., Fernandes, M., Cruz, R., Gonçalves, R., Martins, S., Rodrigues, J., Almeida, J., Pinto, A. & Vieira, A. (2005). Caracterização da personalidade dos doentes asmáticos. *Revista Portuguesa de Pneumologia,* Jan-Fev, Vol.11, No. 1, pp. 7-34.

Fernandes, L., Fonseca, J., Martins, S., Delgado, L., Pereira, A.C., Vaz, M. & Branco, G. (2010). Association of anxiety with asthma: subjective and objective outcome measures. *Psychosomatics*, Jan, Vol. 51, No. 1, pp. 39-46.

Fonseca, J.A., Fernandes, L., Delgado, L., Costa-Pereira, A., Sousa, M., Martins, S., Gomes, S., Moreira, A., Vaz, M. & Castel-Branco, G. (2004). Asthmatic patients with anxiety:

more symptoms and medication but a better adherence and less Exhaled Nitric Oxide. *Journal Investigational Allergology Clinical Immunology*, Vol. 14, (suppl 1).

Ford, D.H. & Urban, H.B. (1998). Contemporary models of psychotherapy. A comparative Analysis (2nd ed). New York: John Wiley.

Ford, D.H. (1987). Humans as self –construction living systems. A developmental perspective on behavior, personality, and health. New York: Erlbaum.

Forsythe, P., Ebeling, C., Gordon, J.R., Befus, A.D. & Vliagoftis, H. (2004). Opposing effects of short- and long-term stress on airway inflammation. *Am J Respir Crit Care Med*, Vol. 169, pp. 220-6.

French, T.M. & Alexander, F. (1941). Psychogenic factors in bronchial asthma. *Psychosom Med Monographs*, Vol. 4, pp. 1941.

Friedman, H.S. & Booth-Kewley, S. (1987). The "disease-prone personality". A meta-analytic view of the construct. *American Psychologist*, Vol. 42, No. 6, pp. 539-555.

Gallagher, R. & Appenzeller, T. (1999). Beyond reductionism. *Science*, Vol. 284, pp. 79.

Garden, G.M. (1993). Psychiatric and social aspects of brittle asthma. *Thorax*, Vol. 48, pp. 501-505.

GINA – Global Initiative for Asthma (2010). *Global Strategy for Asthma Management and Prevention. National Institutes of Health.* National Heart, Lung, and Blood Institute. Available at: www.ginasthma.org.

Goethe, J.W., Maljanian, R., Wolf, S., Hernandez, P. & Cabrera, Y. (2001). The impact of depressive symptoms on the functional status of inner-city patients with asthma. *Ann Allergy Asthma Immunol*, Vol. 87, pp. 205-210.

Goldberg, D.P. & Hillier, V.F. (1979). A Scaled Version of the General Health Questionnaire. *Psychological Medicine*, Vol. 9, pp. 139-145.

Goldstein, D.S. & Dekker, M. (2001). *The autonomic nervous system in health and disease.* Informa Healthcare.

Gonzalez, S., & Steinglass, P. (2002). Application of Multifamily Groups in Chronic Medical Disorders. In: McFarlane, W. *Multifamily Groups in the Treatment of Severe Psychiatric Disorders.* New York: The Guilford Press.

Gonzalez, S., Steinglass, P., & Reiss, D. (1986). *Family- centred interventions for the chronically disabled: The 8-session multiple-family group programme: Treatment manual.* Washington, DC: George Washington University Rehabilitation Research and Training Center.

Goodwin, R.D. & Eaton, W.W. (2003). Asthma and the risk of panic attacks among adults in the community. *Psychological Medicine*, Vol. 33, pp. 879-885.

Graffar, M. (1956). Une méthode de classification sociale d'échantillons de population. *Courier, Vol.* 6, pp. 455-459.

Gregerson, M.B. (2000). The curious 2000-year case of asthma. *Psychosom Med*, Vol. 62, pp. 816-827.

Gustafsson, P.A. & Cederblad, M. (1986). Family therapy in the treatment of severe childhood asthma. *Journal of Psychosomatic Research*, Vol. 30, pp. 369-374.

Hasler, G., Gergen, P.J., Kleinbaum, D.G. & Ajdacic, V. (2005). Asthma and Panic in Young Adults. A 20-Year Prospective Community Study. *American Journal of Respiratory and Critical Care Medicine*, Vol. 171, pp. 1224-1230.

Heaney, L.G., Conway, E., Kelly, C. & Gamble, J. (2005). Prevalence of psychiatric morbidity in a difficult asthma population: relationship to asthma outcome. *Respir Med*, Vol. 99, pp. 1152-1159.

Hibbert, G.A. & Pilsbury, D. (1988). Demonstration and treatment of hyperventilation causing asthma. *Br J Psychiatry*, Vol. 153, pp. 687-9.

Hollaender, J. & Florin, I. (1983). Expressed emotion and airway conductance in children with bronchial asthma. *Journal of Psychosomatic Research*, Vol. 27, pp. 307-311.

Hornsveld, H.K. & Garssen, B. (1996). Double-blind placebo-controlled study of thehyperventilation provocation test and the validity of the hyperventilation syndrome. *Lancet*, Vol. 384, pp. 158.

Horton, D.J., Suda, W.L., Kinsman, R.A., Souhrada, J. & Spector, S.L. (1978). Bronchoconstrictive suggestion in asthma: a role for airways hyperreactivity and emotions. *American Review of Respiratory Disease*; Vol. 117, pp. 1029-1038.

Innes, N.J., Reid, A., Halstead, J., Watkin, S.W. & Harrison, B.D. (1998). Psychosocial risk factors in near-fatal asthma and in asthma deaths. *J R Coll Physicians Lond*, Vol. 32, pp. 430-434.

Irvine, L., Crombie, I.K., Clark, R.A., Slane, P.W., Feyerabend, C., Goodman, K.E. & Cater, J.I. (1999). Advising parents of asthmatic children on passive smoking: Randomised controlled trial. *BMJ*, Vol. 318, pp. 1456-1459.

Isenberg, S.A., Lehrer, P. & Hochron, S.M. (1992). The effects of suggestion and emotional arousal on pulmonary function in asthma: a review and a hypothesis regarding vagal mediation. *Psychosomatic Med*, Vol. 54, pp. 192-216.

Jasnoski, M.B.L., Bell, I.R. & Peterson, R. (1994). What connections exist between shyness, hay fever, anxiety, anxiety sensivity, and panic disorders? *Anxiety Stress Coping*, Vol. 7, pp. 19-34.

Juniper, E.F., Guiyatt, G.H., Cox, F.M., Ferrie, P.J. & King, D.R. (1999a). Mini Asthma Quality of Life. *Eur Respir J*, Vol. 14, pp. 32-38.

Juniper, E.F., O'Byrne, P.M., Guyatt, G.H., Ferrie, P.J. & King, D.R. (1999b). Development and validation of a questionnaire to measure asthma control. *Eur Respir J*, Vol. 14, pp. 902-907.

Kang, D.H., Coe, C.L., McCarthy, D.O., Jarjour, N.N., Kelly, E.A., Rodriguez, R.R., Busse, W.W. (1997). Cytokine profiles of stimulated blood lymphocytes in asthmatic and healthy adolescents across the school year. *Journal of Interferon and Cytokine Research*, Vol. 17, pp. 481-487.

Kelloway, J.S., Wyatt, R., DeMarco, J. & Adlis, S. (2000). Effect of salmentrol on patients adherence to their prescribed refills for inhaled corticosteroids. *Annals of Allergy, Asthma and Immunology*, Vol. 84, pp. 324-328.

Kinsman, R.A., Dirks, J.F. & Jones, N.F. (1982). Psychomaintenance of chronic physical illness. In: Millon, T. & Green, C.J. *Handbook of clinical Health Psychology*. New York: Plenum, pp. 435-465.

Kinsman, R.A., Luparello, T., O'Banion, K. & Spector, S. (1973). Multidimensional Analysis of the Subjective Symptomatology of Asthma. *Psychosomatic Medicine*, Vol. 35, No. 3, pp. 250-266.

Koch, C. & Laurent, G. (1999). Complexity and the nervous system. *Science*, Vol. 284, pp. 96-98.

Koivumaa-Honkanen, H.T., Honkanen, R., Vinamäki, H., Heikkilä, K., Kaprio, J. & Koskenvuo, M. (2000). Self-reported life satisfaction and 20-year mortality in healthy Finnish adults. *Am J Epidemiol*, Vol. 152, pp. 983-991.

Kotses, H., Bernstein, I.L., Bernstein, D.I., Reynolds, R.V.C., Korbee, L., Wigal, J.K., Ganson, E., Stout, C. & Creer, T.L. (1995). A self-management program for adult asthma. Part I: Development and evaluation. *Journal of Allergy and Clinical Immunology*, Vol. 95, pp. 529-540.

Landreville, P. & Veniza, J. (1994). Differences in appraisal and coping between elderly coronary artery disease patients high and low in depressive symptoms. *J Ment Health*, Vol. 3, pp. 79-90.

Lask, B. & Matthew, D. (1979). Childhood asthma. A controlled trial of family psychotherapy. *Archives of Disease in Childhood*, Vol. 54, pp. 116-119.

Lavoie KL, Bouthillier D, Bacon SL, Lemière, C., Martin, J., Hamid, Q., Ludwig, M., Olivenstein, R. & Ernst, P. (2010). Psychological distress and maladaptive coping styles in patients with severe versus moderate asthma. *Chest*, Vol. 137, No. 6, pp. 1324-31.

Lavoie, K.L., Bacon, S.L., Barone, S., Cartier, A., Ditto, B. & Labrecque, M. (2006). What is worse for asthma control and quality of life: depressive disorders, anxiety disorders, or both? *Chest*, Vol. 130, pp. 1039–1047.

Lehrer, P.M. (1998). Emotionally triggered asthma: A review of research literature and some hypotheses for self-regulation therapy. *Applied Psychophysiology and Biofeedback*, Vol. 23, pp. 13-41.

Lehrer, P.M., Feldman, J., Giardino, N., Song, H.S. & Schamaling, K. (2002). Psychological aspects of asthma. *Journal of Consulting and Clinical Psychology*, Vol. 70, No. 3, pp. 691-711.

Lehrer, P.M., Generelli, P. & Hochron, S. (1997). The effect of facial and trapezius muscle tension impedance in asthma. *Applied Psychophysiology and Biofeedbac*, Vol. 22, pp. 43-54.

Lehrer, P.M., Isenberg, S. & Hochron, S.M. (1993). Asthma and emotion: a review. *J Asthma*, Vol. 30, pp. 5-21.

Lehrer, P.M., Vaschillo, E., Vaschillo, B., Lu, S.E., Scardella, A., Siddique, M. & Habib, R.H. (2004). Biofeedback Treatment for Asthma. *Chest*, Vol. 126, pp. 352-361.

Lehrer, P.M., Vaschilo, E., Vaschilo, B., Lu, S.E., Eckeberg, D.L., Edelberg, R., Shih, W.J., Lin, Y., Kuusela, T.A., Tahvanainen, K.U. & Hamer, R.M. (2003). Heart rate variability biofeedback increases baroreflex gain and peak expiratory flow. *Psycosomatic Medicine*, Vol. 65, pp. 796-805.

Levenson, R.W. (1979). Effects of thematically relevant and general stressors on specificity of responding in asthmatic subjects. *Psychosom Med*, Vol. 41, pp. 28-39.

Levitan, H. (1985). Onset of asthma during intense mourning. *Psychosomatics*; Vol. 26, pp. 939-941.

Levy, S. (1984). Behavior and cancer. In: Light, R.J. & Pilemer, D.B. *Summing up: The science of reviewing research*. Cambridge, MA: Harvard University Press.

Luparello, T.J., Lyons, H.A., Bleecker, E.R. & McFadden, E.R. (1968). Influences of suggestion on airway reactivity in asthmatic subjects. *Psychosom Med*, Vol. 30, pp. 819-825.

MacKenzie, J.N. (1986). The production of "rose asthma" by artificial rose. *Am J Med Sci*, Vol. 91, pp. 45-47.

Manto, P.G. (1969). *An investigation of feedback mechanisms in stress-induced changes of autonomic balance*. Dissertação Académica: Rutgers University.

Martin, A.J., Campbell, D.A., Gluya, P.A., Coates, J.R., Ruffin, R.E., Roder, D.M., et al. (1995). Characteristics of near-fatal asthma in childhood. *Pediatric Pulmonology*, Vol. 20, pp. 1-8.

Martins, F. (1995). STAXI. In: Almeida, L., Simões, M. & Gonçalves, M. *Provas Psicológicas em Portugal*. Braga: APPORT.

Mathinson, D.A. (1993). Asthma in adults: diagnosis and treatment. In: Middleton, E., Rees, C.E., Ellis, E.F., Adkinson, N.F., Yunginger, J.W. & Busse, W.W. (Editors). *Allergy: principles and practice*. Vol 2. (4th ed.), pp. 1263-1300. St Louis (MO): Mosby.

Mayer-Gross, W., Slater, E. & Roth, M. (1969). *Clinical Psychiatry* (3rd ed.). London: Baillière, Tindall & Cassell.

McFadden, E.R., Luparello, T., Lyons, H.A. & Bleecker, E. (1969). The mechanism of action of sugestión in the induction of acute asthma attacks. *Psychosom Med*, Vol. 31, pp. 134-143.

McFarlane, W.R., Link, B., Dushay, R., et al. (1995). Psychoeducational multiple family groups: Four-year relapse outcome in schizophrenia. *Family Process*, Vol. 34, pp. 127-144.

McQuaid, E.L., Kopel, S.J. & Nassau, J.H. (2001). Behavioral adjustment in children with asthma: A meta-analysis. *J Dev Behav Pediatr*, pp. 430-490.

Miller, B.D. & Strunk, R.C. (1989). Circumstances surrounding the deaths of children due to asthma. *American Journal of Diseases of Children*, Vol. 143, pp. 1294-1299.

Miller, B.D. (1987). Depression and asthma: a potentially lethal mixture. *J Allergy Clin Immunol*, Vol. 80, pp. 481-486.

Miller, D.J. & Kotses, H. (1995). Classical conditioning of total respiratory resistance in humans. *Psychosomatic Medicine*, Vol. 57, pp. 148-153.

Mrazek, D.A., Schuman, W.B. & Klinnert, M. (1998). Early asthma onset: Risk of emotional and behavioral difficulties. *J Child Psychol Psychiatry*, Vol. 39, No. 2, pp. 247-254.

Neild, J.E. & Cameron, I.R. (1985). Bronchoconstriction in response to suggestion: its prevention by an inhaled anticholinergic agent. *BMJ*, Vol. 290, pp. 674.

Nouwen, A., Freeston, M.H., Labbé, R. & Boulet, R.P. (1999). Psychological factors associated with emergency room visits among asthmatic patients. *Behavior Modification*, Vo. 23, pp. 217-233.

Osowiecki, D.M. & Compas, B.E. (1999). A prospective study of coping, perceived control, and psychological adaptation to breast cancer. *Cogn Ther Res*, Vol. 23, pp. 169-80.

Picado, C., Montserrat, J.N., de Pablo, J., Plaza, V. & Agusti-Vidal, A. (1989). Predisposing factors to death after recovery from a life-threatning asthmatic attack. *J Asthma*, Vol. 26, No. 4, pp. 231-236.

Ponciano, E., Vaz Serra, A. & Relvas, J. (1982). Aferição da escala de auto-avaliação de ansiedade, de Zung, numa amostra de população portuguesa – I. – Resultados da aplicação numa amostra de população normal. *Psiquiatria Clínica*, Vol. 3, No. 4, pp. 191-202.

Ponciano, E., Vaz Serra, A. & Relvas, J. (1982). Aferição da escala de auto-avaliação de ansiedade, de Zung, numa amostra de população portuguesa – I. – Resultados da aplicação numa amostra de população normal. *Psiquiatria Clínica*, Vol. 3, No. 4, pp. 191-202.

Prueter, C. & Norra, C. (2005). Mood disorders and their treatment in patients with epilepsy. *J Neuropsychiatry Clin Neurosci*, Vol. 17, No. 1, pp. 20-8.

Put, C., Demedts, M., van den Bergh, O., Demyttenaere, K. & Verleden, G. (1999). Asthma symptoms: influence of personality versus clinical status. *Eur Respir J*, Vol. 13, pp. 751-756.

Rietveld, S.B.I. & Everaerd, W. (2000). Psychological confounds in medical research: the example of excessive cough in asthma. *Behav Res Ther*, Vol. 38, pp. 791-800.

Rimington, L.D., Davies, D.H., Lowe, D. & Pearson, M.G. (2001). Relationship between anxiety, depression, and morbidity in adult asthma patients. *Thorax*, Vol. 56, pp. 266-271.

Rumbak, M.J., Kelso, T.M., Arheart, K.L. & Self, T.H. (1993). Perception of anxiety as a contributing factor of asthma: indigent. *J Asthma*, Vol. 30, pp. 165-169.

Sandberg, S., Paton, J., Ahola, S., McCann, D.C., McGuinness, D., Hillary, C.R. & Oja, H. (2000). The role of acute and chronic stress in asthma attacks in children. *Lancet*, Vol. 356, No. 9234, pp. 982-7.

Santavirta, N. (1997). Coping, pain and disability in patients with chronic inflammatory and musculoskeletal diseases. Stockholm: Karolinska Institutet.

Santos, S.C. & Silva, D.R. (1997). Adaptação do State-Trait Anxiety Inventory (STAI) Form Y para a população portuguesa: Primeiros dados. *Revista Portuguesa de Psicologia*, Vol. 32, pp. 71-89.

Scharloo, M., Kaptein, A., Weinman, J., Hazes, J.M., Willems, L.N.A. (1998). Illness perceptions, coping and functioning in patients with rheumatoid arthritis, chronic obstructive pulmonary disease and psoriasis. *J Psychosom Res*, Vol. 44, pp. 537-85.

Scott, K.M., Von Korff, M., Ormel, J., Zhang, M.Y., Bruffaerts, R., Alonso, J., Kessler, R.C., Tachimori, H., Karam, E., Levinson, D., Bromet, E.J., Posada-Villa, J., Gasquet, I., Angermeyer, M.C., Borges, G., de Girolamo, G., Herman, A. & Haro, J.M. (2007) Mental disorders among adults with asthma: results from the World Mental Health Survey. *Gen Hosp Psychiatry*, Mar-Apr, Vol. 29, No. 2, pp. 123-33.

Silagy, C. (1999). Advising parents of asthmatic children on passive smoking: Ramdomized controlled trial. *Journal of Paediatrics*, Vol. 135, pp. 650-651.

Silva, D.R. & Campos, R. (1998). Alguns dados normativos do Inventário de Estado-Traço de Ansiedade Forma Y (STAI) de Spielberger para a população portuguesa. *Revista Portuguesa de Psicologia*, Vol. 33, pp. 71-89.

Silverglade, I., Tosi, D.J., Wise, P.S., D'Costa, A. (1994). Irrational beliefs and emotionality in adolescents with and without bronchial asthma. *Journal of General Psychology*, Vol. 121, pp.199-207.

Smith, J.R., Mildenhall, S., Noble, M.J., Shepstone, L., Koutantji, M., Mugford, M. & Harrison, B.D. (2005). The Coping with Asthma Study: a randomised controlled trial of a home based, nurse led psychoeducational intervention for adults at risk of adverse asthma outcomes. *Thorax*, Dec, Vol. 60, No. 12, pp. 1003-11.

Smith, J.R., Mugford, M., Holland, R., Noble, M.J. & Harrison, B.D. (2007). Psycho-educational interventions for adults with severe or difficult asthma: a systematic review. *J Asthma*, Apr, Vol. 44, No. 3, pp. 219-41.

Spielberger, C.D. & London, P. (1990). Blood pressure and injustice. *Psychology Today*, Vol. 1, pp. 48-51.

Spielberger, C.D. (1983). *Manual for the State-Trait Anxiety Inventory STAI (Form Y) ("Self Evaluation Questionnaire")*. Palo Alto: Consulting Psychologists Press, Inc.

Spielberger, C.D. (1988). *State-trait Anger Expression Inventory (STAXI)*. Odessa, FL: Psychological Assessment Resources.

Spinhoven, P., Peski-Oosterbaan, A.S., Van der Dooes, A.J., Willelms, N.J. & Sterk, P.J. (1997). Association of anxiety with perception of induced bronchoconstriction in patients with asthma. *Thorax*, Vol. 52, pp. 152.

Staudenmayer, H., Kinsman, R., Dirks, J.F., Spector, S.L. & Wangaard, C. (1979). Medical outcome in asthmatic patients: effects of airways hyperreactivity and symptom-focused anxiety. *Psychosomatic Medicine*, Vol. 41, pp. 109-118.

Steiner, H., Higgs, C.M.B., Fritz, G.K., Laszlo, G. & Harvey, J.E. (1987). Defense Style and the perception of asthma. *Psychosomatic Med*, Vol. 49, pp. 35-44.

Steinglass, P. (1998). Multiple family discussion groups for patients with chronic medical illness. *Families, Systems and Health*, Vol. 16, pp. 55-70.

Steinglass, P., Ostroff J., & Steinglass A.S. (2002). *Treatment Manual: The Ackerman/memorial Sloan-Kettering multiple family discussion group for cancer patients and their families*. Washington DC: George Washington University Rehabilitation Research and Training Centre.

Stout, C.K.H. & Creer, T.L. (1997). Improving perception of air flow obstruction in asthma patients. *Psychosomatic Med*, Vol. 59, pp. 201-206.

Strunk, R., Mrazek, D.A., Fuhrmann, G.S. & LaBrecque, J.F. (1985). Physiologic and psychological characteristics associated with deaths due to asthma in childhood. *J Am Med Assoc*, Vol. 254, No. 9, pp. 1193-1198.

Strunk, R.C., Nicklas, R.A., Milgrom, H., Ikle, D. (1999). Fatal and near-fatal asthma questionnaire: prelude to a national registry. *J Allergy Clin Immunol*, Vol. 104, pp. 763–768.

Suissa, S., Ernest, P., Benayoun, S., Baltzan, M. & Cai, B. (2000). Low-dose inhaled corticosteroids and the prevention of death from asthma. *N Engl J Med*, Vol. 343, pp. 332-336.

Sullivan, S.D., Elixhauser, A., Buist, S., Luce, B.R., Eisenberg, J. & Weiss, K.B. (1996). National asthma education and prevention program working group report on the cost effectiveness of asthma care. *Am J Respir Care Med*, Vol. 154, pp. 584-595.

Sun, H.W., Wang, J.P., Wang, S.Z., Wang, Y.Y., Song, Y.P., Yang, Z.H. & Wang, L.X. (2010). Effect of educational and psychological intervention on the quality of life of asthmatic patients. *Respir Care*, Vol. 55, No. 6, pp. 725-8.

Taitel, M.S., Kotses, H., Bernstein, I.L., Bernstein, D.I. & Creer, T.L. (1995). A self-management program for adult asthma. Part II: Cost-benefit analysis. *Journal of Allergy and Clinical Immunology*, Vol. 95, pp. 672-676.

ten Brinke, A., Ouwerkerk, M.E., Bel, E.H. & Spinhoven, P. (2001a). Similar psychological characteristics in mild and severe asthma. *Journal of Psychosomatic Research*, Vol. 50, pp. 7-10.

ten Brinke, A., Ouwerkerk, M.E., Zwinderman, A.H., Spinhoven, P. & Bel, E.H. (2001b). Psychopathology in patients with severe asthma is associated with increased health care utilization. *American Journal of Respiratory & Critical Care Medicine*, Vol. 163, pp. 1093-1096.

Thomas, M., Bruton, A., Moffat, M. & Cleland, J. (2011). Asthma and psychological dysfunction. *Prim Care Respir J*, Vol. 15.

Thomas, M., McKinley, R.K., Freeman, E. & Foy, C. (2001). Prevalence of dysfunctional breathing in patients treated for asthma in primary care: cross sectional survey. *BMJ*, Vol. 322, pp. 98-100.

van den Bergh, O., Stegen, K. & van de Woestijne, K.P. (1997). Learning to have psychosomatic complaints in psychosomatic patients. *Psychosomatic Medicine*, Vol. 59, pp. 13-23.

Vila, G., Nollet-Clemencon, C., Blic, J., Mouren-Simeoni, M.C. & Scheinmann, P. (2000). Prevalence of DSM IV anxiety and affective disorders in a pediatric population of asthmatic children and adolescents. *J Affect Disord*, Vol. 58, pp. 223-231.

Wainwright, N.W., Surtees, P.G., Wareham, N.J. & Harrison, B.D. (2007). Psychosocial factors and incident asthma hospital admissions in the EPIC-Norfolk cohort study. *Allergy*, Vol. 62, pp. 554-60.

Wamboldt, M.Z., & Levin, L.B.A. (1995). Utility of Multifamily Psychoeducational Groups for Medically - III Children and Adolescents. *Family Systems Medicine*, Vol. 13, pp. 151-161.

Weng, G., Bhalla, U.S. & Iyengar, R. (1999). Complexity in biological signaling systems. *Science*, Vol. 284, pp. 92-96.

Whitesides, G.M. & Ismagilov, G.M. (1999). Complexity in chemistry. *Science*, Vol. 284, pp. 89-92.

Wilson, S.R., Latini, D., Starr, N.J., Fish, L., Loes, L.M., Page, A. & Kubic, P. (1996). Education of parents of infants and very young children with asthma: a developmental evaluation of the wee wheezers program. *Journal of Asthma*, Vol. 33, No. 4, pp. 239-254.

Wöller, W., Kruse, J., Winter, P., Mans, E.J. & Alberti, L. (1993). Cortisone image and emotional support by key figures in patients with bronchial asthma. *Psychotherapy and Psychosomatics*, 59; 190-196.

Wright, R.J., Rodriguez, M. & Cohen, S. (1998). Review of psychosocial stress and asthma: an integrated biopsychosocial approach. *Thorax*, Vol. 53, pp. 1066-74.

Yellowlees, P.M. & Kalucy, R.S. (1990). Psychobiological aspects of asthma and the consequent research implications. *Chest*, Vol. 97, pp. 628-634.

Yellowlees, P.M. & Ruffin, R.E. (1989). Psychological defenses and coping styles in patients following a life-threatening attack of asthma. *Chest*, Vol. 95, pp. 1298-1303.

Yellowlees, P.M., Haynes, S., Potts, N. & Ruffin, R.E. (1988). Psychiatric morbidity in patients with life-threatening attack of asthma: initial report of a controlled study. *Med J Aust*, Vol. 149, pp. 246-249.

Yorke, J., Fleming, S.L. & Shuldham, C. (2007). Psychological interventions for adults with asthma: a systematic review. *A Respir Med,* Vol. 101, No. 1, pp. 1-14.

Zigmond, A.S.S.R. (1983). The hospital anxiety and depression scale. *Acta Psychiatr Scand,* Vol. 67, pp. 361-370.

Zung, W.W.K. (1971). A rating instrument for anxiety disorders. *Psychosomatics,* Vol. 6, pp. 371-379.

3

Asthma and Health Related Quality of Life in Childhood and Adolescence

Esther Hafkamp-de Groen and Hein Raat
Erasmus MC-University Medical Center Rotterdam
The Netherlands

1. Introduction

Asthma is the most frequent chronic disorder in childhood. Asthma puts a serious burden on children's health related quality of life, despite the availability of effective and safe treatment (Dalheim-Englund et al., 2004; Global Initiative for Asthma, 2010; Masoli et al., 2004; Mohangoo et al., 2005). The overall goal of asthma management is to achieve optimal disease control and health related quality of life improvements (Bateman et al., 2007; Pedersen et al., 2011). The World Health Organization has defined the term health related quality of life as the individual's perception of their position of life in the context of the culture and value systems in which they live and in relation to their goals, expectations and concerns (World Health Organization, 1993). The own perception is important because it emphasises that these are the impairments that patients themselves consider important. As in most medical conditions, the correlation between asthma control and health related quality of life is modest. Therefore, the impact that asthma has on a patient's health related quality of life cannot be inferred from the conventional clinical measures of asthma (e.g. spirometry); it must be measured directly (Juniper et al., 1999a, 1999b).

During the past decade, the use of health related quality of life as an essential outcome measure of childhood asthma treatment and management has increased (Merikallio et al., 2005). This review summarises recent literature on: 1) health related quality of life instruments for childhood asthma, 2) the impact of childhood asthma on children's health related quality of life, 3) the impact of children's asthma on caregiver's health related quality of life and 5) factors associated with health related quality of life in childhood asthma.

2. Health related quality of life instruments and childhood asthma

Several feasible, reliable and validated pediatric health related quality of life questionnaires are standardised and available to measure health related quality of life in asthmatic children (Fiese et al., 2005; Raat et al., 2006). Both generic and asthma-specific questionnaires are used to measure health related quality of life in school aged children. Generic health related quality of life questionnaires intend to measure all dimensions of health-related quality of life (Raat et al., 2006). Frequently applied generic health related quality of life questionnaires are: the Child Health Questionnaire (CHQ) (Gorelick et al., 2003), the Pediatric Quality of Life Inventory (PedsQL) (Varni et al., 2005), the TNO-AZL (Preschool) Children's Quality of Life questionnaire (TAPQoL/TACQoL) (Bunge et al., 2005), the Infant-Toddler Quality of

Life (ITQOL) questionnaire (Spuijbroek et al., 2011) and the KIDSCREEN/DISABKIDS questionnaires (Petersen et al., 2005). Asthma-specific health related quality of life questionnaires focus on those dimensions that are likely to be affected by asthma disease or treatment. The most prominent asthma-specific health related quality of life questionnaires are the Pediatric Asthma Quality of Life Questionnaire (PAQLQ) (Juniper et al., 1996; Raat et al. 2005), the How Are You (HAY) (Le Coq et al., 2000) instrument and the Childhood Asthma Questionnaire (CAQ) (Christie et al., 1993).

If children are unable to report about their own experience reliably, parents are appropriate sources of information about health related quality of life (Petsios et al., 2011). One study suggests that fathers may be better proxy reporters than mothers (Petsios et al., 2011). The correlation between child and parent reported quality of life improves with increasing age of the child (Annett et al., 2003). Although the agreement between child self-report and parent proxy report on health related quality of life has been showed as satisfactory, according to Petsios et al. (2011), parents may overestimate health related quality of life of their children with asthma. This has to be taken into account when interpreting results from parent reported health related quality of life questionnaires, in comparison with child self-reports.

The PAQLQ is the most frequently used disease-specific health related quality of life instrument with regard to childhood asthma. Therefore, using this instrument has the benefit for researchers that results can more easily be compared with previous findings. However, using the existing health related quality of life instruments may have some limitations. A recent study has investigated whether asthma-specific health related quality of life questionnaires actually include all relevant aspects of asthma-specific health related quality of life for children with asthma (Annett et al., 2003). They have found disagreement between distinct health related quality of life questionnaires on components of asthma-specific health related quality of life: only some components of the asthma symptoms domain and of the activity limitations domain are part of all questionnaires. Furthermore, according to Van den Bemt et al. (2010), not all essential components of asthma-specific health related quality of life, according to childhood asthma, are part of existing asthma-specific health related quality of life questionnaires.

When classifying health related quality of life questionnaires into standardised and individualised health related quality of life instruments, another limitation is revealed. In standardised health related quality of life instruments the questions and range of answers are predetermined and the same for all patients. As opposed to standardised health related quality of life instruments, individualised health related quality of life instruments allow patients to define their quality of life in relation to their goals and expectations. Carr & Higginson (2001) conclude that standardised health related quality of life questionnaires have limited ability to capture the health related quality of life of individual asthma patients.

The most appropriate approach to measure health related quality of life in asthmatic children would be to use a combination of parental and self-reports of both generic and asthma-specific health related quality of life by validated questionnaires (Raat et al., 2006). Whether such health related quality of life measures are truly patient centred and to what extent they actually represent the quality of life of individual or groups of asthmatic children should always be taken into account when one interprets study results (Carr & Higginson, 2001).

3. Impact of asthma on children's health related quality of life

Asthma might have physical, emotional and psychosocial impact on children's lives (Grootenhuis et al., 2007; Juniper, 1997; Merikallio et al., 2005; Sawyer et al., 2004). Important components of health related quality of life are the effects on, and consequences of asthma on peer relationships (e.g., being bullied), the dependence on medication, shortness of breath, cough, limitations in activities and limitations due to the response on cigarette smoke exposure (Van den Bemt et al., 2010). Compared to preschool children without asthma symptoms, preschool children with asthma symptoms have significantly lower health related quality of life scores for lung problems, sleeping, appetite, communication and positive mood health related quality of life scales (Mohangoo et al., 2005).

Most studies have focused on severity of symptoms to examine the impact of asthma symptoms on children's health related quality life; the results are conflicting (Everhart & Fiese, 2009). For example, disease severity is not consistently associated with children's health related quality of life in some studies (Erickson et al., 2002; Vila et al., 2003), whereas others report that children with moderate or severe asthma have a worse level of functioning in several domains of their health related quality of life compared to children with mild asthma (Annett et al., 2001; Merikallio et al., 2005; Mohangoo et al., 2007, 2011; Sawyer et al., 2000) suggesting there may be a 'dose-response' relationship between the frequency and intensity of children's asthma symptoms and their health related quality of life. Mohangoo et al. (2007, 2011) evaluated health related quality of life in infants and adolescents with asthma-like symptoms, such as attacks of wheezing and shortness of breath (Mohangoo et al., 2007, 2011). Asthma-like symptoms during the first year of life are associated with impaired health related quality of life at the age of 12 months. Also, the presence of at least four wheezing attacks during the past year was associated with impaired adolescents' health related quality of life. Frequent wheezing attacks mostly affect adolescents' general health, bodily pain, self esteem and mental health (Mohangoo et al., 2007). Previous studies have also found that wheezing attacks more often have a physical impact than a psychosocial impact (Merikallio et al., 2005).

As described earlier, one of the main goals of asthma management is to achieve good asthma control. Asthma control has been defined as the minimisation of night time and daytime symptoms, activity limitation, rescue bronchodilator use and airway narrowing (Global Initiative for Asthma, 2010). Poorly controlled asthma symptoms impair health related quality of life in children (Guilbert et al., 2011). An important issue is whether proper asthma management improves quality of life in asthma patients, and whether poor health related quality of life makes disease management harder. Studies have found that poor health related quality of life is predictive of subsequent asthma-related emergency department visits, which implicates poor asthma control (Magid et al, 2004). Pont et al. (2004) show that proper asthma management improves health related quality of life.

In short, children experience asthma as an interruption in daily life that influences them physically, emotionally and socially.

4. Impact of children's asthma on caregiver's health related quality of life

With childhood asthma, the family and particularly the primary caregiver may face a considerable burden. While there are several questionnaires for assessing parental/caregiver's health related quality of life not directly related to asthma (Osman &

Silverman, 1996), there is only one instrument to examine the specific impact of childhood asthma on parental/caregiver functioning: The Pediatric Asthma Caregiver's Quality of Life Questionnaire (PACQLQ) (Juniper et al., 1996).

Whereas some studies find no association between caregiver's health related quality of life and children's asthma symptoms (Annett et al., 2003), duration of asthma illness and asthma pre-treatment severity (Vila et al., 2003), other studies report that caregiver's and child's health related quality of life are significantly associated with each other (Dean et al., 2009, 2010; Garro, 2011; Halterman et al., 2004). Halterman et al. (2004) find that higher symptom levels with regard to childhood asthma are associated with lower parental health related quality of life. Further, when children's symptoms improve, parents show higher health related quality of life.

It should be considered how childhood asthma affects caregiver's health related quality of life. Caregivers of asthmatic children appear to be more compromised in their resistance to stress, mood, emotional stability, amount of spare time and leisure activities (Garro, 2011). Caregivers of children with uncontrolled asthma report significantly higher absenteeism than their controlled counterparts (Dean et al., 2009, 2010).

Both caregiver's health related quality of life, caregiver's perception of the child's asthma symptoms, and the child's health related quality of life may be important in diagnosis and control of established asthma in childhood (Skoner, 2002). While giving attention to the caregiver's health related quality of life, it should be taken into account that the profile of health related quality of life impairment is different in asthmatic children and in their parents (Farnik et al., 2010). Where activity limitation seems to be the most impaired domain in children, asthma symptom perception and emotional health appear to be the most affected health related quality of life domains in parents.

In addition to evaluation of the asthmatic child, the integral assessment of asthma requires the evaluation of caregiver's health related quality of life. Giving attention to caregiver's health related quality of life is needed in clinical practice in order to avoid possible interferences of the caregiver's distress in the optimization of child's asthma treatment outcomes (Majani et al., 2005).

5. Factors associated with health related quality of life in asthmatic children

As we described earlier, the frequency and severity of asthma attacks and effects of asthma management or treatment are associated with children's health related quality of life. Researchers have also investigated other variables in association to health related quality of life in childhood asthma (Annett et al., 2003; Erickson et al., 2002; Mrazek, 1992; Sawyer et al., 2000, 2001). Hospital admissions, absences from school, limitations of sport and other activities, sleeping problems (and fatigue) are associated with health related quality of life in asthmatic children (Mrazek, 1992). Erickson et al. (2002) show that both asthma morbidity and health related quality of life are related to socioeconomic status. Also, household income is most consistently associated with the health related quality of life of asthmatic children and their caregivers. Sawyer et al. (2001) report the impact of family functioning on health related quality of life in children with asthma. They have found that the degree to which children are upset by their asthma is related to general functioning of their families, and their symptom levels are associated with several dimensions of family functioning (Sawyer et al., 2000, 2001). Children living in families with more clearly defined roles, greater interest and concern for the well-being of each other and clearer rules have been found to be less bothered by their asthma symptoms (Sawyer et al., 2000). A study by Annett *et al.* (2003) didn't find an association between health related quality of life of asthmatic children and family functioning, measured by the degree of cohesion among family members.

Results suggest that several factors may impact health related quality of life of asthmatic children. Important predictors of the health related quality of life of asthmatic children are socioeconomic status and family functioning. These findings implicate the need of specific attention to health related quality of life in asthmatic children from families with low socioeconomic status and poor family functioning.

6. Conclusion

Health care workers should be aware of the impact of asthma on children's life, their families and the factors associated with the health related quality of life of these children. Routine use of an health related quality of life questionnaire to evaluate health related quality of life in children with asthma symptoms and their caregivers should be recommended in health care. Specific application, for example, can be found in preventive child health care and in primary health care to prevent impairment of health related quality of life due to asthma symptoms and to realise adequate management of asthma symptoms. Attention should be given to health related quality of life in asthmatic children from families with low socioeconomic status and poor family functioning. Generally, a combination of parental and self-reports of both general and asthma-specific patient centred health related quality of life questionnaires should be applied. Further research should focus on which factors are responsible for the greatest burden on asthmatic children's health related quality of life and their caregivers' health related quality of life and how such risk factors should be prevented and managed.

7. References

Annett, RD.; Bender, BG.; Lapidus, J.; DuHamel, TR. & Lincoln, A. (2001). Predicting children's quality of life in an asthma clinical trial: What did children's reports tell us? *J Pediatr*, Vol.139, No.6, pp. 854-861, ISSN 0022-3476

Annett, RD.; Bender, BG.; DuHamel, TR. & Lapidus, J. (2003). Factors influencing parent reports on quality of life for children with asthma. *J Asthma*, Vol.40, No.5, pp. 577-587, ISSN 0277-0903

Bateman, E.D.; Bousquet, J.; Keech, ML.; Busse, WW.; Clark, TJ. & Pedersen, SE. (2007). The correlation between asthma control and health status: the GOAL study. *Eur Respir J*, Vol.29, No.1, pp. 56-63, ISSN 0903-1936

Bunge, EM.; Essink-Bot, ML.; Kobussen, MP.; Van Suijlekom-Smit, LW.; Moll, HA. & Raat, H. (2005). Reliability and validity of health status measurement by the TAPQOL. *Arch Dis Child*, Vol.90, No.4, pp. 351-358, ISSN 1468-2044

Carr, AJ. & Higginson, IJ. (2001). Are quality of life measures patient centred? *BMJ*, Vol.322, No.7298, pp. 1357-1360, ISSN 0959-8138

Christie, MJ.; French, D.; Sowden, A. & West, A. (1993). Development of child-centred disease-specific questionnaires for living with asthma. *Psychosom Med*, Vol.55, No.6, pp. 541-548, ISSN 0033-3174

Dalheim-Englund, AC.; Rydström, I.; Rasmussen, BH.; Moller, C. & Sandman, PO. (2004). Having a child with asthma-quality of life for Swedish parents. *J Clin Nurs*, Vol.13, No.3, pp. 386-395, ISSN 0962-1067

Dean, BB.; Calimlim, BC.; Kindermann, SL.; Khandker, RK. & Tinkelman, D. (2009). The impact of uncontrolled asthma on absenteeism and health-related quality of life. *J Asthma*, Vol.46, No.9, pp. 861-866, ISSN 1532-4303

Dean, BB.; Calimlim, BC.; Sacco, P.; Aguilar, D.; Maykut, R. & Tinkelman, D. (2010). Uncontrolled asthma: assessing quality of life and productivity of children and their caregivers using a cross-sectional Internet-based survey. *Health Qual Life Outcomes*, Vol.8, pp. 96, ISSN 1477-7525

Erickson, SR.; Munzenberger, PJ. & Plante, MJ.; Kirking, DM.; Hurwitz, ME. & Vanuya, RZ. (2002). Influence of sociodemographics on the health-related quality of life of pediatric patients with asthma and their caregivers. *J Asthma*, Vol.39, No.2, pp. 107-117, ISSN 0277-0903

Everhart, RS. & Fiese, BH. (2009). Asthma severity and child quality of life in pediatric asthma: A systematic review. *Patient Educ Couns*, Vol.75, No.2, pp. 162-168, ISSN 0738-3991

Farnik, M.; Pierzchała, W.; Brozek, G.; Zejda, JE. & Skrzypek, M. (2010). Quality of life protocol in the early asthma diagnosis in children. *Pediatr Pulmonol*, Vol.45, No.11, pp. 1095-1102, ISSN 1099-0496

Fiese, BH.; Wamboldt, FS. & Anbar, RD. (2005). Family asthma management routines: connections to medical adherence and quality of life. *J Pediatrics*, Vol.146, No.2, pp. 171-176, ISSN 0022-3476

Garro A. (2011). Health-related quality of life (HRQOL) in Latino families experiencing pediatric asthma. *J Child Health Care*, (Epub ahead of print), ISSN 1741-2889

Global Initiative for Asthma (GINA) Executive Committee. (2010). Global strategy for asthma management and prevention, In: Global Initiative for Asthma (GINA), Available from: www.ginasthma.org

Gorelick, MH.; Scribano, PV.; Stevens, MW. & Schultz, TR. (2003). Construct validity and responsiveness of the Child

Health Questionnaire in children with acute asthma. *Ann Allergy Asthma Immunol*, Vol.90, No.6, pp. 622-628, ISSN 1081-1206

Grootenhuis, MA.; Koopman, HM.; Verrips, EG.; Vogels, AG. & Last, BF. (2007). Health-related quality of life problems of children aged 8-11 years with a chronic disease. *Dev Neurorehabil*, Vol.10, No.1, pp. 27-33, ISSN 1751-8423

Guilbert, TW.; Garris, C.; Jhingran, P.; Bonafede, M.; Tomaszewski, KJ.; Bonus, T.; Hahn, RM. & Schatz, M. (2011). Asthma that is not well-controlled is associated with increased healthcare utilization and decreased quality of life. *J Asthma*, Vol.48, No.2, pp. 126-132, ISSN 1532-4303

Halterman, JS.; Yoos, HL.; Conn, KM.; Callahan, PM.; Montes, G.; Neely, TL. & Szilagyi, PG. (2004). The impact of childhood asthma on parental quality of life. *J Asthma*, Vol.41, No.6, pp. 645-653, ISSN 0277-0903

Juniper, EF.; Guyatt, GH.; Feeny, DH.; Ferrie, PJ.; Griffith, LE. & Townsend, M. (1996). Measuring quality of life in children with asthma. *Qual Life Research*, Vol.5, No.1, pp. 35-46, ISSN 0962-9343

Juniper, EF.; Guyatt, GH.; Feeny, DH.; Ferrie, PJ.; Griffith, LE. & Townsend, M. (1996). Measuring quality of life in the parents of children with asthma. *Qual Life Research*, Vol.5, No.1, pp. 27-34, ISSN 0962-9343

Juniper, EF. (1997). How important is quality of life in pediatric asthma? *Pediatr Pulmonology*, Suppl.15, pp. 17-21, ISSN 1054-187X

Juniper, EF.; Jenkins, C.; Price, MJ., Thwaites RMA. & James MH. (1999). Quality of life of asthma patients treated with salmeterol/fluticasone propionate combination product and budesonide (abstract). *Eur Respir J*, Vol.14, Suppl.30, pp. 370s

Juniper, EF.; Svensson, K.; O'Byrne, PM.; Barnes, PJ.; Bauer, CA.; Lofdahl, CG.; Postma, DS.; Pauwels, RA.; Tattersfield, AE. & Ullman, A. (1999). Asthma quality of life during 1 year of treatment with budesonide with or without formoterol. *Eur Respir J*, Vol.14, No.5, pp. 1038-104, ISSN 0903-1936

Le Coq, EM.; Colland, VT.; Boeke, AJ.; Boeke, P.; Bezemer, DP. & Van Eijk, JT. (2000). Reproducibility, construct validity, and responsiveness of the "How Are You?" (HAY), a self-report quality of life questionnaire for children with asthma. *J Asthma* , Vol.37, No.1, pp. 43-58, ISSN 0277-0903

Magid, DJ.; Houry, D.; Ellis, J.; Lyons, E. & Rumsfeld, JS. (2004). Health-related quality of life predicts emergency department utilization for patients with asthma. *Ann Emerg Med*, Vol.43, No.5, pp. 551-557, ISSN 1097-6760

Majani, G.; Baiardini, I.; Giardini, A.; Pasquali, M.; Tiozzo, M.; Tosca, M.; Cosentino, C.; La Grutta, S.; Marseglia, GL. &

Canonica, GW. (2005). Impact of children's respiratory allergies on caregivers. *Monaldi Arch Chest Dis*, Vol.63, No.4, pp. 199-203, ISSN 1122-0643

Masoli, M.; Fabian, D.; Holt, S. & Beasley, R. (2004). Global Initiative for Asthma (GINA) Program. The global burden of asthma: executive summary of the GINA Dissemination Committee report. *Allergy*, Vol.59, No.5, pp. 469-478, ISSN 0105-4538

Merikallio, VJ.; Mustalahti, K., Remes, ST., Valovirta, EJ. & Kaila, M. (2005). Comparison of quality of life between asthmatic and healthy school children. *Pediatr Allergy Immunol*, Vol.16, No.4, pp. 332-340, ISSN 0905-6157

Mohangoo, AD.; Essink-Bot, ML.; Juniper, EF.; Moll, HA.; De Koning, HJ. & Raat, H. (2005). Health-related quality of life in preschool children with wheezing and dyspnea: Preliminary results from a random general population sample. Qual Life Research, Vol. 14, No.8, pp. 1931-1936, ISSN 0962-9343

Mohangoo, AD.; De Koning, HJ.; Mangunkusumo, RT. & Raat, H. (2007). Health-Related Quality of Life in Adolescents with Wheezing Attacks. *J Adolesc Health*, Vol.41, No.5, pp. 464-471, ISSN 1879-1972

Mohangoo, AD.; De Koning, HJ.; De Jongste, JC.; Landgraf, JM.; Van der Wouden, JC.; Jaddoe, VW.; Hofman, A.; Moll, HA.; Mackenbach, JP. & Raat, H. (2011). Asthma-like symptoms in the first year of life and health-related quality of life at age 12 months: the Generation R study. *Qual Life Research*, In Press (Accepted: 2011-06-14), ISSN 1573-2649

Mrazek D. (1992). Psychiatric complications of pediatric asthma. *Ann Allergy*, Vol.69, No.4, pp. 285-293, ISSN 0003-4738

Osman, L. & Silverman, M. (1996). Measuring quality of life for young children with asthma and their families. *Eur Respir J*, Suppl.21, pp. 35s-41s, ISSN 0904-1850

Pedersen, SE.; Hurd, SS.; Lemanske, RF. (Jr); Becker, A.; Zar, HJ.; Sly, PD.; Soto-Quiroz, M.; Wong, G. & Bateman, ED. (2011). Global strategy for the diagnosis and management of asthma in children 5 years and younger. *Pediatr Pulmonol*, Vol.46, No.1, pp. 1-17, ISSN 1099-0496

Petersen, C.; Schmidt, S.; Power, M. & Bullinger, M. (2005). Development and pilot-testing of a health-related quality of life chronic generic module for children and adolescents with chronic health conditions: a European perspective. *Qual Life Research*, Vol.14, No.4, 1065-1077, ISSN 0962-9343

Petsios, K.; Priftis, KN.; Tsoumakas, C.; Hatziagorou, E.; Tsanakas, JN.; Galanis, P.; Antonogeorgos, G. & Matziou, V. (2011). Level of parent-asthmatic child agreement on health-related quality of life. *J Asthma*, Vol.48, No.3, pp. 286-297, ISSN 1532-4303

Pont, LG.; Van der Molen, T.; Denig, P.; Van der Werf, GT. & Haaijer-Ruskamp, FM. (2004). Relationship between guideline treatment and health-related quality of life in asthma. *Eur Respir J*, Vol.23, No.5, pp. 718-722, ISSN 0903-1936

Raat, H.; Bueving, H.J.; De Jongste, J.C.; Grol, MH.; Juniper, EF. & Van der Wouden, JC. (2005). Responsiveness, longitudinal- and cross-sectional construct validity of the Pediatric Asthma Quality of Life Questionnaire (PAQLQ) in Dutch children with asthma. *Qual Life Research*, Vol.14, No.1, pp. 265-272, ISSN 0962-9343

Raat, H.; Mohangoo, A.D. & Grootenhuis, M.A. (2006). Pediatric health-related quality of life questionnaires in clinical trials. *Curr Opin Allergy Clin Immunol*, Vol.6, No.3, pp. 180-185, ISSN 1528-4050

Sawyer, MG.; Spurrier, N.; Whaites, L.; Kennedy, D.; Martin, AJ. & Baghurst, P. (2000). The relationship between asthma severity, family functioning, and the health related quality of life of children with asthma. *Qual Life Research*, Vol.9, No.10, pp. 1105-1115, ISSN 0962-9343

Sawyer, MG.; Spurrier, N.; Kennedy, D. & Martin, J. (2001). The relationship between the quality of life of children with asthma and family functioning. *J Asthma*, Vol.38, No.3, pp. 279-284, ISSN

Sawyer, MG.; Reynolds, KE.; Couper, JJ.; French, DJ.; Kennedy, D.; Martin, J.; Staugas, R.; Ziaian, T. & Baghurst, PA. (2004). Health-related quality of life of children and adolescents with chronic illness – a two year prospective study. *Qual Life Research*, Vol.13, No.7, pp. 1309-1319, ISSN 0962-9343

Skoner D. (2002). Outcome measures in childhood asthma. *Pediatrics*, Vol.109, Suppl.2, pp. 393-398, ISSN 1098-4275

Spuijbroek, AT.; Oostenbrink, R.; Landgraf, JM.; Rietveld, E.; De Goede-Bolder, A.; Van Beeck, EF.; Van Baar, M.; Raat, H. & Moll, HA. (2011). Health-related quality of life in preschool children in five health conditions. *Qual Life Research*, Vol.20, No.5, pp. 779-786, ISSN 1573-2649

Van den Bemt, L.; Kooijman, S.; Linssen, V.; Lucassen, P.; Muris, J.; Slabbers, G. & Schermer, T. (2010). How does asthma influence the daily life of children? Results of focus group interviews. *Health Qual Life Outcomes*, Vol.8, pp. 5, ISSN 1477-7525

Varni, JW.; Burwinkle, TM.; Sherman, SA.; Hanna, K.; Berrin, SJ.; Malcarne, VL. & Chambers, HG. (2005). Health-related quality of life of children and adolescents with cerebral palsy: hearing the voices of the children. *Dev Med Child Neurol*, Vol.47, No.9, pp. 592-597, ISSN 0012-1622

Vila, G.; Hayder, R.; Bertrand, C.; Falissard, B.; De Blic, J.; Mouren-Simeoni, MC. & Scheinmann, P. (2003). Psychopathology and quality of life for adolescents with asthma and their parents. *Psychosomatics*, Vol.44, No.4, pp. 319-328, ISSN 0033-3182

World Health Organization (WHO), Division of Mental Health. (1993). Measurement of Quality of Life in Children. Available from: www.who.int/mental_health/media/en/663.pdf

Part 2

Treatment Strategies

4

Microbiota and Allergy:
From Dysbiosis to Probiotics

Anne-Judith Waligora-Dupriet and Marie-José Butel
EA 4065 Département Périnatalité, Microbiologie, Médicament, Faculté des Sciences Pharmaceutiques et Biologiques, Université Paris Descartes, Sorbonne Paris Cité, France

1. Introduction

The update theory of hygiene implicates the gut microbiota in the increasing prevalence of allergy. Indeed, changes have been observed in the establishment of the gut microbiota over the last fifteen years, and dysbiosis has been demonstrated in allergic subjects by numerous clinical studies comparing the microbiota in subjects from countries with high and low prevalence of allergy, or subjects with or without allergic diseases. These results support the use of pro- and prebiotics to treat or prevent allergic diseases; however, randomized controlled trials, mainly concerning atopic dermatitis, rhinitis and asthma, provide conflicting data. The mechanism of action of probiotics has not been elucidated. Nevertheless, it appears that lactobacilli and bifidobacteria may mediate immune responses in a strain-specific way, and the interactions involved seem to include dendritic cells and detection of microbe-associated molecular patterns. Although these functional foods are promising, numerous issues, including the bacterial strains and doses to use, remain to be determined.

1.1 The update theory of hygiene implicates the gut microbiota

Over recent decades, the incidence of allergic diseases has been increasing in industrialized country whereas it is stable in developing countries (Mannino *et al.*, 1998). This dichotomy and the large differences in the prevalence of allergy between genetically similar populations suggest that environmental factors make a large contribution to the development of allergies (Asher *et al.*, 2010). Numerous studies agree on the importance of the T-helper CD4 lymphocyte population balance (Th1, Th2, Th17, T regulatory cells), and an imbalance towards Th2 is considered to be a major factor for the onset of allergic disease. Imbalances of this type have long been associated with the absence of triggers of the Th1 immune response during childhood. Indeed, the increase in incidence of allergic diseases in industrialized countries coincides with widespread vaccination, antibiotic usage, declining family size, improvements in household amenities, and higher standards of personal cleanliness, all of which have reduced the opportunity for cross infection between children over the past century (the hygiene hypothesis, proposed by Strachan in 1989). However, the reduction of Th1 responses as a consequence of modern lifestyle cannot alone explain the high prevalence of allergic diseases in industrialized countries. Moreover, epidemiologic studies show that the morbidity of autoimmune diseases, which are associated with a Th1 or Th17 profiles, are increasing and that helminthiasis, associated with a Th2 profile, are not associated with an increased risk of allergic disease (Bach, 2002). Recent work implicates therefore inadequate stimulation of either various regulatory T cell subsets, or Toll-like receptor (Okada et al., 2010;Akdis et al., 2004).

Commensal bacteria of the intestinal microbiota play a crucial role in development of the intestinal immune system and modulation of the T helper cell balance. Rautava et al. extended this "hygiene hypothesis" and suggested that the initial composition of the infant gut microbiota may be a key determinant in the development of atopic disease (Rautava et al., 2004). Indeed, neonates are biased towards T helper type 2 responses with reference to adults (Adkins et al., 2004;Protonotariou et al., 2004), and the first bacteria to colonize the infant's gut are the first stimuli for post-natal maturation of the T-helper balance. The immature Th2-dominant neonatal response undergoes environment-driven maturation via microbial contact during the early postnatal period resulting in a gradual inhibition of the Th2 response and an increase of the Th1 response and prevention of allergic diseases. This hypothesis is consistent with various observations: the delayed colonization of the digestive tract associated with changes in lifestyle over the last 15 years (Campeotto et al., 2007;Adlerberth and Wold, 2009); and evidence that caesarian section (Kero et al., 2002;Laubereau et al., 2004), prematurity (Agosti et al., 2003), and exposure to antibiotics during pregnancy (McKeever et al., 2002) —all factors which modify establishment of the gut microbiota— are associated with a higher risk of atopic disease.

2. The gut microbiota and its functions

The composition of microbial communities in the gut was first investigated through culture-based studies, leading to estimates of 400 to 500 different species in the adult human intestinal tract (Manson et al., 2008). The dominant microbiota (10^9-10^{11} CFU.g^{-1}) is composed of obligate anaerobes, including Gram-negative bacilli such as *Bacteroides*, Gram-positive bacilli such as *Bifidobacterium, Eubacterium,* and Gram-positive cocci. The subdominant microbiota (10^6-10^8 CFU.g^{-1}) is composed of facultative anaerobes including various species of enterobacteria, notably *Escherichia coli*, and species of the *Enterococcus* and *Lactobacillus* genera. With population densities of below 10^6 CFU.g^{-1}, this microbiota is often extremely variable and transient.

The use of culture-independent approaches has provided novel insights into the gut microbiota community (Manson et al., 2008). Many of the techniques used are based on analysis of 16S rRNA gene sequences, and studies have exploited combinations of 16S rRNA gene libraries, DNA microarrays, 16S rRNA gene fingerprinting, fluorescent *in* situ hybridization, and quantitative PCR. These culture-independent techniques have shown that the intestinal microbiota community is more complex than previously described. The proportion of bacteria in the adult intestine that can be cultured varies between 15 and 85% (Eckburg et al., 2005); over 1200 bacterial species have been characterized (Rajilic-Stojanovic et al., 2007), and current estimates are that there are up to 1000 bacterial species per individual and over 5000 different species in total in human intestines (Zoetendal et al., 2008). Most of the gut microbiota are from only four major phyla (Tap et al., 2009). *Firmicutes* and *Bacteroidetes* are the most abundant, and *Actinobacteria* - including bifidobacteria - and *Proteobacteria* are less abundant despite representing more than 1% of the total microbiota. Adult fecal microbiota has been demonstrated to be individual-specific and relatively stable over time (Rajilic-Stojanovic *et al.*, 2009). However, even though each individual harbors a unique microbiota, a number of microbial species are present in all individuals, consistent with the existence of a universal phylogenetic core to the human intestinal microbiota (Rajilic-Stojanovic *et al.*, 2009;Tap *et al.*, 2009).

The intestinal ecosystem develops rapidly during the neonatal stage of life. The intestine is sterile at birth and is colonized by bacteria following contact with the maternal microbiota and the surrounding environment. Little is known about the factors that lead to the establishment of particular bacterial strains. Colonizing bacteria originate mainly from the mother; the maternal gut microbiota is a major source and other sources include the microbiota of the vagina, perineum, and skin. Breast milk has also been demonstrated to be a source of lactic acid bacteria (Martin *et al.*, 2009;Gueimonde *et al.*, 2007). Infants encounter numerous bacteria in the environment including the microbiota of food and the microbiota of the skin of parents, siblings and nurses. Consequently, the number of bacterial species, mainly obligate anaerobes, increases with time in the infant gut. As a result of the diversity of exposure, there is substantial inter-individual variability in the composition and patterns of bacterial colonization during the first weeks of life (Penders *et al.*, 2006c;Palmer *et al.*, 2007;Vaishampayan *et al.*, 2010). However, by the end of the first year of life, the bacterial composition in the gut converges toward an adult-like microbiota profile (Palmer *et al.*, 2007). Various external factors can affect the pattern of bacterial colonization (for review see (Adlerberth and Wold, 2009;Vael and Desager, 2009;Campeotto *et al.*, 2007). Infants born by cesarean section are deprived of contact with their mother's gut and vaginal microbiota, which decreases bacterial diversity and colonization by obligate anaerobes, particularly bifidobacteria and *Bacteroides*. The mode of infant feeding also strongly affects bacterial establishment, with a dominant colonization by bifidobacteria being a characteristic distinguishing breastfed from formula-fed infants. However, improvements in infant formulas have led to there now being only minor differences in colonization according to feeding method (Adlerberth and Wold, 2009;Campeotto *et al.*, 2007). Finally, the establishment of gut microbiota in infants in industrialized countries appears to have been affected in modern times, most likely due to improved hygiene and general cleanliness in these countries, resulting in reduced bacterial exposure (Adlerberth and Wold, 2009;Campeotto *et al.*, 2007).

Although the gut microbiota community was for several decades mostly studied to elucidate pathogenic relationships, it is now clear that most microorganism-host interactions in the gut are, in fact, commensal or even mutualistic (Bik, 2009;Dethlefsen *et al.*, 2007). This complex ecosystem has various major functions (Fujimura *et al.*, 2010). Colonic fermentation of non-digestible dietary residues and endogenous mucus supplies energy and nutritive products to the bacteria. It also plays a role in the trophic functions of the intestinal epithelium (Wong *et al.*, 2006). The barrier effect, which involves secretion of antimicrobial molecules, competition for nutrients, and attachment to ecological niches, refers to a resistance to colonization by exogenous or opportunistic bacteria present at a low level in the gut (Stecher and Hardt, 2008). Finally, the gut microbial community has a major immune function. The contribution of the gut microbiota to immune system maturation has been demonstrated by the description of major abnormalities of the immune system in germ-free mice (Smith *et al.*, 2007). Intestinal IgA-secreting plasma cells are rare in germ-free animals, and the Peyer's patches are smaller and contain fewer lymphoid follicles than those in conventional mice. The T cell content of the mucosal immune system is also low in germ-free animals, and particularly the CD4+ cells of the lamina propria. Spleen and lymph nodes are relatively structureless with abnormal B- and T- cell zones. These morphologic features are associated with substantial functional abnormalities, such as hypogammaglobulinemia, a Th2 cell shift and defects in oral tolerance induction (Round *et al.*, 2010). Recent reviews have highlighted how the microbiota elicits innate and adaptive immune mechanisms that cooperate to protect the host and maintain intestinal homeostasis (Hooper and Macpherson, 2010;Garrett *et al.*, 2010). Colonization of germ-free mice by a single species of bacteria e.g. *Bacteroides fragilis* (Mazmanian *et al.*, 2005) or segmented filamentous bacteria (Gaboriau-Routhiau *et al.*, 2009), has been shown to be sufficient to restore the development of a multifaceted adaptive immune response. The capacity to stimulate steady-state gut T cell responses appears to be restricted to a small number of bacteria (Gaboriau-Routhiau *et al.*, 2009) and certain strains. Indeed, the immunostimulatory properties of *Bifidobacterium* are strain-specific (Medina *et al.*, 2007;Menard *et al.*, 2008) and only some strains of *Bifidobacterium* are able to induce Foxp3+ regulatory cells or be associated with protection from respiratory and oral allergy in mice (Lyons *et al.*, 2010). *B. infantis* restored the susceptibility to oral tolerance induction in germ-free mice only if the inoculation was at the neonatal stage (Sudo *et al.*, 1997). This suggests that there is a 'time window of opportunity' during the neonatal phase, consistent with observations with probiotics (Feleszko *et al.*, 2007).

3. Microbiota and allergy

The extended version of the hygiene hypothesis implicating the gut microbiota is supported by several clinical studies which have shown a relationship between allergic disease and gut microbiota. In particular, they have shown that the composition of the bacterial community in the feces differ between children who live in countries with high and low prevalence of allergy, as well between children with or without allergic diseases.

3.1 Is gut microbiota different between healthy individuals and allergic subjects? Case-control studies

Numerous studies have addressed the composition of the microbiota in healthy and allergic subjects. Some of the first studies (Bjorksten *et al.*, 1999;Sepp *et al.*, 1997) compared the microbiota between two-year old children in countries with high (Sweden) and low (Estonia) incidence of allergic diseases. Irrespective of country of residence, allergic children were colonized by fewer lactobacilli but had higher counts of aerobic bacteria, especially *Enterobacteriaceae* and staphylococci and lower counts of *Bacteroides*. A prospective study (Bjorksten *et al.*, 2001) found that children who developed atopic dermatitis and/or positive skin prick test results during the two first years of life were less often colonized with enterococci during the first month of life and with bifidobacteria during the first year of life. Furthermore, allergic infants had higher counts of clostridia at 3 months of age and lower counts of *Bacteroides* at 12 months. The prevalence of colonization with *Staphylococcus aureus* was also higher in allergic children than the reference group at 6 months old.

Case-control studies confirmed differences of the gut microbiota composition between allergic and healthy subjects but the differences identified concerned various particular genera and species, including *Bifidobacterium, Clostridium, Bacteroides, Lactobacillus* and *Enterobacteriaceae*. Indirect methods suggested an association between allergy and

Clostridium difficile. Allergic infants had higher fecal concentrations of the rarely detected i-caproic acid, which has been associated with the presence of *Clostridium difficile* (Bottcher *et al.*, 2000) and higher *C. difficile* IgG antibody levels at one year than non-allergic infants (Woodcock *et al.*, 2002). However, counting bacteria by FISH analysis indicated that colonization by *Clostridium* sp. was lower in allergic than reference subjects (Mah *et al.*, 2006) and no significant difference in *Clostridium* counts were found between preschool controls and children with allergy-associated atopic eczema/dermatitis syndrome (AAEDS) and non-allergic atopic eczema/dermatitis syndrome (NAAEDS) (Kendler *et al.*, 2006)

Numerous other studies reported quantitative differences in colonization with *Bifidobacterium*, a dominant genus in infant fecal microbiota which may have beneficial effects (Ventura *et al.*, 2004). The prevalence of *Bifidobacterium* has been found to be similar in healthy and allergic subjects, whatever the allergic disease (Stsepetova *et al.*, 2007;Waligora-Dupriet *et al.*, 2011), and for atopic dermatitis (Gore *et al.*, 2008), and wheezing (Murray *et al.*, 2005). However, the findings of one study are discordant (Sepp *et al.*, 2005) with none of the 5-year-old children with atopic dermatitis and only one child with bronchial asthma colonized with bifidobacteria. Besides, low levels of bifidobacterial colonization have been observed in infants suffering from atopic dermatitis (Kirjavainen *et al.*, 2001;Watanabe *et al.*, 2003;Mah *et al.*, 2006) and in infants suffering from atopic dermatitis and wheezing; note that these results have been contradicted by studies comparing healthy subjects with wheezing infants without other symptoms (Murray *et al.*, 2005) and with patients suffering from both atopic dermatitis and food allergy (Penders *et al.*, 2006a).

3.2 Does dysbiosis precede allergic symptoms? Prospective studies

Some prospective studies report that modifications of the composition of the intestinal microbiota can be detected before any atopic syndrome, suggesting that bacteria implicated in the maturation of the immune system may be important. The bacterial fatty acid profile in fecal samples differed significantly between 3-week-old infants in whom atopy was and was not developing. The stools of atopic subjects had more clostridia and tended to have fewer bifidobacteria than those of non atopic subjects, resulting in a reduced ratio of bifidobacteria to clostridia (Kalliomaki *et al.*, 2001a). The Koala Birth Cohort Study in the Netherlands confirmed these results by showing that gut dysbiosis precedes the manifestation of atopic symptoms and atopic sensitization (Penders *et al.*, 2007). In particular, *C. difficile* was associated with all atopic symptoms and sensitization. The presence of *Escherichia coli* was associated with a higher risk of developing (non-atopic) eczema, this risk increasing with increasing *E. coli* counts; infants colonized with *C. difficile* were at higher risk of developing atopic dermatitis, recurrent wheeze and allergic sensitisation. As *E. coli* was only associated with eczema and *C. difficile* was associated with all atopic outcomes, the underlying mechanisms may be different. Colonization with clostridia, including *C. difficile*, was associated with allergy development up to age 2 years in several studies (Kalliomaki *et al.*, 2001a;Bjorksten *et al.*, 2001;Penders *et al.*, 2007) but not in others (Adlerberth *et al.*, 2007;Sjogren *et al.*, 2009;Songjinda *et al.*, 2007). Fecal colonization at age 3 weeks with *Clostridium coccoides* subcluster XIVa species has been described as an early indicator of possible asthma later in life (Vael *et al.*, 2008;Vael *et al.*, 2011). However, Verhulst *et al.* (2008) found an association between antibiotics, anaerobic bacteria and wheezing during the first year of life, but increasing levels of *Clostridium* were protective against wheezing. These studies considered different *Clostridium* species and the genus *Clostridium* is a very heterogeneous group comprising several different clusters (Stackebrandt *et al.*, 1999). Indeed, it seems unlikely that all members of this genus exert the same effects on the human immune system (Penders *et al.*, 2007).

Children not developing allergy before age 2 years have been shown to be more frequently colonized with bifidobacteria than children developing allergy (Bjorksten *et al.*, 2001), but this decreased prevalence of *Bifidobacterium* in children suffering allergies was not confirmed in all studies (Songjinda *et al.*, 2007;Penders *et al.*, 2006a;Adlerberth *et al.*, 2007). Differences in patterns of colonization by bifidobacteria species have also been observed but no clear consensus exists. Young *et al* (2004) compared the populations of bifidobacteria in feces from children aged 25 to 35 days in Ghana (which has a low prevalence of atopy), New Zealand, and the United Kingdom (high-prevalence countries): almost all fecal samples from Ghana contained *Bifidobacterium longum* subsp *infantis* whereas those from the children living in the other countries did not. The authors suggested that place of birth influences the patterns of bifidobacterial species present. *B. adolescentis* has been found in the fecal microbiota of both allergic infants (Ouwehand *et al.*, 2001;He *et al.*, 2001) and non-allergic infants (Sjogren *et al.*, 2009). Similarly, *B. catenulatum/pseudocatenulatum* has been isolated from both allergic (Gore *et al.*, 2008) and non-allergic infants (Stsepetova *et al.*, 2007). Some authors report that restricted *Bifidobacterium* diversity is linked with allergy (Stsepetova *et al.*, 2007) but again, this was not confirmed in other studies at the species (Sjogren *et al.*, 2009;Waligora-Dupriet *et al.*, 2011) or strain level (Waligora-Dupriet *et al.*, 2011). It has been suggested that the intrinsic properties of bacterial strains may be pertinent. Indeed, *in vitro*, bifidobacterial species differentially affected expression of cell surface markers and cytokine production by dendritic cells harvested from cord blood. *B. bifidum*, *B. longum*, and *B. pseudocatenulatum*, species commonly detected in children in New Zealand and the United Kingdom increased the expression of the dendritic-cell activation marker CD83 and induce IL-10 production, whereas *B. infantis*, a species commonly isolated in Ghana, does not (Young *et al*, 2004). By contrast, heat-inactivated *B. longum* subsp *longum* and *B. adolescentis*, known as adult-type bifidobacteria, were significantly stronger inducers of pro-inflammatory cytokine (IL-12 and TNF-alpha) production by a murine macrophage cell line than *B. bifidum*, *B. breve*, and *B. longum* subsp *infantis* usually isolated from infants (He *et al.*, 2002). The Th1 stimulation profile induced by *B. adolescentis* (Karlsson *et al.*, 2004;He *et al.*, 2002) may intensify pathology in allergic infants (He *et al.*, 2002). However, the properties of intestinal bifidobacteria are highly strain-dependent (Matto *et al.*, 2004), and this is particularly true of immunostimulatory properties (Menard *et al.*, 2008;Medina *et al.*, 2007).

Bacteroidaceae are also associated with allergic development, although, as for clostridia and bifidobacteria, findings are contradictory. Indeed, *Bacteroides* colonization of the gut was not found to be linked to allergy in several studies (Adlerberth *et al.*, 2007;Kalliomaki *et al.*, 2001a; Bjorksten *et al.*, 2001; Sjogren *et al.*, 2009), but colonization with the *B. fragilis* group at age 3 weeks has been associated with a higher risk of developing asthma later in life (Vael *et al.*, 2008;Vael *et al.*, 2011). A high level of *Bacteroides* colonization positively correlated with IgE in children with atopic dermatitis (Kirjavainen *et al.*, 2002). Moreover, fecal *Bacteroides* strains induced high levels of Th2 cytokine production by peripheral blood monocyte cells from patients suffering from Japanese Cedar Pollinosis (Odamaki *et al.*, 2007).

Discrepancies between studies might be the consequence of the methods used to study the gut microbiota. Indeed, in the same study, some differences were observed with FISH but that were not detected by bacterial cultivation (Kalliomaki *et al.*, 2001a). These discrepancies are such that it is not possible to conclude about the association of particular species, genera or groups with the development of allergy, although it seems that the diversity of the gut microbiota is a major determinant in allergy risk. Interestingly, a large recent study did not find any relationships between the presence of various particular bacteria and allergy development up to 18 months of age (Adlerberth *et al.*, 2007), but showed that infants who developed allergy had a lower diversity in their gut microbiota at one week of age (Wang *et al.*, 2008).

Despite prospective studies showing that modifications of the gut microbiota composition can be detected before any atopic syndrome, these epidemiological studies cannot demonstrate which of these factors appears first. Atopy could be linked to a mucosal state favoring some bacterial populations to the detriment of others. In a mouse model of food allergy, mice with high and low anaphylaxis scores showed differences in intestinal microbiota composition: high responders exhibited less staphylococcus colonization (Rodriguez *et al.*, 2011). The composition of the intestinal bacteria fluctuated significantly during the pollen season in adults with IgE-dependent pollinosis, with colonization by the *Bacteroides fragilis* group increasing with pollen dispersal, especially at the end of the pollen season (Odamaki *et al.*, 2007). It is clear that the cause-and-effect relationship between the composition of the microbiota and allergic diseases remains to be determined.

4. Probiotics and allergic diseases

Despite discrepancies between studies, there is mounting evidence of a relationship between the intestinal microbiota and allergy. It therefore follows that a modulation of the gut microbiota may help prevent allergic diseases and this notion supports the use of probiotics, prebiotics and synbiotics. Probiotics are currently defined as "live microorganisms which when administered in adequate amounts confer a health benefit on the host" (FAO/WHO, 2001; FAO/WHO 2001, 2002). The most widely used probiotics are lactic acid bacteria, specifically *Lactobacillus* and *Bifidobacterium* species (Williams, 2010). The yeast *Saccharomyces boulardii* is also used. Although the efficacy of probiotics is sometimes debatable, they offer substantial potential benefits to health and are safe for human use.

The mechanisms of action of "probiotic" strains in allergic diseases may include modulation of the gut microbiota, maturation of the gut barrier, stimulation of the immune system and immunomodulation. However, the effects of probiotics described in experimental models need to be confirmed for human use through randomized controlled trials. We conducted bibliographic searches in the PubMed/Medline database for the following terms (all field): allergy AND probiotic*", and results limited to randomized controlled trials identified 99 publications.

4.1 Clinical impact of probiotics in atopic/allergic diseases
4.1.1 Probiotics in the treatment of atopic dermatitis

Fifty studies have evaluated clinical consequences of probiotics in the treatment of atopic dermatitis (AD) in infants and children, and between them have studied about 1100 subjects. AD is a chronic highly pruritic inflammatory skin disease including IgE- and non-IgE-mediated mechanisms. It commonly occurs during early infancy but can persist or even start in adulthood. It includes a wide clinical spectrum from minor forms to major symptoms including erythrodermic rash and can be associated with other atopic diseases such as food allergy, asthma, and allergic rhinitis. To evaluate the effects of probiotics on AD, a rigorous definition of study participants is necessary. The diagnosis of AD is currently based on diagnostic criteria scales developed by Hanifin and Rafka in 1980 and by the "United Kingdom Working party" in 1994 (*in* Roguedas-Contios and Misery, 2011). It is equally important that diseases outcome measures used in treatment studies are both valid and reliable. Three of the various eczema outcome measures have been shown to be reliable: SCORing Atopic Dermatitis (SCORAD), the Eczema Area and Severity Index (EASI) and the Patient Oriented Eczema Measure (POEM). SCORAD is commonly used in studies of probiotics. It combines an estimation of the intensity and extent of the eczema with a subjective itch. However, it assesses a clinical state of the disease at a particular time point without taking into account overall severity or evolution of the disease (Société Française de Dermatologie, 2005). Some quality of life scales are also used, for example the Infant Dermatitis Quality Of Life (IDQOL), Dermatitis Family Impact (DFI), and Dermatitis Family Impact Questionnaire (DFIQ) scores (Gerasimov *et al.*, 2010; Weston *et al.*, 2005) scores.

The age range of subjects included varies between studies: around weaning (median 5 months old) (Brouwer *et al.*, 2006;Isolauri *et al.*, 2000;Kirjavainen *et al.*, 2003;Viljanen *et al.*, 2005b;Gruber *et al.*, 2007), around 1 year old (Weston *et al.*, 2005;Folster-Holst *et al.*, 2006), and around 5 years old (Rosenfeldt *et al.*, 2003, 2004; Sistek *et al.*, 2006; Woo *et al.*, 2010). Seven of these publications describe effects of *Lactobacillus rhamnosus* GG LGG in infants but report contradictory results (Brouwer *et al.*, 2006;Isolauri *et al.*, 2000;Kirjavainen *et al.*, 2003;Viljanen *et al.*, 2005b;Gruber *et al.*, 2007;Folster-Holst *et al.*, 2006;Nermes *et al.*, 2011). Two of them (Isolauri *et al.*, 2000;Kirjavainen *et al.*, 2003) showed a significant decrease of the SCORAD score, but both these studies included only small groups of infants (27 and 35). Moreover, the heat-inactivated LGG used in Kirjavainen's study induced adverse gastrointestinal symptoms and diarrhea leading to the recruitment of patients being stopped after the pilot phase (Kirjavainen *et al.*, 2003). Six other studies, similar in terms of subjects included and protocol, did not find any improvement in SCORAD scores following LGG supplementation (Folster-Holst *et al.*, 2006;Brouwer *et al.*, 2006;Gruber *et al.*, 2007;Viljanen *et al.*, 2005b;Nermes *et al.*, 2011;Rose *et al.*, 2010). Other probiotic strains have been studied, and *Bifidobacterium lactis* Bb12 (Isolauri *et al.*, 2000), *L. sakei* KCTC 10755B0 and *L. fermentum* VRI-003 (Weston *et al.*, 2005) induced significant decreases in SCORAD scores. In the last of these studies, the effects of *L. fermentum* VRI-003 were found to persist two months after the end of supplementation. Four studies used a *L. rhamnosus* strain (not LGG) alone (Brouwer *et al.*, 2006) or mixed with *L. reuteri* (Rosenfeldt *et al.*, 2003) or with other *Lactobacillus sp.* and *Bifidobacterium sp.* (Viljanen *et al.*, 2005b;Sistek *et al.*, 2006). These studies did not detect significant SCORAD score improvement although in the crossover study of Rosenfeldt *et al* (2003), which included children older than those in the other studies, patients felt better according to their subjective evaluations. Nevertheless, a pronounced decrease in SCORAD score was observed in patients with a positive skin prick-test response and increased IgE levels (Viljanen *et al.*, 2005b;Rosenfeldt *et al.*, 2003;Sistek *et al.*, 2006). The administration of a probiotic mixture containing *L. acidophilus* DDS-1, *B. lactis* UABLA-12, and fructo-oligosaccharide was associated with a significant clinical improvement in children with AD and in particular a large decrease in SCORAD score and increase in quality of life score relative to the placebo group (Gerasimov *et al.*, 2010). This was not the case with a mixture of *B. breve* M-16V and galacto-/fructooligosaccharide (Immunofortis) (van der Aa *et al.*, 2010), even though this synbiotic mixture seemed to prevent asthma-like symptoms in infants with

AD (van der Aa *et al.*, 2011). To conclude, investigations of probiotics for the treatment of AD provide promising results, but are not conclusive, as confirmed by meta-analyzes (Lee *et al.*, 2008;Osborn and Sinn, 2007) such that they do not provide sufficient basis to recommend the use of such products.

4.1.2 Probiotics in the treatment of rhinitis and respiratory allergic diseases

Eleven studies have evaluated clinical effects of probiotics in the treatment of allergic diseases of the respiratory tract, *i.e.* rhinitis and asthma, and altogether included about 890 subjects.

Lactobacillus paracasei-33, whether or not heat-inactivated, improved quality of life of patients with allergic rhinitis: both frequency and intensity of symptoms were significantly lower in the LP-33 group than the placebo group, after the 30-day treatment (Wang *et al.*, 2004;Peng & Hsu, 2005). Likewise, *Lactobacillus casei* DN114 001 decreased the occurrence of rhinitis episodes and improved the health status of children with allergic rhinitis (Giovannini *et al.*, 2007). For patients with Japanese cedar pollen allergy, LGG and *Lactobacillus gasseri* TMC0356 reduced nasal symptoms (Kawase *et al.*, 2009), and *B. longum* BB536 was able to relieve eye symptoms (Ishida *et al.*, 2005;Xiao *et al.*, 2007). The degree of eosinophil infiltration into the respiratory mucosa correlates directly with the intensity of allergic rhinitis and can be used as an objective marker of the disease. A mixture of *L. acidophilus* NCFMTM and *B. lactis* Bl-04 reduced nasal eosinophil infiltration (Ouwehand *et al.*, 2009) as did *Bacillus clausii* which also reduced the number of days on which antihistamine was used in children with allergic rhinitis due to pollen sensitization (Ciprandi *et al.*, 2005a). However, *L. rhamnosus* ATCC53103 was not beneficial to teenagers and young adults allergic to birch pollen or ingested apple and who had intermittent symptoms of atopic allergy and/or mild asthma (Helin *et al.*, 2002). Similarly, *L. casei* Shirota was not found to reduce symptoms of Japanese cedar pollen allergy (Tamura *et al.*, 2007), although the strain did reduce serum concentrations of IL-5, IL-6, IFN-γ and specific IgE in subjects with allergic rhinitis (Ivory *et al.*, 2008). In children with recurrent wheeze and an atopic family history, LGG had no clinical effect on asthma-related events, and only a small effect on allergic sensitization (Rose *et al.*, 2010); likewise, long-term consumption of fermented milk containing *L. casei* had no detectable effect in asthmatic children (Giovannini *et al.*, 2007)

4.1.3 Probiotics in the primary prevention of allergic diseases

The prevention of allergy through an early administration of probiotics is appealing.

Four studies investigating probiotic supplementation begun during pregnancy. The first study to be published was by the team of Isolauri and reported promising results on preventive effects of LGG (Kalliomaki *et al.*, 2001b). LGG was given prenatally to 132 mothers who had at least one first-degree relative (or partner) with atopic eczema, allergic rhinitis, or asthma, and postnatally for 6 months to their infants. Two years later, the frequency of atopic eczema in infants given probiotics was half that of those on placebo (Kalliomaki *et al.*, 2001b). The reduction was greatest for infants who were exclusively breastfed, and therefore who did not receive the probiotic directly until 3 months of age (LGG being given to the mother) (Rautava *et al.*, 2002a). Administration of probiotics to the mother during pregnancy and breast-feeding appeared to be a safe and effective method for enhancing the immunoprotective potential of breast milk and preventing atopic eczema in the infant. The protective effect of LGG extended beyond infancy until 7 years old

(Kalliomaki *et al.*, 2003; 2007). Infants most likely to benefit from probiotics might be those with an elevated cord blood IgE concentration (Rautava *et al.*, 2002a), despite such high IgE levels not appearing as a risk factor for atopic diseases (Bergmann *et al.*, 1998). However, LGG had no impact on sensitization: there was no difference between LGG and placebo groups at 2, 4 and 7 year old as concerns the numbers of infants with high levels of specific IgE and/or positive prick test results (Kalliomaki *et al.*, 2001b; 2003; 2007).

The preventive effect of LGG was not confirmed in a similar study by Kopp *et al.* (2008) with 94 mother-infant couples. The discrepancies between the data of Kalliomaki *et al* and the data of Kopp *et al* cannot be explained by the minor differences between the study designs, but could be linked to the study populations. The German cohort (Kopp *et al*) was at higher risk of allergy than the Finnish cohort (Kalliomaki *et al*), the infants had older siblings, and the genetic contexts were different. Two other preventive studies considered prenatal and postnatal supplementation with probiotics. An investigation of *L reuteri* ATCC55730 supplementation for infants with a family history of allergic disease did not confirm a preventive effect against infant eczema but found a decreased prevalence of IgE-associated eczema during the second year. The effect was larger in the subgroup of children of allergic mothers (Abrahamsson *et al.*, 2007). Infants receiving *L rhamnosus* HN001 had a significantly lower risk of eczema than infants receiving placebo, but this was not the case for *B animalis* subsp *lactis* and there was no significant effect of these two strains on atopy (Wickens *et al.*, 2008). Taylor *et al* (2006a; 2006b; 2007a; 2007b) and of Soh *et al* (2009) studied newborns given, from birth to 6 months of life, *L. acidophilus* LAVRI-A1 (178 infants) and a mixture of *L. rhamnosus* LPR and *B. longum* BL999 (253 infants), respectively, and did not find any reduction of the risk of AD in high-risk infants as assessed from the numbers of patients affected, SCORAD score or IgE sensitization. Moreover, *L. acidophilus* was associated with increased allergen sensitization (Taylor *et al.*, 2007a). Likewise, supplementation with LGG during pregnancy and early infancy did not alter the severity of atopic dermatitis in affected children and was associated with an increased rate of recurrent episodes of wheezing and bronchitis (Kalliomaki *et al.*, 2003; 2007; Kopp *et al.*, 2008).

4.2 Mechanisms of probiotic action in atopic/allergic diseases in human

Although no unambiguous clinical benefits were observed in several studies, probiotics may nevertheless have useful effects on microbiota composition, the immune system and the gut barrier in infants and in children.

4.2.1 Effects of probiotics on microbiota composition

Any effects of probiotic microorganisms on health and well-being may potentially be due, at least in part, to modulation of the intestinal microbiota. However, few of the studies on probiotics and allergic diseases assessed the consequences of probiotic use on gut microbiota composition. From the available evidence, it seems that probiotics have no impact on microbiota. In the treatment of rhinitis with *L. acidophilus* NCFMTM, fecal probiotic cell counts correlated positively with fecal acetic, propionic and butyric acid concentrations (Ouwehand *et al.*, 2009), suggesting that the presence of *L. acidophilus* NCFMTM increases microbial fermentation in the colon. However, the colonization pattern did not differ between groups that consumed the probiotic strains and placebo. Similarly, no modification of the gut microbiota was observed following LGG supplementation in infants with AD (Kirjavainen *et al*, 2003). The fecal microbiota fluctuated in subjects with Japanese cedar pollinosis during the pollen season and supplementation with BB536 yogurt modulated the microbiota in a manner that may possibly contribute to the alleviation of allergic symptoms (Odamaki *et al*, 2007).

4.2.2 Gut immunity and barrier effect
Probiotics may modulate local immune systems. Treatment with LGG resulted in a trend towards elevated fecal IgA levels, and this effect was significant in IgE-associated cow-milk allergy infants, suggesting maturation of intestinal immunity and triggering of a mechanism to protect the gut from the offending food (Viljanen *et al.*, 2005a). In older subjects with a mature immune system and suffering from allergic rhinitis, fecal IgA concentrations increased in the placebo group during the pollen season; this increase was prevented by *L. acidophilus* NCFMTM (Ouwehand *et al.*, 2009).

Probiotics have also been reported to decrease the levels of fecal inflammatory markers, but this is controversial: findings differ between studies and strains used. Treatment of AD with LGG was associated with a decrease of TNF-α and α-antitrypsin levels suggesting that LGG may alleviate inflammation in the gut. Indeed, TNF-α is a proinflammatory cytokine for both Th1- and Th2-type cells, and a marker of local inflammation. The presence of α-antitrypsin indicates protein loss in the intestine and is a marker of mucosal integrity. These results were not confirmed in the studies by Folster-Holt *et al* (2006) and Brouwer *et al* (2006) who did not observe any differences in α-antitrypsin, or calprotectin, or eosinophilic cationic protein levels between infants receiving or not receiving LGG. Accumulation of eosinophilic cationic protein at sites of allergic inflammation demonstrates local eosinophil degranulation in the gut. Specific lactobacilli (*L. rhamnosus* 19070-2 and *L reuteri* DSM 12246) might reverse increased small intestinal permeability (such permeability is involved in the pathogenesis of atopic dermatitis) thereby stabilizing the intestinal barrier function and decreasing gastrointestinal symptoms in children with AD (Rosenfeldt *et al.*, 2004).

4.2.3 Th1/Th2 balance
Certain strains of *Lactobacillus* and *Bifidobacterium* can modulate cytokine production.

Bacillus clausii modulated the cytokine pattern in the nasal mucosa in allergic children with recurrent respiratory infections. In particular, *B. clausii* restored physiological Th1 polarization and induced T-regulatory cell responses, as documented by increased levels of IL-10 and tumor growth factor (TGF)-β after treatment (Ciprandi *et al.*, 2005b). TGF-β is a regulatory cytokine which may be responsible for a decrease in local inflammation (Shull *et al.*, 1992). Interestingly, Rautava *et al* (2002b) observed high TGF-β2 concentrations in breast-milk from mothers who had received LGG for prevention of allergic disease. The authors concluded that, first, direct supplementation of infant after birth is not necessary, and second that probiotics could increase the protective effects of breast milk.

The effects on the Th1-Th2 balance of probiotic strains used for the treatment of AD in early infancy have been evaluated in several studies. Pohjavuori *et al.* (2004) were able to demonstrate greater IFN-γ production in anti-CD3/anti-CD28-stimulated *in vitro* peripheral blood mononuclear cells (PBMC) from infants treated with LGG than placebo. A different modulatory effect was observed with a mix of four bacterial strains including LGG: a significant increase in secretion of IL-4 in infants with cow milk allergy. By contrast, production of the predominant Th1 cytokine INF-γ, and the Th2 cytokines IL-4 or IL-5 after polyclonal or specific anti-CD3/anti-CD28 stimulation, was unaffected by supplementation with *L rhamnosus, LGG* (Brouwer *et al.*, 2006) or a lactobacillus mix (Rosenfeldt *et al.*, 2003). A decrease in circulating IgA-, IgG- and IgM-secreting cells and an increase in memory B cells during LGG supplementation has been described (Nermes *et al.*, 2011).

The oral administration of particular probiotic strains to patients with atopic dermatitis can modulate the cytokine pattern *in vivo* at site other than the intestine. *L. casei* Shirota reduced serum concentrations of IL-5, IL-6, IFN-γ and specific IgE in subjects with allergic rhinitis (Ivory *et al.*, 2008) but was not found to be effective in reducing the symptoms of Japanese cedar pollen allergy (Tamura *et al.*, 2007). Probiotics can be involved in both antagonistic and synergistic relationships with each other, and with members of the gut ecosystem. Indeed, mixtures of bacteria induced a response in human dendritic cells different to those of the component bacteria in isolation: antagonistic immunosuppressive effects were observed with certain strains of *Lactobacillus* and *Bifidobacterium* but synergistic effects were observed when these *Lactobacillus* and *Bifidobacterium* strains were combined with *E. coli* and *K. pneumoniae* strains (Zeuthen *et al.*, 2006).

5. Conclusion

Despite some promising results, the role of probiotics in the treatment and the prevention of allergy and related diseases has not been clearly demonstrated. Indeed, clinical trials provide various contradictory findings that do not allow probiotic supplementation to be included in the guidelines for the management of allergic diseases. These conflicting data may be however attributable to the differences between studies. The populations studied have been very diverse in terms of size, age, sensitization and allergic disease, environment, and genetic background. Study designs included different probiotics in term of strains, preparations (alive/ killed; one strain/mixture/synbiotics), doses, duration of supplementation, and period of administration (prental/postnatal). In addition to these issues, progress in our basic knowledge of probiotic strains, in strain selection, and in understanding their mechanisms of action is needed to give credibility to the health claims made for probiotics and especially for the design of efficacious therapeutic agents.

6. References

Abrahamsson, T.R., Jakobsson, T., Bottcher, M.F., Fredrikson, M., Jenmalm, M.C., Bjorksten, B., and Oldaeus, G. (2007) Probiotics in prevention of IgE-associated eczema: a double-blind, randomized, placebo-controlled trial. *J Allergy Clin Immunol* 119: 1174-1180. ISSN: 0091-6749

Adkins, B., Leclerc, C., and Marshall-Clarke, S. (2004) Neonatal adaptive immunity comes of age. *Nat Rev Immunol* 4: 553-564. ISSN: 1474-1733

Adlerberth, I., Strachan, D.P., Matricardi, P.M., Ahrne, S., Orfei, L., Aberg, N. *et al.* (2007) Gut microbiota and development of atopic eczema in 3 European birth cohorts. *J Allergy Clin Immunol* 120: 343-350. ISSN: 0091-6749

Adlerberth, I., and Wold, A.E. (2009) Establishment of the gut microbiota in Western infants. *Acta Paediatr* 98: 229-238. ISSN: 0803-5253

Agosti, M., Vegni, C., Gangi, S., Benedetti, V., and Marini, A. (2003) Allergic manifestations in very low-birthweight infants: a 6-year follow-up. *Acta Paediatr Suppl* 91: 44-47. ISSN: 0803-5253

Akdis, M., Verhagen, J., Taylor, A., Karamloo, F., Karagiannidis, C., Crameri, R. *et al.* (2004) Immune responses in healthy and allergic individuals are characterized by a fine balance between allergen-specific T regulatory 1 and T helper 2 cells. *J Exp Med* 199: 1567-1575. : 0022-1007

Asher, M.I., Stewart, A.W., Mallol, J., Montefort, S., Lai, C.K., Ait-Khaled, N., and Odhiambo, J. (2010) Which population level environmental factors are associated with asthma, rhinoconjunctivitis and eczema? Review of the ecological analyses of ISAAC Phase One. *Respir Res* 11: 8. ISSN: 1465-9921

Bach, J.F. (2002) The effect of infections on susceptibility to autoimmune and allergic diseases. *N Engl J Med* 347: 911-920. ISSN: 0028-4793

Bergmann, R.L., Bergmann, K.E., and Wahn, U. (1998) Can we predict atopic disease using perinatal risk factors? *Clin Exp Allergy* 28: 905-907. ISSN: 0954-7894

Bik, E.M. (2009) Composition and function of the human-associated microbiota. *Nutr Rev* 67 Suppl 2: S164-S171. ISSN: 0029-6643

Bjorksten, B., Naaber, P., Sepp, E., and Mikelsaar, M. (1999) The intestinal microflora in allergic Estonian and Swedish 2-year-old children. *Clin Exp Allergy* 29: 342-346. ISSN: 0954-7894

Bjorksten, B., Sepp, E., Julge, K., Voor, T., and Mikelsaar, M. (2001) Allergy development and the intestinal microflora during the first year of life. *J Allergy Clin Immunol* 108: 516-520. ISSN: 0091-6749

Bottcher, M.F., Nordin, E.K., Sandin, A., Midtvedt, T., and Bjorksten, B. (2000) Microflora-associated characteristics in faeces from allergic and nonallergic infants. *Clin Exp Allergy* 30: 1590-1596. ISSN: 0954-7894

Brouwer, M.L., Wolt-Plompen, S.A., Dubois, A.E., van der, H.S., Jansen, D.F., Hoijer, M.A. *et al.* (2006) No effects of probiotics on atopic dermatitis in infancy: a randomized placebo-controlled trial. *Clin Exp Allergy* 36: 899-906. ISSN: 0954-7894

Campeotto, F., Waligora-Dupriet, A.J., Doucet-Populaire, F., Kalach, N., Dupont, C., and Butel, M.J. (2007) [Establishment of the intestinal microflora in neonates]. *Gastroenterol Clin Biol* 31: 533-542. ISSN: 0399-8320

Ciprandi, G., Vizzaccaro, A., Cirillo, I., and Tosca, M.A. (2005a) *Bacillus clausii* effects in children with allergic rhinitis. *Allergy* 60: 702-703. ISSN: 0105-4338

Ciprandi, G., Vizzaccaro, A., Cirillo, I., and Tosca, M.A. (2005b) *Bacillus clausii* exerts immuno-modulatory activity in allergic subjects: a pilot study. *Eur Ann Allergy Clin Immunol* 37: 129-134. ISSN: 1764-1384

Dethlefsen, L., McFall-Ngai, M., and Relman, D.A. (2007) An ecological and evolutionary perspective on human-microbe mutualism and disease. *Nature* 449: 811-818. ISSN: 0028-0836

Eckburg, P.B., Bik, E.M., Bernstein, C.N., Purdom, E., Dethlefsen, L., Sargent, M. *et al.* (2005) Diversity of the human intestinal microbial flora. *Science* 308: 1635-1638. ISSN: 0036-8075

FAO/WHO. Health and nutritional properties of probiotics in food includion powder milk with live lactic acid bacteria. 30 (suppl 2), S23-S33. 2001. Argentina. http://www.who.int/foodsafety/publications/fs_management/probiotics/en/index.html

FAO/WHO Working group. Guidelines for the evaluation of probiotics in food. 2002. London, 30 avril-1er mai. http://www.who.int/entity/foodsafety/publications/fs_management/probiotics 2/en/index.html

Feleszko, W., Jaworska, J., Rha, R.D., Steinhausen, S., Avagyan, A., Jaudszus, A. *et al.* (2007) Probiotic-induced suppression of allergic sensitization and airway inflammation is associated with an increase of T regulatory-dependent mechanisms in a murine model of asthma. *Clin Exp Allergy* 37: 498-505. ISSN: 0954-7894

Folster-Holst, R., Muller, F., Schnopp, N., Abeck, D., Kreiselmaier, I., Lenz, T. *et al.* (2006) Prospective, randomized controlled trial on *Lactobacillus rhamnosus* in infants with moderate to severe atopic dermatitis. *Br J Dermatol* 155: 1256-1261. ISSN: 0007-0963

Fujimura, K.E., Slusher, N.A., Cabana, M.D., and Lynch, S.V. (2010) Role of the gut microbiota in defining human health. *Expert Rev Anti Infect Ther* 8: 435-454. ISSN: 1478-7210

Gaboriau-Routhiau, V., Rakotobe, S., Lecuyer, E., Mulder, I., Lan, A., Bridonneau, C. *et al.* (2009) The key role of segmented filamentous bacteria in the coordinated maturation of gut helper T cell responses. *Immunity* 31: 677-689. ISSN:1074-7613

Garrett, W.S., Gordon, J.I., and Glimcher, L.H. (2010) Homeostasis and inflammation in the intestine. *Cell* 140: 859-870. ISSN: 0092-8674

Gerasimov, S.V., Vasjuta, V.V., Myhovych, O.O., and Bondarchuk, L.I. (2010) Probiotic supplement reduces atopic dermatitis in preschool children: a randomized, double-blind, placebo-controlled, clinical trial. *Am J Clin Dermatol* 11: 351-361. ISSN: 1175-0561

Giovannini, M., Agostoni, C., Riva, E., Salvini, F., Ruscitto, A., Zuccotti, G.V., and Radaelli, G. (2007) A randomized prospective double blind controlled trial on effects of long-term consumption of fermented milk containing Lactobacillus casei in pre-school children with allergic asthma and/or rhinitis. *Pediatr Res* 62: 215-220. ISSN: 0031-3998

Gore, C., Munro, K., Lay, C., Bibiloni, R., Morris, J., Woodcock, A. *et al.* (2008) *Bifidobacterium pseudocatenulatum* is associated with atopic eczema: A nested case-control study investigating the fecal microbiota of infants. *J Allerg Clin Immunol* 121: 135-140. ISSN 0091-6749

Gruber, C., Wendt, M., Sulser, C., Lau, S., Kulig, M., Wahn, U. *et al.* (2007) Randomized, placebo-controlled trial of *Lactobacillus rhamnosus GG* as treatment of atopic dermatitis in infancy. *Allergy* 62: 1270-1276. ISSN 0105-4338

Gueimonde, M., Laitinen, K., Salminen, S., and Isolauri, E. (2007) Breast milk: a source of bifidobacteria for infant gut development and maturation? *Neonatology* 92: 64-66. ISSN: 1661-7800

He, F., Morita, H., Ouwehand, A.C., Hosoda, M., Hiramatsu, M., Kurisaki, J. *et al.* (2002) Stimulation of the secretion of pro-inflammatory cytokines by *Bifidobacterium* strains. *Microbiol Immunol* 46: 781-785. ISSN: 0385-5600

He, F., Ouwehand, A.C., Isolauri, E., Hashimoto, H., Benno, Y., and Salminen, S. (2001) Comparison of mucosal adhesion and species identification of bifidobacteria isolated from healthy and allergic infants. *FEMS Immunol Med Microbiol* 30: 43-47. ISSN: 0928-8244

Helin, T., Haahtela, S., and Haahtela, T. (2002) No effect of oral treatment with an intestinal bacterial strain, *Lactobacillus rhamnosus* (ATCC 53103), on birch-pollen allergy: a placebo-controlled double-blind study. *Allergy* 57: 243-246. ISSN 0105-4338

Hooper, L.V., and Macpherson, A.J. (2010) Immune adaptations that maintain homeostasis with the intestinal microbiota. *Nat Rev Immunol* 10: 159-169. ISSN: 1474-1733

Ishida, Y., Nakamura, F., Kanzato, H., Sawada, D., Yamamoto, N., Kagata, H. *et al.* (2005) Effect of milk fermented with *Lactobacillus acidophilus* strain L-92 on symptoms of Japanese cedar pollen allergy: a randomized placebo-controlled trial. *Biosci Biotechnol Biochem* 69: 1652-1660. ISSN: 0916-8451

Isolauri, E., Arvola, T., Sutas, Y., Moilanen, E., and Salminen, S. (2000) Probiotics in the management of atopic eczema. *Clin Exp Allergy* 30: 1604-1610. ISSN 0954-7894

Ivory, K., Chambers, S.J., Pin, C., Prieto, E., Arques, J.L., and Nicoletti, C. (2008) Oral delivery of *Lactobacillus casei* Shirota modifies allergen-induced immune responses in allergic rhinitis. *Clin Exp Allergy* 38: 1282-1289. ISSN 0954-7894

Kalliomaki, M., Kirjavainen, P., Eerola, E., Kero, P., Salminen, S., and Isolauri, E. (2001a) Distinct patterns of neonatal gut microflora in infants in whom atopy was and was not developing. *J Allergy Clin Immunol* 107: 129-134. ISSN 0091-6749

Kalliomaki, M., Salminen, S., Arvilommi, H., Kero, P., Koskinen, P., and Isolauri, E. (2001b) Probiotics in primary prevention of atopic disease: a randomised placebo-controlled trial. *Lancet* 357: 1076-1079. ISSN: 0140-6736

Kalliomaki, M., Salminen, S., Poussa, T., Arvilommi, H., and Isolauri, E. (2003) Probiotics and prevention of atopic disease: 4-year follow-up of a randomised placebo-controlled trial. *Lancet* 361: 1869-1871. ISSN: 0140-6736

Kalliomaki, M., Salminen, S., Poussa, T., and Isolauri, E. (2007) Probiotics during the first 7 years of life: a cumulative risk reduction of eczema in a randomized, placebo-controlled trial. *J Allergy Clin Immunol* 119: 1019-1021. ISSN 0091-6749

Karlsson, H., Larsson, P., Wold, A.E., and Rudin, A. (2004) Pattern of cytokine responses to gram-positive and gram-negative commensal bacteria is profoundly changed when monocytes differentiate into dendritic cells. *Infect Immun* 72: 2671-2678. ISSN: 0019-9567

Kawase, M., He, F., Kubota, A., Hiramatsu, M., Saito, H., Ishii, T. *et al.* (2009) Effect of fermented milk prepared with two probiotic strains on Japanese cedar pollinosis in a double-blind placebo-controlled clinical study. *Int J Food Microbiol* 128: 429-434. ISSN: 0168-1605

Kendler, M., Uter, W., Rueffer, A., Shimshoni, R., and Jecht, E. (2006) Comparison of fecal microflora in children with atopic eczema/dermatitis syndrome according to IgE sensitization to food. *Pediatr Allergy Immunol* 17: 141-147. ISSN: 0905-6157

Kero, J., Gissler, M., Gronlund, M.M., Kero, P., Koskinen, P., Hemminki, E., and Isolauri, E. (2002) Mode of delivery and asthma -- is there a connection? *Pediatr Res* 52: 6-11. ISSN: 0031-3998

Kirjavainen, P.V., Apostolou, E., Arvola, T., Salminen, S.J., Gibson, G.R., and Isolauri, E. (2001) Characterizing the composition of intestinal microflora as a prospective treatment target in infant allergic disease. *FEMS Immunol Med Microbiol* 32: 1-7. ISSN: 0928-8244

Kirjavainen, P.V., Arvola, T., Salminen, S.J., and Isolauri, E. (2002) Aberrant composition of gut microbiota of allergic infants: a target of bifidobacterial therapy at weaning? *Gut* 51: 51-55. ISSN: 0017-5749

Kirjavainen, P.V., Salminen, S.J., and Isolauri, E. (2003) Probiotic bacteria in the management of atopic disease: underscoring the importance of viability. *J Pediatr Gastroenterol Nutr* 36: 223-227. ISSN: 0277-2126

Kopp, M.V., Hennemuth, I., Heinzmann, A., and Urbanek, R. (2008) Randomized, double-blind, placebo-controlled trial of probiotics for primary prevention: no clinical effects of *Lactobacillus* GG supplementation. *Pediatrics* 121: e850-e856. ISSN: 0031-4005

Laubereau, B., Filipiak-Pittroff, B., von, B.A., Grubl, A., Reinhardt, D., Wichmann, H.E., and Koletzko, S. (2004) Caesarean section and gastrointestinal symptoms, atopic dermatitis, and sensitisation during the first year of life. *Arch Dis Child* 89: 993-997. ISSN: 0003-9888

Lee, J., Seto, D., and Bielory, L. (2008) Meta-analysis of clinical trials of probiotics for prevention and treatment of pediatric atopic dermatitis. *J Allergy Clin Immunol* 121: 116-121. ISSN 0091-6749

Lyons, A., O'Mahony, D., O'Brien, F., MacSharry, J., Sheil, B., Ceddia, M. *et al.* (2010) Bacterial strain-specific induction of Foxp3+ T regulatory cells is protective in murine allergy models. *Clin Exp Allergy* 40: 811-819. ISSN 0954-7894

Mah, K.W., Bjorksten, B., Lee, B.W., Van Bever, H.P., Shek, L.P., Tan, T.N. *et al.* (2006) Distinct pattern of commensal gut microbiota in toddlers with eczema. *Int Arch Allergy Immunol* 140: 157-163. ISSN: 1018-2438

Mannino, D.M., Homa, D.M., Pertowski, C.A., Ashizawa, A., Nixon, L.L., Johnson, C.A. *et al.* (1998) Surveillance for asthma--United States, 1960-1995. *MMWR CDC Surveill Summ* 47: 1-27. ISSN: 0892-3787

Manson, J.M., Rauch, M., and Gilmore, M.S. (2008) The commensal microbiology of the gastrointestinal tract. *Adv Exp Med Biol* 635: 15-28. ISSN: 0065-2598

Martin, R., Jimenez, E., Heilig, H., Fernandez, L., Marin, M.L., Zoetendal, E.G., and Rodriguez, J.M. (2009) Isolation of bifidobacteria from breast milk and assessment of the bifidobacterial population by PCR-denaturing gradient gel electrophoresis and quantitative real-time PCR. *Appl Environ Microbiol* 75: 965-969.ISSN: 0099-2240

Matto, J., Malinen, E., Suihko, M.L., Alander, M., Palva, A., and Saarela, M. (2004) Genetic heterogeneity and functional properties of intestinal bifidobacteria. *J Appl Microbiol* 97: 459-470. ISSN: 1364-5072

Mazmanian, S.K., Liu, C.H., Tzianabos, A.O., and Kasper, D.L. (2005) An immunomodulatory molecule of symbiotic bacteria directs maturation of the host immune system. *Cell* 122: 107-118. ISSN: 0092-8674

McKeever, T.M., Lewis, S.A., Smith, C., and Hubbard, R. (2002) The importance of prenatal exposures on the development of allergic disease: a birth cohort study using the West Midlands General Practice Database. *Am J Respir Crit Care Med* 166: 827-832. ISSN: 1073-449X

Medina, M., Izquierdo, E., Ennahar, S., and Sanz, Y. (2007) Differential immunomodulatory properties of *Bifidobacterium longum* strains: relevance to probiotic selection and clinical applications. *Clin Exp Immunol* 150: 531-538. ISSN: 0009-9104

Menard, O., Butel, M.J., Gaboriau-Routhiau, V., and Waligora-Dupriet, A.J. (2008) Gnotobiotic mouse immune response induced by *Bifidobacterium* sp. strains isolated from infants. *Appl Environ Microbiol* 74: 660-666. ISSN: 0099-2240

Murray, C.S., Tannock, G.W., Simon, M.A., Harmsen, H.J., Welling, G.W., Custovic, A., and Woodcock, A. (2005) Fecal microbiota in sensitized wheezy and non-sensitized non-wheezy children: a nested case-control study. *Clin Exp Allergy* 35: 741-745. ISSN 0954-7894

Nermes, M., Kantele, J.M., Atosuo, T.J., Salminen, S., and Isolauri, E. (2011) Interaction of orally administered *Lactobacillus rhamnosus* GG with skin and gut microbiota and humoral immunity in infants with atopic dermatitis. *Clin Exp Allergy* 41: 370-377. ISSN 0954-7894

Odamaki, T., Xiao, J.Z., Iwabuchi, N., Sakamoto, M., Takahashi, N., Kondo, S. *et al.* (2007) Fluctuation of fecal microbiota in individuals with Japanese cedar pollinosis during the pollen season and influence of probiotic intake. *J Investig Allergol Clin Immunol* 17: 92-100. ISSN: 1018-9068

Okada, H., Kuhn, C., Feillet, H., and Bach, J.F. (2010) The 'hygiene hypothesis' for autoimmune and allergic diseases: an update. *Clin Exp Immunol* 160: 1-9. ISSN: 0009-9104

Osborn, D.A., and Sinn, J.K. (2007) Probiotics in infants for prevention of allergic disease and food hypersensitivity. *Cochrane Database Syst Rev*: CD006475. ISSN: 1469-493X

Ouwehand, A.C., Isolauri, E., He, F., Hashimoto, H., Benno, Y., and Salminen, S. (2001) Differences in *Bifidobacterium* flora composition in allergic and healthy infants. *J Allergy Clin Immunol* 108: 144-145. ISSN 0091-6749

Ouwehand, A.C., Nermes, M., Collado, M.C., Rautonen, N., Salminen, S., and Isolauri, E. (2009) Specific probiotics alleviate allergic rhinitis during the birch pollen season. *World J Gastroenterol* 15: 3261-3268. ISSN: 1007-9327

Palmer, C., Bik, E.M., DiGiulio, D.B., Relman, D.A., and Brown, P.O. (2007) Development of the human infant intestinal microbiota. *PLoS Biol* 5: e177. ISSN: 1544-9173

Penders, J., Stobberingh, E.E., Thijs, C., Adams, H., Vink, C., van, R.R., and van den Brandt, P.A. (2006a) Molecular fingerprinting of the intestinal microbiota of infants in whom atopic eczema was or was not developing. *Clin Exp Allergy* 36: 1602-1608. ISSN 0954-7894

Penders, J., Thijs, C., Vink, C., Stelma, F.F., Snijders, B., Kummeling, I. *et al.* (2006b) Factors influencing the composition of the intestinal microbiota in early infancy. *Pediatrics* 118: 511-521. ISSN: 0031-4005

Penders, J., Thijs, C., van den Brandt, P.A., Kummeling, I., Snijders, B., Stelma, F. *et al.* (2007) Gut microbiota composition and development of atopic manifestations in infancy: the KOALA Birth Cohort Study. *Gut* 56: 661-667. ISSN: 0017-5749

Peng, G.C., and Hsu, C.H. (2005) The efficacy and safety of heat-killed *Lactobacillus paracasei* for treatment of perennial allergic rhinitis induced by house-dust mite. *Pediatr Allergy Immunol* 16: 433-438. ISSN: 0905-6157

Pohjavuori, E., Viljanen, M., Korpela, R., Kuitunen, M., Tiittanen, M., Vaarala, O., and Savilahti, E. (2004) *Lactobacillus* GG effect in increasing IFN-gamma production in infants with cow's milk allergy. *J Allergy Clin Immunol* 114: 131-136. ISSN 0091-6749

Protonotariou, E., Malamitsi-Puchner, A., Rizos, D., Papagianni, B., Moira, E., Sarandakou, A., and Botsis, D. (2004) Age-related differentiations of Th1/Th2 cytokines in newborn infants. *Mediators Inflamm* 13: 89-92. ISSN: 0962-9351

Rajilic-Stojanovic, M., Heilig, H.G., Molenaar, D., Kajander, K., Surakka, A., Smidt, H., and De Vos, W.M. (2009) Development and application of the human intestinal tract chip, a phylogenetic microarray: analysis of universally conserved phylotypes in the abundant microbiota of young and elderly adults. *Environ Microbiol* 11: 1736-1751. ISSN:1462-2912

Rajilic-Stojanovic, M., Smidt, H., and De Vos, W.M. (2007) Diversity of the human gastrointestinal tract microbiota revisited. *Environ Microbiol* 9: 2125-2136. ISSN:1462-2912

Rautava, S., Kalliomaki, M., and Isolauri, E. (2002a) Probiotics during pregnancy and breast-feeding might confer immunomodulatory protection against atopic disease in the infant. *J Allergy Clin Immunol* 109: 119-121. ISSN 0091-6749

Rautava, S., Kalliomaki, M., and Isolauri, E. (2002b) Probiotics during pregnancy and breast-feeding might confer immunomodulatory protection against atopic disease in the infant. *J Allergy Clin Immunol* 109: 119-121. ISSN 0091-6749

Rautava, S., Ruuskanen, O., Ouwehand, A., Salminen, S., and Isolauri, E. (2004) The hygiene hypothesis of atopic disease--an extended version. *J Pediatr Gastroenterol Nutr* 38: 378-388. ISSN: 0277-2126

Rodriguez, B., Prioult, G., Bibiloni, R., Nicolis, I., Mercenier, A., Butel, M.J., and Waligora-Dupriet, A.J. (2011) Germ-free status and altered caecal subdominant microbiota are associated with a high susceptibility to cow's milk allergy in mice. *FEMS Microbiol Ecol* 76: 133-144. ISSN: 0168-6496

Roguedas-Contios, A.M., and Misery, L. (2011) What is Intrinsic Atopic Dermatitis? *Clin Rev Allergy Immunol.* ISSN: 1080-0549

Rose, M.A., Stieglitz, F., Koksal, A., Schubert, R., Schulze, J., and Zielen, S. (2010) Efficacy of probiotic *Lactobacillus* GG on allergic sensitization and asthma in infants at risk. *Clin Exp Allergy* 40: 1398-1405. ISSN 0954-7894

Rosenfeldt, V., Benfeldt, E., Nielsen, S.D., Michaelsen, K.F., Jeppesen, D.L., Valerius, N.H., and Paerregaard, A. (2003) Effect of probiotic *Lactobacillus* strains in children with atopic dermatitis. *J Allergy Clin Immunol* 111: 389-395. ISSN 0091-6749

Rosenfeldt, V., Benfeldt, E., Valerius, N.H., Paerregaard, A., and Michaelsen, K.F. (2004) Effect of probiotics on gastrointestinal symptoms and small intestinal permeability in children with atopic dermatitis. *J Pediatr* 145: 612-616. ISSN: 0022-3476

Round, J.L., O'Connell, R.M., and Mazmanian, S.K. (2010) Coordination of tolerogenic immune responses by the commensal microbiota. *J Autoimmun* 34: J220-J225. ISSN: 0896-8411

Sepp, E., Julge, K., Mikelsaar, M., and Bjorksten, B. (2005) Intestinal microbiota and immunoglobulin E responses in 5-year-old Estonian children. *Clin Exp Allergy* 35: 1141-1146. ISSN 0954-7894

Sepp, E., Julge, K., Vasar, M., Naaber, P., Bjorksten, B., and Mikelsaar, M. (1997) Intestinal microflora of estonian and swedish infants. *Acta Paediat* 86: 956-961. ISSN: 0803-5253

Shull, M.M., Ormsby, I., Kier, A.B., Pawlowski, S., Diebold, R.J., Yin, M. *et al.* (1992) Targeted disruption of the mouse transforming growth factor-beta 1 gene results in multifocal inflammatory disease. *Nature* 359: 693-699. ISSN: 0028-0836

Sistek, D., Kelly, R., Wickens, K., Stanley, T., Fitzharris, P., and Crane, J. (2006) Is the effect of probiotics on atopic dermatitis confined to food sensitized children? *Clin Exp Allergy* 36: 629-633. ISSN 0954-7894

Sjogren, Y.M., Jenmalm, M.C., Bottcher, M.F., Bjorksten, B., and Sverremark-Ekstrom, E. (2009) Altered early infant gut microbiota in children developing allergy up to 5 years of age. *Clin Exp Allergy* 39: 518-526. ISSN 0954-7894

Smith, K., McCoy, K.D., and Macpherson, A.J. (2007) Use of axenic animals in studying the adaptation of mammals to their commensal intestinal microbiota. *Semin Immunol* 19: 59-69. ISSN: 1044-5323

Société Française de Dermatologie (2005) Conférence de consensus "Prise en charge de la dermatite atopique de l'enfant". *Ann Dermatol Venereol* 132: 1S19-1S33. ISSN: 0151-9638

Soh, S.E., Aw, M., Gerez, I., Chong, Y.S., Rauff, M., Ng, Y.P. *et al.* (2009) Probiotic supplementation in the first 6 months of life in at risk Asian infants--effects on eczema and atopic sensitization at the age of 1 year. *Clin Exp Allergy* 39: 571-578. ISSN 0954-7894

Songjinda, P., Nakayama, J., Tateyama, A., Tanaka, S., Tsubouchi, M., Kiyohara, C. *et al.* (2007) Differences in developing intestinal microbiota between allergic and non-allergic infants: a pilot study in Japan. *Biosci Biotechnol Biochem* 71: 2338-2342. ISSN: 0916-8451

Stackebrandt, E., Kramer, I., Swiderski, J., and Hippe, H. (1999) Phylogenetic basis for a taxonomic dissection of the genus *Clostridium. FEMS Immunol Med Microbiol* 24: 253-258. ISSN: 0928-8244

Stecher, B., and Hardt, W.D. (2008) The role of microbiota in infectious disease. *Trends Microbiol* 16: 107-114. ISSN: 0966-842X

Strachan, D.P. (1989) Hay fever, hygiene, and household size. *BMJ* 299: 1259-1260. ISSN: 0959-8138

Stsepetova, J., Sepp, E., Julge, K., Vaughan, E., Mikelsaar, M., and De Vos, W.M. (2007) Molecularly assessed shifts of *Bifidobacterium* ssp. and less diverse microbial communities are characteristic of 5-year-old allergic children. *FEMS Immunol Med Microbiol* 51: 260-269. ISSN: 0928-8244

Sudo, N., Sawamura, S., Tanaka, K., Aiba, Y., Kubo, C., and Koga, Y. (1997) The requirement of intestinal bacterial flora for the development of an IgE production system fully susceptible to oral tolerance induction. *J Immunol* 159: 1739-1745. ISSN: 0022-1767

Tamura, M., Shikina, T., Morihana, T., Hayama, M., Kajimoto, O., Sakamoto, A. *et al.* (2007) Effects of probiotics on allergic rhinitis induced by Japanese cedar pollen: randomized double-blind, placebo-controlled clinical trial. *Int Arch Allergy Immunol* 143: 75-82. ISSN: 1018-2438

Tap, J., Mondot, S., Levenez, F., Pelletier, E., Caron, C., Furet, J.P. *et al.* (2009) Towards the human intestinal microbiota phylogenetic core. *Environ Microbiol* 11: 2574-2584. ISSN: 1462-2912

Taylor, A., Hale, J., Wiltschut, J., Lehmann, H., Dunstan, J.A., and Prescott, S.L. (2006a) Evaluation of the effects of probiotic supplementation from the neonatal period on innate immune development in infancy. *Clin Exp Allergy* 36: 1218-1226. ISSN 0954-7894

Taylor, A.L., Dunstan, J.A., and Prescott, S.L. (2007a) Probiotic supplementation for the first 6 months of life fails to reduce the risk of atopic dermatitis and increases the risk of allergen sensitization in high-risk children: a randomized controlled trial. *J Allergy Clin Immunol* 119: 184-191. ISSN 0091-6749

Taylor, A.L., Hale, J., Hales, B.J., Dunstan, J.A., Thomas, W.R., and Prescott, S.L. (2007b) FOXP3 mRNA expression at 6 months of age is higher in infants who develop atopic dermatitis, but is not affected by giving probiotics from birth. *Pediatr Allergy Immunol* 18: 10-19. ISSN: 0905-6157

Taylor, A.L., Hale, J., Wiltschut, J., Lehmann, H., Dunstan, J.A., and Prescott, S.L. (2006b) Effects of probiotic supplementation for the first 6 months of life on allergen- and vaccine-specific immune responses. *Clin Exp Allergy* 36: 1227-1235. ISSN 0954-7894

Vael, C., and Desager, K. (2009) The importance of the development of the intestinal microbiota in infancy. *Curr Opin Pediatr* 21: 794-800. ISSN: 1040-8703

Vael, C., Nelen, V., Verhulst, S.L., Goossens, H., and Desager, K.N. (2008) Early intestinal Bacteroides fragilis colonisation and development of asthma. *BMC Pulm Med* 8: 19. ISSN: 1471-2466

Vael, C., Vanheirstraeten, L., Desager, K.N., and Goossens, H. (2011) Denaturing gradient gel electrophoresis of neonatal intestinal microbiota in relation to the development of asthma. *BMC Microbiol* 11: 68. ISSN: 1471-2180

Vaishampayan, P.A., Kuehl, J.V., Froula, J.L., Morgan, J.L., Ochman, H., and Francino, M.P. (2010) Comparative metagenomics and population dynamics of the gut microbiota in mother and infant. *Genome Biol Evol* 2: 53-66. ISSN: 1759-6653

van der Aa, L.B., Heymans, H.S., van Aalderen, W.M., Sillevis Smitt, J.H., Knol, J., Ben, A.K. *et al.* (2010) Effect of a new synbiotic mixture on atopic dermatitis in infants: a randomized-controlled trial. *Clin Exp Allergy* 40: 795-804. ISSN 0954-7894

van der Aa, L.B., van Aalderen, W.M., Heymans, H.S., Henk Sillevis, S.J., Nauta, A.J., Knippels, L.M. *et al.* (2011) Synbiotics prevent asthma-like symptoms in infants with atopic dermatitis. *Allergy* 66: 170-177. ISSN 0105-4338

Ventura, M., van, S.D., Fitzgerald, G.F., and Zink, R. (2004) Insights into the taxonomy, genetics and physiology of bifidobacteria. *Antonie van Leeuwenhoek* 86: 205-223. ISSN: 0003-6072

Verhulst, S.L., Vael, C., Beunckens, C., Nelen, V., Goossens, H., and Desager, K. (2008) A longitudinal analysis on the association between antibiotic use, intestinal microflora, and wheezing during the first year of life. *J Asthma* 45: 828-832. ISSN: 0277-0903

Viljanen, M., Kuitunen, M., Haahtela, T., Juntunen-Backman, K., Korpela, R., and Savilahti, E. (2005a) Probiotic effects on faecal inflammatory markers and on faecal IgA in food allergic atopic eczema/dermatitis syndrome infants. *Pediatr Allergy Immunol* 16: 65-71. ISSN: 0905-6157

Viljanen, M., Savilahti, E., Haahtela, T., Juntunen-Backman, K., Korpela, R., Poussa, T. *et al.* (2005b) Probiotics in the treatment of atopic eczema/dermatitis syndrome in infants: a double-blind placebo-controlled trial. *Allergy* 60: 494-500. ISSN 0105-4338

Waligora-Dupriet, A.J., Campeotto, F., Romero, K., Mangin, I., Rouzaud, G., Menard, O. *et al.* (2011) Diversity of gut *Bifidobacterium* species is not altered between allergic and non-allergic French infants. *Anaerobe.* ISSN: 1075-9964

Wang, M., Karlsson, C., Olsson, C., Adlerberth, I., Wold, A.E., Strachan, D.P. *et al.* (2008) Reduced diversity in the early fecal microbiota of infants with atopic eczema. *J Allergy Clin Immunol* 121: 129-134. ISSN 0091-6749

Wang, M.F., Lin, H.C., Wang, Y.Y., and Hsu, C.H. (2004) Treatment of perennial allergic rhinitis with lactic acid bacteria. *Pediatr Allergy Immunol* 15: 152-158. ISSN: 0905-6157

Watanabe, S., Narisawa, Y., Arase, S., Okamatsu, H., Ikenaga, T., Tajiri, Y., and Kumemura, M. (2003) Differences in fecal microflora between patients with atopic dermatitis and healthy control subjects. *J Allergy Clin Immunol* 111: 587-591. ISSN 0091-6749

Weston, S., Halbert, A., Richmond, P., and Prescott, S.L. (2005) Effects of probiotics on atopic dermatitis: a randomised controlled trial. *Arch Dis Child* 90: 892-897. ISSN: 0003-9888

Wickens, K., Black, P.N., Stanley, T.V., Mitchell, E., Fitzharris, P., Tannock, G.W. *et al.* (2008) A differential effect of 2 probiotics in the prevention of eczema and atopy: a double-blind, randomized, placebo-controlled trial. *J Allergy Clin Immunol* 122: 788-794. ISSN 0091-6749

Williams, N.T. (2010) Probiotics. *Am J Health Syst Pharm* 67: 449-458. ISSN: 1079-2082

Wong, J.M., de, S.R., Kendall, C.W., Emam, A., and Jenkins, D.J. (2006) Colonic health: fermentation and short chain fatty acids. *J Clin Gastroenterol* 40: 235-243. ISSN: 0192-0790

Woo, S.I., Kim, J.Y., Lee, Y.J., Kim, N.S., and Hahn, Y.S. (2010) Effect of *Lactobacillus sakei* supplementation in children with atopic eczema-dermatitis syndrome. *Ann Allergy Asthma Immunol* 104: 343-348. ISSN: 1081-1206

Woodcock, A., Moradi, M., Smillie, F.I., Murray, C.S., Burnie, J.P., and Custovic, A. (2002) *Clostridium difficile*, atopy and wheeze during the first year of life. *Pediatr Allergy Immunol* 13: 357-360. ISSN: 0905-6157

Xiao, J.Z., Kondo, S., Yanagisawa, N., Miyaji, K., Enomoto, K., Sakoda, T. *et al.* (2007) Clinical efficacy of probiotic *Bifidobacterium longum* for the treatment of symptoms of Japanese cedar pollen allergy in subjects evaluated in an environmental exposure unit. *Allergol Int* 56: 67-75. ISSN: 1323-8930

Young, S.L., Simon, M.A., Baird, M.A., Tannock, G.W., Bibiloni, R., Spencely, K. *et al.* (2004) Bifidobacterial species differentially affect expression of cell surface markers and cytokines of dendritic cells harvested from cord blood. *Clin Diagn Lab Immunol* 11: 686-690. ISSN: 1071-412X

Zeuthen, L.H., Christensen, H.R., and Frokiaer, H. (2006) Lactic acid bacteria inducing a weak interleukin-12 and tumor necrosis factor alpha response in human dendritic cells inhibit strongly stimulating lactic acid bacteria but act synergistically with gram-negative bacteria. *Clin Vaccine Immunol* 13: 365-375. ISSN: 1556-6811

Zoetendal, E.G., Rajilic-Stojanovic, M., and De Vos, W.M. (2008) High-throughput diversity and functionality analysis of the gastrointestinal tract microbiota. *Gut* 57: 1605-1615. ISSN: 0017-5749

β_2-Adrenoceptor Agonists and Allergic Disease: The Enhancing Effect of β_2-Adrenoceptor Agonists on Cytokine-Induced TSLP Production by Human Lung Tissue Cells

Akio Matsuda and Kyoko Futamura
Department of Allergy and Immunology,
National Research Institute for Child Health and Development, Tokyo,
Japan

1. Introduction

1.1 β_2-adrenoceptor agonists and asthma

The adrenergic receptors (adrenoceptors) are a member of the G protein-coupled receptor superfamily of membrane proteins that are targets of the catecholamines, norepinephrine and epinephrine. To date, two main groups of adrenoceptors, α and β, with several subtypes have been identified. Many types of cells possess these receptors, and the binding of an agonist will generally cause a sympathetic response. Among them, β2-adrenoceptor agonists (β2-agonists) are widely used as bronchodilators in the treatment of bronchial asthma because of their potent bronchodilating effects on airway smooth muscle. In addition to being bronchodilators, they may also have anti-inflammatory properties, including inhibition of granulocyte functions (Yasui et.al., 2006). However, concerns have been raised regarding the use of β2-agonists on a regular daily basis rather than only as needed for rescue therapy. More specifically, continuous and repetitive β_2-agonist monotherapy has been considered to be associated with an increase in the degree of allergic inflammation (Cockcroft et.al., 1995), poor asthma outcomes (Paris et.al., 2008) and an increase in the risk of asthma death (Crane et.al., 1989; Nelson et.al., 2006). Although the precise molecular mechanisms underlying these undesirable effects of β_2-agonists are not fully understood, several studies have independently demonstrated that β_2-agonists have the potential to increase Th2 cytokine-mediated inflammation both *in vivo* and *in vitro*. For instance, Coqueret et.al. demonstrated that ovalbumin-sensitized mice treated with a daily injection of salbutamol showed increased anti-ovalbumin IgE levels in their serum, probably due to increased production of Th2 cytokines (Coqueret et.al., 1994). Panina-Bordignon et.al. demonstrated that β_2-agonists prevented Th1 development by selectively inhibiting IL-12 production (Panina-Bordignon et.al., 1997). More recently, Loza et.al. demonstrated that human Th2 cells express β_2-adrenergic receptor and that β_2-agonists augmented the accumulation of Th2 cells in human peripheral blood lymphocyte cultures subjected to bystander stimuli (Loza et.al., 2007). These findings suggest a mechanism by which β_2-agonist monotherapy may favor Th2 immune responses, which are believed to be involved in the pathogenesis of asthma.

1.2 TSLP and asthma

Thymic stromal lymphopoietin (TSLP) is an IL-7-like cytokine which was originally identified in the supernatant of a murine thymic stromal cell line (Friend et.al., 1994). Increasing evidence suggests that TSLP plays important roles in the pathogenesis of allergic diseases such as asthma and atopic dermatitis (Al-Shami te.al., 2005; Yoo et.al., 2005). The most clinically relevant role of TSLP is mediated by dendritic cells (DCs) through induction of OX40 ligand expression on DCs (Ito et.al., 2005; Liu, 2007a). Naïve T cells receiving antigen-presentation from TSLP-primed DCs develop into Th2 cells that produce IL-4, -5, -13 and TNF-α but not IL-10 (Ito et.al., 2005; Liu, 2007a; Soumelis et.al., 2002). These Th2 cells are now referred as to "inflammatory Th2 cells" in consideration of their potential for releasing the proinflammatory cytokine, TNF-α, in addition to Th2 cytokines (Orihara et.al.; 2008). Furthermore, mice with transgenic overexpression of TSLP in the lung develop severe airway inflammation, including massive infiltration by inflammatory cells, goblet cell hyperplasia and airway hyperresponsiveness (Zhou et.al., 2005). Mice with transgenic overexpression of TSLP in skin keratinocytes develop severe dermatitis with itching, which is similar to the clinical features of atopic dermatitis in humans (Yoo et.al., 2005). On the other hand, mice lacking the TSLP receptor exhibit strong Th1 responses and fail to develop an inflammatory lung response to antigens (Al-Shami te.al., 2005). Thus, TSLP is an important cytokine that is necessary and sufficient for initiation of allergic inflammation.

2. The enhancing effect of β_2-adrenoceptor agonists on cytokine-induced TSLP production by human lung tissue cells

2.1 Cytokine-induced production of TSLP by lung tissue cells

It is widely accepted that TSLP is expressed predominantly in epithelial cells of the lung, intestine and skin keratinocytes (Soumelis et.al., 2002; Liu et.al., 2007b). We confirmed an earlier report (kato et.al., 2007) that a combination of IL-4 and TNF-α synergistically induced TSLP production by normal human bronchial epithelial cells (NHBE) (Fig. 1A). Unlike NHBE, lung mesenchymal cells such as bronchial smooth muscle cells (BSMC) and normal human lung fibroblasts (NHLF) produced TSLP in response to TNF-α, but not IL-4 alone. However, like NHBE, those cells produced greater amounts of TSLP as a result of synergistic effects between IL-4 and TNF-α (Fig. 1B and 1C). Of note, these mesenchymal cells produce appreciable amounts of TSLP compared to NHBE, suggesting the possibility that lung mesenchymal cells are, like epithelial cells, important cellular sources of TSLP.

2.2 Effects of β_2-agonists on cytokine-induced TSLP production

We next examined the effects of β_2-agonists on the cytokine-induced TSLP production by the human lung tissue cells. Although β_2-agonists act mainly on airway smooth muscle as bronchodilators, they are also known to express anti-inflammatory effects on granulocytes (Yasui et.al., 2006), epithelial cells (Koyama et.al., 1999) and fibroblasts (Spoelstra et.al., 2002). As shown in Fig 2A, when NHBE were stimulated with a combination of IL-4 and TNF-α, simultaneous addition of various concentrations of two long-acting β_2-agonists, i.e., salmeterol and formoterol, and a short-acting β_2-agonist, salbutamol, showed significant enhancement of the cytokine-induced TSLP production. Optimal concentrations of these β_2-agonists were employed, and then the mRNA expression of TSLP in NHBE was measured by quantitative real-time PCR. TSLP mRNA expression was significantly enhanced by 10^{-10} M salmeterol, 10^{-10}

β₂-Adrenoceptor Agonists and Allergic Disease: The Enhancing Effect of β₂-Adrenoceptor
Agonists on Cytokine-Induced TSLP Production by Human Lung Tissue Cells

89

M formoterol and 10^{-8} M salbutamol (Fig. 2B), suggesting that the enhancing effects of β₂-agonists on TSLP production were transcriptionally-regulated. It should be noted that β₂-agonists enhanced TSLP production by airway smooth muscle cells and lung fibroblasts as well as bronchial epithelial cells (Fig. 2C and 2D). We suppose that the production of TSLP by these lung tissue cells is particularly important because dendritic cells have to migrate through these airway interstitial cells to lymphopoietic tissues in order to present antigen information to naïve T cells. Therefore, enhanced TSLP production by lung tissue cells in response to β₂-agonists may lead to exacerbation of allergic airway inflammation, and this may partly explain the undesirable clinical effects of continuous β₂-agonist monotherapy.

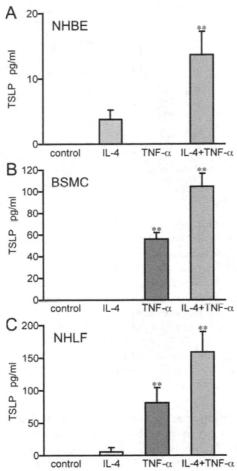

Fig. 1. Cytokines induce production of TSLP by lung tissue cells. NHBE (**A**), BSMC (**B**) and NHLF (**C**) were treated with 10 ng/ml IL-4 alone, 10 ng/ml TNF-α alone and a combination of both for 48 h. TSLP concentrations in the culture supernatants were quantified by ELISA. Data are shown as the mean ± SD of quadruplicate samples and are representative of at least three separate experiments. ** $p < .01$ compared with unstimulated control. Reprinted from Futamura et. Al., 2010.

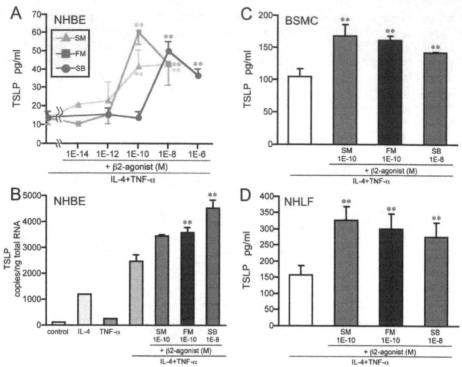

Fig. 2. β_2-agonists enhance cytokine-induced TSLP production by lung tissue cells. (**A**) NHBE were treated with different concentrations of two long-acting β_2-agonists, salmeterol (SM) and formoterol (FM), or a short-acting β_2-agonist, salbutamol (SB), in the presence of 10 ng/ml IL-4 and 10 ng/ml TNF-α for 48 h. TSLP concentrations in the culture supernatants were quantified by ELISA. (**B**) NHBE were treated with cytokines at 10 ng/ml in the presence and absence of the indicated concentrations of each β_2-agonist (SM, FM, SB) for 6 h. The copy numbers of TSLP mRNA are shown. BSMC (**C**) and NHLF (**D**) were treated with the indicated concentrations of each β_2-agonist (SM, FM, SB) in the presence of 10 ng/ml IL-4 and 10 ng/ml TNF-α for 48 h. TSLP concentrations in the culture supernatants were quantified by ELISA. All data are shown as the mean ± SD of quadruplicate samples and are representative of at least three separate experiments. ** $p < .01$ compared with IL-4 plus TNF-α. Reprinted from Futamura et. Al., 2010.

2.3 Effects of cAMP-elevating agents on cytokine-induced TSLP production

It is well known that binding of β_2-agonists to β_2-adrenoceptors activates adenylate cyclase, resulting in generation of intracellular cAMP. We therefore examined the role of intracellular cAMP in the enhancement of TSLP production. The cells were stimulated with three cAMP-elevating agents, i.e., 8-bromoadenosine cyclic monophosphate, dibutyryl adenosine cyclic monophosphate (hereinafter referred to as 8-Br cAMP and db cAMP, respectively) and forskolin (an adenylate cyclase activator). All three agents caused significant enhancement of cytokine-induced TSLP production by the lung tissue cells (Fig. 3). These results suggest that the enhancing effects of β_2-agonists on TSLP production were mediated via upregulation of intracellular cAMP in these cells.

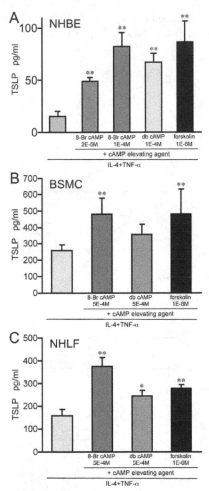

Fig. 3. Intracellular cAMP-elevating agents enhance cytokine-induced TSLP production by
lung tissue cells. NHBE (**A**), BSMC (**B**) and NHLF (**C**) were treated with 10 ng/ml IL-4 and
10 ng/ml TNF-α in the presence and absence of the indicated concentrations of each cAMP-
elevating agent (8-Br cAMP, db cAMP, forskolin) for 48 h. TSLP concentrations in the
culture supernatants were quantified by ELISA. Data are shown as the mean ± SD of
quadruplicate samples and are representative of at least three separate experiments. * p < .05
and ** p < .01 compared with IL-4 plus TNF-α. Reprinted from Futamura et. Al., 2010.

2.4 Effects of corticosteroid on cytokine-induced TSLP production

According to the recently updated guidelines for asthma management, the preferred treatment
regimen for patients with intermittent asthma is an inhaled short-acting β₂-agonist, and the
next step regimen is additional treatment with an inhaled corticosteroid. Therefore, we
examined the effects of a corticosteroid, fluticasone, on the β₂-agonist-induced increase in
TSLP production. Simultaneous addition of various concentrations of fluticasone caused dose-
dependent, significant inhibition of both cytokine-induced (closed squares) and salmeterol-

enhanced (closed triangles) TSLP production by NHBE (Fig. 4A, upper graph). Similar results were obtained in experiments using NHLF (Fig. 4A, lower graph) and BSMC (data not

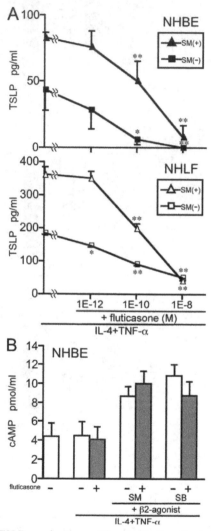

Fig. 4. Fluticasone inhibits TSLP production without affecting the intracellular cAMP level. (**A**) NHBE (upper graph) and NHLF (lower graph) were treated with 10 ng/ml IL-4 and 10 ng/ml TNF-α with and without 10⁻¹⁰ M salmeterol (SM) for 48 h. The effects of simultaneous addition of the indicated concentrations of fluticasone on the TSLP production are shown. Data are shown as the mean ± SD of quadruplicate samples and are representative of at least three separate experiments. * p < .05 and ** p < .01 compared to without fluticasone. (**B**) NHBE were treated with 10 ng/ml IL-4 and 10 ng/ml TNF-α with and without a β₂-agonist (10⁻¹⁰ M SM, 10⁻⁸ M SB) for 5 min. The effects of simultaneous addition of 10⁻⁸ M fluticasone on the intracellular cAMP levels are shown. Data are shown as the mean ± SD of triplicate samples and are representative of three separate experiments. Reprinted from Futamura et. al., 2010.

β₂-Adrenoceptor Agonists and Allergic Disease: The Enhancing Effect of β₂-Adrenoceptor
Agonists on Cytokine-Induced TSLP Production by Human Lung Tissue Cells

93

shown). Importantly, simultaneous treatment at the highest concentration of fluticasone (10^{-8} M), which can still considered to be clinically feasible, almost completely abrogated not only the cytokine-induced TSLP production but also the enhancement by the β₂-agonists.

2.5 Corticosteroid inhibition of TSLP production is not due to direct inhibition of cAMP signaling

In order to clarify how corticosteroids might inhibit TSLP production, we examined the effects of fluticasone and β₂-agonists on the intracellular cAMP level in NHBE. Addition of salmeterol or salbutamol significantly increased the cAMP level after 5 minutes of incubation. Addition of 10^{-8} M fluticasone showed no effect on the intracellular cAMP level whether in the presence or absence of a β₂-agonist (Fig. 4B), indicating that corticosteroid inhibition of TSLP production is not due to direct inhibition of cAMP signaling. These results also suggest that corticosteroids inhibit TSLP synthesis by acting on the downstream signaling pathway of cAMP.

To date, several mechanisms have been proposed to explain the synergistic action between corticosteroids and β₂-agonists: induction and protection of β₂-adrenoceptors by corticosteroids (Barnes, 2002), enhancement of translocation of glucocorticoid receptors into the nucleus by β₂-agonists (Usami et.al., 2005) and post-transcriptional regulation to suppress expression of inflammatory genes (Kaur et.al., 2008). Our results may shed new light on the mechanisms by which combination therapy using an inhaled β₂-agonist and an inhaled corticosteroid shows synergistic clinical efficacy in patients with asthma.

3. Future challenges

It remains to be clarified whether the enhancing effect of β₂-agonists on cytokine production is specific to TSLP or not. Koyama et. al. demonstrated that TNF-α-induced production of granulocyte-macrophage colony-stimulating factor (GM-CSF), CCL5 and IL-8 by a human bronchial epithelial cell line, BEAS-2B, was significantly inhibited by procaterol, a β₂-agonist (Koyama et. al., 1999). We confirmed that the cytokine-induced production of GM-CSF and CCL5, but not IL-8, by NHBE was significantly suppressed by β₂-agonist treatment (data not shown). On the other hand, it was reported that rhinovirus-induced IL-6 production by NHBE was increased by salmeterol (Edwards et. Al., 2007), and we also found that the cytokine-induced production of IL-6 as well as TSLP by NHBE was significantly enhanced by simultaneous treatment with β₂-agonists (data not shown). Thus, β₂-agonists are able to crucially modulate the production of various inflammatory mediators through mechanisms that need to be further elucidated.

4. Conclusion

In this study, we focused on the effects of β₂-agonists on the *in vitro* synthesis of TSLP, which is a key cytokine in the development of allergic diseases. We found that β₂-agonists significantly enhanced cytokine-induced TSLP production by cultured primary human lung tissue cells. This enhancement may be partly responsible for the undesirable clinical effects of continuous β₂-agonist monotherapy, and our other findings suggest that combination therapy with a corticosteroid might effectively inhibit TSLP-mediated allergic inflammation.

5. Acknowledgements

We would like to thank Dr. Kanami Orihara of the Department of Allergy and Immunology, National Research Institute for Child Health and Development, for her contribution in this work. This work was supported in part by grants from the National Institute of Biomedical Innovation (ID05-24 and ID05-41) and a grant from the Japan Health Science Foundation (KH51046).

6. References

Al-Shami, A.; Spolski, R.; Kelly, J.; Keane-Myers, A. & Leonard, W.J. (2005) A role for TSLP in the development of inflammation in an asthma model. J Exp Med 202:829-839.

Barnes, P.J. (2002) Scientific rationale for inhaled combination therapy with long-acting beta2-agonists and corticosteroids. Eur Respir J 19:182-191.

Cockcroft, D.W.; O'Byrne, P.M.; Swystun, V.A. & Bhagat, R. (1995) Regular use of inhaled albuterol and the allergen-induced late asthmatic response. J Allergy Clin Immunol 96:44-49.

Coqueret, O.; Petit-Frere, C.; Lagente, V.; Moumen, M.; Mencia-Huerta, J.M. & Braquet, P. (1994) Modulation of IgE production in the mouse by beta 2-adrenoceptor agonist. Int Arch Allergy Immunol 105:171-176.

Crane, J.; Pearce, N.; Flatt, A.; Burgess, C.; Jackson, R.; Kwong, T.; Ball, M. & Beasley, R. (1989) Prescribed fenoterol and death from asthma in New Zealand, 1981-83: case-control study. Lancet 1(8644):917-922.

Edwards, M.R.; Haas, J.; Panettieri, R.A.Jr.; Johnson, M. & Johnston, S.L. (2007) Corticosteroids and beta2 agonists differentially regulate rhinovirus-induced interleukin-6 via distinct Cis-acting elements. J Biol Chem 282:15366-15375.

Friend, S.L.; Hosier, S.; Nelson, A.; Foxworthe, D.; Williams, D.E. & Farr, A. (1994) A thymic stromal cell line supports in vitro development of surface IgM+ B cells and produces a novel growth factor affecting B and T lineage cells. Exp Hematol 22:321-328.

Futamura, K.; Orihara, K.; Hashimoto, N.; Morita, H.; Fukuda, S.; Sagara, H.; Matsumoto, K.; Tomita, Y.; Saito, H. & Matsuda, A. (2010) beta2-adrenoceptor agonists enhance cytokine-induced release of thymic stromal lymphopoietin by lung tissue cells. Int Arch Allergy Immunol 152:353-361

Ito, T.; Wang, Y.H.; Duramad, O.; Hori, T.; Delespesse, G.J.; Watanabe, N.; Qin, F.X.; Yao, Z.; Cao, W. & Liu, Y.J. (2005) TSLP-activated dendritic cells induce an inflammatory T helper type 2 cell response through OX40 ligand. J Exp Med 202:1213-1223.

Kato, A.; Favoreto, S. Jr.; Avila, P.C. & Schleimer, R.P. (2007) TLR3- and Th2 cytokine-dependent production of thymic stromal lymphopoietin in human airway epithelial cells. J Immunol 179:1080-1087.

Kaur, M.; Chivers, J.E.; Giembycz, M.A. & Newton, R. (2008) Long-acting beta2-adrenoceptor agonists synergistically enhance glucocorticoid-dependent transcription in human airway epithelial and smooth muscle cells. Mol Pharmacol 73:203-14.

β₂-Adrenoceptor Agonists and Allergic Disease: The Enhancing Effect of β₂-Adrenoceptor
Agonists on Cytokine-Induced TSLP Production by Human Lung Tissue Cells

95

Koyama, S.; Sato, E.; Masubuchi, T.; Takamizawa, A.; Kubo, K.; Nagai, S. & Isumi, T. (1999)
    Procaterol inhibits IL-1beta- and TNF-alpha-mediated epithelial cell eosinophil
    chemotactic activity. Eur Respir J 14:767-775.

Liu, YJ. (2007a) Thymic stromal lymphopoietin and OX40 ligand pathway in the initiation
    of dendritic cell-mediated allergic inflammation. J Allergy Clin Immunol 120:238-
    244.

Liu, Y.J.; Soumelis, V.; Watanabe, N.; Ito, T.; Wang, Y.H.; de Waal-Malefyt, Rd. R.; Omori,
    M.; Zhou, B. & Ziegler, S.F. (2007b) TSLP: an epithelial cell cytokine that regulates T
    cell differentiation by conditioning dendritic cell maturation. Annu Rev Immunol
    25:193-219.

Loza, M.J.; Peters, S.P.; Foster, S.; Khan, I.U. & Penn, R.B. (2007) beta-Agonist enhances type
    2 T-cell survival and accumulation. J Allergy Clin Immunol 119:235-244.

Nelson, H.S.; Weiss, S.T.; Bleecker, E.R.; Yancey, S.W. & Dorinsky, P.M. (2006) The
    Salmeterol Multicenter Asthma Research Trial: a comparison of usual
    pharmacotherapy for asthma or usual pharmacotherapy plus salmeterol. Chest
    129:15-26.

Orihara, K.; Nakae, S.; Pawankar, R. & Saito, H. (2008) Role of regulatory and
    proinflammatory T-cell populations in allergic diseases. WAO (World Allergy
    Organization) Journal 1:9-14.

Panina-Bordignon, P.; Mazzeo, D.; Lucia, P.D.; D'Ambrosio, D.; Lang, R.; Fabbri, L.; Self, C.
    & Sinigaglia, F. (1997) Beta2-agonists prevent Th1 development by selective
    inhibition of interleukin 12. J Clin Invest 100:1513-1519.

Paris, J.; Peterson, E.L.; Wells, K.; Pladevall, M.; Burchard, E.G.; Choudhry, S.; Lanfear,
    D.E. & Williams, L.K. (2008) Relationship between recent short-acting beta-
    agonist use and subsequent asthma exacerbations. Ann Allergy Asthma Immunol
    101:482-487.

Soumelis, V.; Reche, P.A.; Kanzler, H.; Yuan, W.; Edward, G.; Homey, B.; Gilliet, M.; Ho, S.;
    Antonenko, S.; Lauerma, A.; Smith, K.; Gorman, D.; Zurawski, S.; Abrams, J.;
    Menon, S.; McClanahan, T.; de Waal-Malefyt, Rd. R.; Bazan, F.; Kastelein, R.A. &
    Liu, Y.J. (2002) Human epithelial cells trigger dendritic cell mediated allergic
    inflammation by producing TSLP. Nat Immunol 2002;3: 673-680.

Spoelstra, F.M.; Postma, D.S.; Hovenga, H.; Noordhoek, J.A. & Kauffman, H.F. (2002)
    Additive anti-inflammatory effect of formoterol and budesonide on human lung
    fibroblasts. Thorax 57:237-241.

Usmani, O.S.; Ito, K.; Maneechotesuwan, K.; Ito, M.; Johnson, M.; Barnes, P.J. & Adcock, I.M.
    (2005) Glucocorticoid receptor nuclear translocation in airway cells after inhaled
    combination therapy. Am J Respir Crit Care Med 172:704-712.

Yasui, K.; Kobayashi, N.; Yamazaki, T.; Agematsu, K.; Matsuzaki, S.; Nakata, S. & Baba, A.
    (2006) Differential effects of short-acting beta2-agonists on human granulocyte
    functions. Int Arch Allergy Immunol 139:1-8.

Yoo, J.; Omori, M.; Gyarmati, D.; Zhou, B.; Aye, T.; Brewer, A.; Comeau, M.R.; Campbell,
    D.J. & Ziegler, S.F. (2005) Spontaneous atopic dermatitis in mice expressing an
    inducible thymic stromal lymphopoietin transgene specifically in the skin. J Exp
    Med 202:541-549.

Zhou, B.; Comeau, M.R.; De Smedt, T.; Liggitt, H.D.; Dahl, M.E.; Lewis, D.B.; Gyarmati, D.;
        Aye, T.; Campbell, D.J. & Ziegler, S.F. (2005) Thymic stromal lymphopoietin as a
        key initiator of allergic airway inflammation in mice. Nat Immunol 6:1047-1053.

6

Natural Products and Dermatological Hypersensitivity Diseases

Clayton MacDonald and Marianna Kulka

Institute for Nutriscience and Health, National Research Council,
Canada

1. Introduction

The management of dermatological hypersensitivity diseases is a lifelong struggle for most patients. Often, patients are advised to avoid triggers and aggregating factors that lead to flare ups which eventually becomes second nature to them. However, when the symptoms of these conditions become unbearable and conventional medicine no longer provides relief, an increasing proportion of allergy patients are looking to alternative treatments for comfort. Natural products are compounds isolated from natural sources (usually plants or animals) that have potentially beneficial bioactivity. However, many types of compounds can be defined as natural bioactives including synthesized molecules that are based upon naturally occurring compounds. As such, we will define the term "natural bioactive" as any compound whose parent compound structure occurs in nature. Medical research is exploring these compounds as potential treatment sources for a myriad of conditions, including the dermatological hypersensitivity diseases. With the growing interest in natural health products it could be possible that disease sufferers, by self exploring alternative treatments, are potentially leading the search towards the next new approved and medically accepted treatment.

2. Current treatments and management in dermatological hypersensitivity diseases

The management of atopic and hypersensitivity diseases are initially addressed by life style modifications. With all hypersensitivity diseases, be it food allergies, contact hypersensitivity, or allergic asthma, suffers quickly become aware of their disease triggers and begin a lifelong course of avoidance (Custovic *et al.*, 1998). Unknown triggers can be identified medically using a skin prick/patch test. This involves a controlled dermal exposure to the known and the most frequent allergens, and triggers are identified from the resultant skin reactions (Li, 2002). Pharmacological treatments are added into the treatment schedule as the severity of disease progresses, following well-developed treatment ladders (algorithms) (Schmitt *et al.*, 2008). As the patient moves into the stronger classes of treatments in these schedules, the associated side effects become more severe, influencing treatment decisions, ultimately compliance rate and exploration of alternative treatments.

2.1 Life style modifications and diet
The effect of diet on allergies and atopic diseases mitigation has been well studied, but has produced conflicting results (Allan & Devereux, 2011; Devereaux & Yusuf, 2003; Finch *et al.*,

2010; Wichers, 2009). In children with a family history of atopic diseases, research has been focused towards the effects of maternal diet during pregnancy, lactation, and then subsequently in the infant when and which foods are introduced. Of particular interest is the effect of probiotics on the development of allergies which will be discussed below (section 4.2.4). In patients with food allergies triggers are eliminated from the diet, however other foods have been suggested which might be beneficial to allergy suffers. Some of these compounds include poly-unsaturated fatty acids (PUFA); Vitamins C (Chang *et al.*, 2009), D, E, Zinc, Selenium. However, these findings have been meet with mixed results (Finch *et al.*, 2010).

2.2 Medical treatment

Medical treatments are initiated as the severity of symptoms become worse and the disease becomes intolerable (Schmitt *et al.*, 2008). For each condition, drug classes have been recommended to be added in a specific order/time in the treatment schedule. However, due to the nature of these conditions treatment is individually tailored depending on patient response and their tolerance of the side effects. These patients follow a defined treatment plan consisting of pharmacological classes, based on their indications and complications. When treatment is initiated for a patient, the success of treatment always needs to balance with the side effect the treatment has on patient quality of life. (R. Finkel *et al.*, 2009). The following is a brief overview of some conventional treatments for hypersensitivity disease such as steriods and anti-histamines. Some of these compounds originated from natural sources but have been modified extensively to improve both their efficacy and potency. As such, these medications are not strictly considered "naturally sourced." In section 3 below, we will address "naturally sourced" treatments for comparison.

2.2.1 Corticosteroids

Corticosterioids are a class of steroid hormones that are frequently used as a first line treatment in many immunological and dermatological diseases (Richard Finkel, 2009). They can be classified as short to long acting (1-55+ hours) and are applied topically or systematically. They are very effective at mitigating inflammation; however, their side effects limit their long term use. Many of the new treatments are being sought as corticosteroids sparing alternatives (Del Rosso & Friedlander, 2005).

Mechanism of Action: Corticosteroids bind intracellular receptors forming dimers that bind to the glucocorticoid response element of the promoter region of steroid responsive genes, which up regulates 10-100 genes (Bolognia *et al.*, 2008). They also act by inhibiting nuclear factor kB (NF-κB) which dramatically decreases the inflammatory response through the down regulation of certain cytokines, cell adhesion molecules and other inflammatory mediators. (Ex: TNFα, GM-CSF, several interleukins (ex. Il-1, IL-2, IL-6, Il-8); Intercellular adhesion molecule-1 and E-selectin; cyclooxygenase, etc). (D'Acquisto *et al.*, 2002; Richard Finkel, 2009)

Topical Benefits: Reduced itching, improvements in sleep, appearance of skin, self-esteem and quality of life (Miller & Eichenfield, 2006):. *Side effects*(Miller & Eichenfield, 2006) Short Term – stinging on application (for potent preparations); Medium to Long Term – local complications (i.e. skin thinning, striate, glaucoma from periocular use, contact sensitization and tolerance), etc. ; Systemic effects – suppression of the hypothalamic-pituitary-adrenal axis, Cushing's syndrome, decreased immunity.

Systemic Benefits (Miller & Eichenfield, 2006)*:* Relief from itching, skin redness and infiltration and reduced oozing; *Side Effects*(Miller & Eichenfield, 2006): Short term – increased appetite, psychosis and dyspepsia; Long term - hypertension, osteoporosis, adrenal suppression, striate and muscle atrophy, Cushing's Syndrome, decreased immunity.

2.2.2 Emollients

Emollients are creams designed to alleviate the symptoms of pruritus in dermatitis (Bolognia *et al.*, 2008). They are normally applied daily and act by coating the skin and creating an artificial barrier. They are composed of either water free or water-in-oil ointments with urea (10-20%) or lactic acid (5-12%). The underlying principle of this treatment is to 'correct' the barrier defect of the skin in AD. *Benefits:* Reduce skin dryness, itching and penetration of skin by irritants and allergens; prevention of skin cracking; possible reduced need for topical corticosteroids, possible enhanced response when used with topical corticosteroids. *Side Effects:* Possible stinging on application (R. Finkel *et al.*, 2009).

2.2.3 Topical calcineurin inhibitors

These compounds are among the newest class of immunomodulatory compounds that have been approved for use in inflammatory skin diseases (2000) (Grassberger *et al.*, 2004). Members of this class include Pimecrolimus, Tacrolimus and Ascomycin. All originated as natural products isolated from the fermentation products of the bacteria *Streptomyces sp.* *(Richard Finkel, 2009)*. This class has the advantage of treating AD refractory to corticosteroids and reducing the amount of corticosteroids required in severe cases (Spergel & Leung, 2006).

Mechanism of Action: Inhibits calcineurin phosphatase by binding to FK506 binding protein which then complexes to calcineurin preventing its activation (Assmann *et al.*, 2000). Activated calcineurin dephosphorylates the cytoplasmic subunit of the nuclear factor of activated T cells (NFAT), which then translocates to the nucleus where it forms a complex that assists in transcription of numerous cytokines (ex. Th1: IL2, INFY; Th2: IL4, IL5) (Grassberger *et al.*, 1999; Sakuma *et al.*, 2001).

Indications: (Bolognia et al., 2008)

Pimecrolmus – Mild to moderate atopic dermatitis, other inflammatory dermatoses

Tacrolimus – Moderate to severe atopic dermatitis, other inflammatory dermatoses

Benefits: Reduced itching and improvements in sleep, appearance of skin, self-esteem and quality of life (Grassberger *et al.*, 2004; Miller & Eichenfield, 2006)

Adverse Effects

Short term – mild stinging or burning upon application; normally improves after a week

Long term – (>5 years) – Tacrolimus: safety unknown, use with caution with excess exposure to UV light; Pimecrolimus: safety profile based on 5 years of use appears good.

2.2.4 Immunomodulators

This class of drugs/compounds function by attenuating the immune response underlying the hypersensitivity reaction. Some of these compounds have been used as immunosuppressants in transplant medicine while others are either components of the immune system or a new class of treatments known as 'biological agents' which are artificially created monoclonal antibody designed to target errant members of the immune system (R. Finkel *et al.*, 2009). Interestingly some of the immunosuppressants have their origin as natural products including: cyclosporine (isolotaed from fungus *Tolypocladium inflatum*), mycophenolate mofetil (isolated from fungus *Penicillium stoloniferum*) tacrolimus (isolated from *Streptomyces tsukubaensis*) as well as others (R. Finkel *et al.*, 2009).

Interferon γ

Was investigated for use in atopic dermatitis due to its pathological dysregulation, and was found to be effective in short term (Hanifin *et al.*, 1993) and long term studies (Stevens *et al.*, 1998). However, its low response rate and high costs deter its regular use and implementation.

Biological Agents – Monoclonal Antibodies

These agents are biologically engineered antibodies directed against specific targets in the immune system. Some of these agents have made it to market for specific conditions (see table1). Omalizumab is a humanized mouse monocolonal antibody targeting the IgE Fc Region. It binds free IgE but not IgE bound to FcεRI on masts cells, so in this way it sequesters free IgE without activating bound IgE and causing mast cell degranulation (Presta *et al.*, 1993). Omalizumab has been approved by the FDA for use in severe recalcitrant asthma (Strunk & Bloomberg, 2006) and has been investigated for severe cases of atopic dermatitis with positive results (Lane *et al.*, 2006).

AGENT	TARGET / MOA	CONDITION
Alefacept, Efalizumab	T-cell activation, T-cell trafficking	Psoriasis
Etanercept, Infliximab, Adalimumab	TNFα	Psoriasis
Anakinra	IL-1	Rheumatoid arthritis
Rituximab	CD20 (B-cells)	B-cell mediated skin diseases

Table 1. Examples of Biological Agents employed in Dermatological Conditions

Immunosuppresants: Cyclosporine, methotrexate, Mycophenolate mofetil

These drugs act by modulating different functions of the immune system and decreasing their activity. These drugs while very potent in activity require caution in use, because of associated side effects including nephro- , neuro-, and hepatictoxicity (R. Finkel *et al.*, 2009).

2.2.5 Other medical treatments

Anti-Microbial:

This class of pharmaceuticals are commonly used against infections caused by pathological secondary barrier defects in the epidermis. Infections can be caused by intense scratching leading to excoriations or due to immune suppression from other treatments. Common infections associated with atopic dermatitis include bacterial (*S. aurues)*, viral (*Molluscum contagiosum, HSV*) and fungal (*Candida sp., Malassezia sp.*) (Bolognia *et al.*, 2008).

Retinoids

Retinoids are related to Vitamin A and act by binding nuclear receptors (RAR, RXR) which directly and indirectly up regulate gene expression responsible for immune and inflammatory responses and proliferation and differentiation of epithelial cells (Bolognia *et al.*, 2008). Retinoids require careful consideration before use due to side effects including local effects, systemic, psychological but more importantly teratogenic effects (David *et al.*, 1988).

Anti-Histamines

This class of drugs has multiple therapeutic targets including allergic and inflammatory conditions, motion sickness and nausea, gastric acid secretion and others (Richard Finkel, 2009). They play a role in urticaria prevention (Jauregui *et al.*, 2007) and symptomatic treatment in other mast cell conditions (Herman & Vender, 2003; Montoro *et al.*, 2007) especially for edema control and pruritus.

Mast Cell Stabilizers

Members of this class of drugs include cromolyn and nedocromil, and are used in mast cell mediated allergic conditions. They function by inhibiting the IgE mediated release of histamine by stabilization of the membrane (Corin, 2000).

2.2.6 Other treatments

In addition to medicinal treatments prescribed by practitioners are a series of physical and alternative treatments. Very popular with dermatological treatment is the use of UV light and tanning beds, especially for psoriasis. Although the mechanism of action is unknown, it is thought that UV activates Psoralen which inhibits cellular proliferation. In certain conditions practitioners may prescribe Ichthyotherapy in which small fish (doctor fish) are employed to remove dead skin from lesions. Coal tar (mixture of hydrocarbons) is used as an emollient and remains a popular treatment in many dermatological centers (Bolognia *et al.*, 2008).

3. The use of Complementary and Alternative Medicine (CAM)

Complementary and Alternative Medicine (CAM): Group of diverse medical and health care interventions, practices, products or disciplines that are not generally considered as part of conventional medicine (NCCAM, 2011)

Complementary Medicine: Any of a range of medical therapies that fall beyond the scope of scientific medicine but may be used alongside it in the treatment of disease and ill health (NCCAM, 2011)

Alternative Medicine: Medical therapies that are used in lieu of conventional therapy (NCCAM, 2011),

(Note: There are many definitions that have been put forward for CAM, these are the ones designated by the National Center for Complementary and Alternative Medicine (USA)).

Recognition of the rising interest and potential importance of Traditional Medicine (TM) and CAM lead the WHO to survey its membership on their respective national attitudes and regulatory status of this branch of health care. They found in 2005 that 71% of respondents have laws, legislative mandates and National regulatory bodies in place for TM/CAM (WHO, 2005). In 1991, the United States created the Office of Alternative Medicine to scientifically scrutinize alternative health practices for the benefit of public and health professionals knowledge. By 1998, due to increasing interest of the subject, this department was expanded into the National Center for Complementary and Alternative Medicine as a member institute of the United States Institutes of Health. It was from this department that a systematic classification of Complementary and Alternative Medicines was formed and grouped into 5 categories (Molassiotis *et al.*, 2005), see Table 1. It is from the biological based therapies and the Alternative Medical systems that sources of natural products are being explored for as potential disease treatments and being entered into clinical trials. It should be noted that treatments from the other groups have entered clinical trials for certain conditions with mixed results including massage (Schachner *et al.*, 1998), acupuncture (Salameh *et al.*, 2008), meditation (Chida *et al.*, 2007), prayer and others.

CLASSIFICATION		EXAMPLES
I	Alternative Medical Systems	Traditional Chinese Medicine, Ayruveda
II	Mind-Body Interventions	Meditation, Prayer, Healing or Support Groups
III	Biological Based Therapies	Herbs, Dietary Supplements, Vitamins
IV	Manipulation and Body Based	Massage, Chiropractive, Osteopathy
V	Energy Therapies	Qi Gong, Reiki

Table 2. Classification of CAM devised by Center for Complementary and Alternative Medicine

3.1 Demographics of CAM use in industrialized nations

There has been a well-recognized trend in the increasing use of CAM among the general public (Harris & Rees, 2000; Su & Li, 2011). In the 2002 US National Health Interview Survey (NHIS) of 31,044 adults, 36% of adults reported using CAM in the previous 12 months, and if a life time prevalence was included, this figure rose to 50% (Barnes *et al.*, 2004). The results from the 2007 survey saw the 12 month prevalence figure rise to 38.6% and among those positive respondents, the most common CAM was listed as 'natural products' (Barnes *et al.*, 2008). Earlier smaller scale national surveys conducted by Eisenberg *et al.* found prevalence rates of 33.8% in 1990 and 42.1% in 1997, although these values are higher (possibly due to the small samples size) it is generally agreed that CAM use is continually increasing (Eisenberg *et al.*, 1998). The NHIS surveys identified some demographic characteristics common among users which have been confirmed from other studies. CAM use is more prevalent among women, adults with higher education, those who engaged in leisure time and physical activity, those who had one or more existing health conditions and have made frequent medical visits in the past year (Barnes *et al.*, 2008; Eisenberg *et al.*, 1998; Metcalfe *et al.*, 2010; Sirois & Gick, 2002). Other identified factors are higher socioeconomic status, being married, those who wished to take a more active role in health care decision making and most interestingly those with a chronic health condition (Metcalfe *et al.*, 2010; Wiles & Rosenberg, 2001). The popularity of CAM use is also recognized in other industrialized countries ; the rates for Canada are estimated at 12-20% (Gavin & Boon, 2005) and 46% in Germany and 49% in France where alternative treatments are well engrained in the national consciousness (Fisher & Ward, 1994). The trend of increasing CAM can be identified from Germany (West) with its 12 months prevalence almost doubling since the 1970's (See Figure

1) (Dixon *et al.*, 2003). It should be kept in perspective when looking at the trends of TM/CAM use that (as defined by the WHO) up to 80% of the world's population uses TM/CAM as their sole source of health care in the places where Western health care is inaccessible ((World Health Organization., 2009).

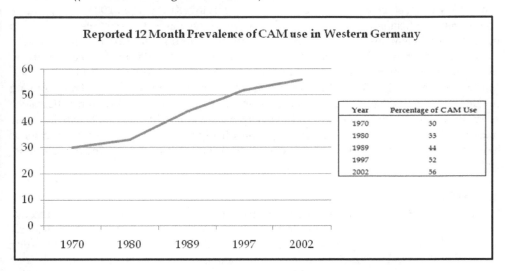

Fig. 1. Reported Use of CAM in Western Germany from 1970s to 2002

3.2 Patient and user attitude toward CAM

There have been many attempts to identify the reasons and motivations as to why members of the public are exploring alternative options for their well-being and health care. A large European study of 956 Cancer patients in 12 countries, found a prevalence rate of CAM use of 38.2% (Range of 14.8% to 73.1%). From those who reported using CAM therapy they were investigated first, for their motivation and second, how found out about them. The most common motivation for CAM use was to increase their body's ability to fight disease (50.7%), followed by improved physical well-being (40.6%), and improvement of emotional well-being (35.2%). Sources of information about CAM were identified as friends (56.5%), family (29.1%), media (28.4%) and only 18.6% said their physician was the source (Molassiotis *et al.*, 2005). Use of CAM is associated with greater number of physical symptoms and with symptoms of greater intensity, longer disease duration (Sirois & Gick, 2002). The reasons for people to explore alternative treatment are varied, but what should be recognized is that are they exploring them. By having members of the public vetting these treatments in terms of personal satisfaction gives health care workers a unique opportunity by looking at the usage trends in members of the public as potential treatments sources.

3.3 Health care practitioners attitude towards CAM

The number of visits to practitioners of alternative therapies is now higher than the number of visits to all US primary care physicians (Pagan & Pauly, 2005). Physician and health care professionals response to CAM has been varied with differences depending on country, region, age, experience and even sex. In a literature review by Sewitch *et al* found that characteristics of physicians whom are more likely to recommend CAM are younger, female, less experienced; while those less likely to recommend CAMs were older, male, more experienced physicians (Sewitch & Rajput, 2010). Older physicians are less likely to use CAMs themselves or recommend it to their family (Kurtz *et al.*, 2003). It should be noted that physicians are the most skeptical and least likely to recommend CAMs to patients, of all members of the health care profession. Rural health care providers offered CAM more frequently than their urban colleagues (Brems *et al.*, 2006). Between 60-80% of surveyed physicians express interest in CAM therapy (Corbin Winslow & Shapiro, 2002; Milden & Stokols, 2004) but few as 14% have recommended it their patients. Among physicians there is prejudice about the different types if CAMs, established practices such as acupuncture, chiropractor tend to be surveyed as the most likely to be beneficial to the patient; While reiki, bioelectromagnetics, aromatherapy have been ranked by doctors as having the least potential to be beneficial or event harmful to the patient (Levine *et al.*, 2003).

3.4 CAM and allergies

In a German study of 351 subjects with hypersensitivity (hay fever, asthma, atopic eczema, food allergies), 93 (26%) were found to be users of CAM. Of the 93 users, 94% previously were treated conventionally before starting CAM while 3 users used CAM before starting conventional treatment. Of those treated conventionally the majority (85%) were treated more than 10 years before trying CAM, they also score the efficacy of conventional medicine lower in their experience. Their reported motivations for using CAM were: conviction that CAM has less side effects (78%), wish to try everything (72%), unsatisfying results from conventional medicine (66%), and belief CAM is more natural (61%) (Schafer *et al.*, 2002) . In a review of 7 surveys of dermatological patients who used CAM they found life time prevalence of 35-65% (Ernst, 2000); among all the surveys they found severity of illness and length of disease had the greatest influence on CAM use. In Europe approximately 30% of patients with allergies report using CAM and this rises to approximately 50% of patients whom required in-patient treatment (Schafer, 2004). The use CAM is related to the severity of the symptoms of their conditions, patients who identify with having poor control are more likely to explore alternative treatments.

4. Search for natural products

Natural products are compounds that have been isolated from a living organism that have been found to be biologically active. A large proportion of the medicines in our current pharmacopeia have either originate as natural products or are inspired by a natural product using it chemical structure as framework on which to build on (Newman & Cragg, 2007). These compounds are being explore for, from all facets of nature including CAMs, our foodstocks, and on an increasing scale the marine sources. The remainder of the chapter will explore some of the natural products undergoing clinical trials for the treatment of Atopic dermatitis. Atopic dermatitis was selected due to its complex pathology, its association with the atopic march and the availability of an animal model which will be discussed below. The test compounds will be discussed below in the context of atopic dermatitis; however some of them are being tested in other related dermatological conditions.

4.1 Clinical trials

Any medicinal compound before entering into an approved treatment system (i.e. National Pharmacopeia) requires rigorous study and clinical trials, which have a defined set of trial steps, before they can be approved for use by National Regulatory bodies. In the United States this task is mandated by the Food and Drug Administration (FDA), in Canada by Health Canada and in the European Union by the European Medicines Agency (Rawson, 2000). All drug approvals required an evidence based approach to qualify their efficacy, evaluate the potential toxicity, and to prevent any unforeseen harm to patients. It is interesting to note that estimates now have the cost of marketed drugs from the R&D stage to consumer use at 500 million to 1 billion dollars and at a time frame of up to 10-15 years (DiMasi et al., 2003). Only about 1 out of 1000 drugs from the animal testing stage (or preclinical phase) make it into clinical trials and from there only 1 in 5-10 eventually become approved. In this manner only 21 new drugs were approved by the FDA in 2010, 25 in 2009 and 21 in 2008 (Kaitin & DiMasi, 2011). However if natural compounds are identified from CAM treatment sources already employed by members of the public they may provide new treatment options which can enter rigorous evidence based trials which have already been vetted by members of the public.

Pre-Clinical Studies / Phase 0: Pre-clinical studies are conducted as *In vitro* (cell culture) and *In Vivo* (animal studies) as initial investigations into suspected potential biological activity. Phase 0 studies are human trials using microdoses to determine if its biological effects are what is expected (Yση α Pανι, 2009)

Phase I: Small scale study of 20-100 healthy subjects, testing the safety, pharmacodynamics and pharmacokinetics of the study compound (Streiner & Normam, 2009), consists usually of either single or multiple ascending doses trials.

Phase II: Following the safety approval of drugs in Phase I, these are a small studies of 50-300 diseased subjects , designed to assess dosing requirements, efficacy, (Streiner & Normam, 2009) and safety profiles in people with the condition.

Phase III: Randomized controlled multicenter trials on large group of diseased patients with the target condition, this study are used to determine if the study compound has targeted therapeutic effects (R. Finkel et al., 2009).

Phase IV: These studies occur after the drug has enter the market and is known as Post-Marketing Surveillance. They determine if any adverse events happen in large group of patients which were not previously identified. This phase is important is identifying any rare adverse events which occur in large treatment populations. This monitoring is responsible from removing from market approved drug which later have been found to be potentially harmful, examples are Troglitazone (Cohen, 2006; Gale, 2006) and Vioxx (Karha & Topol, 2004).

4.2 Atopic Dermatitis

Atopic dermatitis (AD) has been recognized since at least the 1500s (Wallach et al., 2005) with its first formal medical description in 1933(Wise & Sulzberger, 1933). This condition is currently a popular target of medical research due to its increasing incidence (Peroni et al., 2008; H. Williams, 1992), distressing rash and intense pruritic symptoms(Hanifin & Rajka, 1980), leading to general negative effects on the patients quality of life (Kiebert et al., 2002) and its being refractory to treatment, along with a host of other reasons . With is long recognition in recent medical history, has led to many treatment options being made available. If any new product is found to possess immunomodulatory effects they tend to be investigated as possible treatments for AD. The remainder of this chapter will look at Natural Products and Natural Preparations undergoing clinical trials for the treatment of AD.

PHASE	PARAMETERS
Pre-Clinical	In-Vitro (Cell Culture) and In Vivo (Animal Studies), determines biological activity, toxicity, etc
I	Small group health subjects; Pharmacokinetic and Pharmacodynamic properties, Single Ascending Dose, Multiple Ascending Doses
II	Small group diseased subjects, determine dosing requirements, drug efficacy
III	Larger group diseased subjects; Randomized Controlled Multicenter trials
IV	Post Marketing Surveillance Trial

Table 3. Phases of Clinical Trials

4.2.1 Animal Models: NC/Nga mice

One of the advantages of research into treatment for atopic dermatitis has been the development of an animal model that has been accepted to be representative of the disease (Suto et al., 1999). Using this model, researchers are able to easily test products prior to proceeding to human clinical trials. NC/Nga mice are a strain that originated from the Japanese fancy mice (Nishiki-Nezumi), established as an inbred strain in 1955 (Matsuda et al., 1997). Researchers noticed the development of spontaneous dermatitis like lesions that appeared just before or after weaning but the cause and pathogenesis had been unclear. A study was conducted to compare these lesions to those of human Atopic Dermatitis (Suto et al., 1999). Mice raised in specific pathogen free (SPF) air controlled bioclean rooms did not develop lesion, but when moved to air uncontrolled rooms, spontaneously several different type of lesions developed after 8 weeks. These mice developed clinical signs similar to AD: itching, erythema and hemorrhage, edema, superficial erosion, deep excoriation, scaling and dryness of the skin, and retarded growth. Infectious causes were ruled out by co-rearing with BALB/c mice which did not develop lesions. The histopathological changes which were consistent with Atopic Dermatitis as well as clinical labs values such as IgE hyperproduction (Matsuda et al., 1997), overproduction of Th2 specific cytokines (Suto et al., 1999; Vestergaard et al., 1999). A literature search conducted in May 2011 resulted in 245 and 185 articles when the following keywords were used together: NC/Nga Mice, Atopic Dermatitis.

4.2.2 Animal trials

The following is a list of compounds (albeit not exhaustive) investigated using the NC/Nga mice model as potential treatments for Atopic Dermatitis. All were oral feeding studies in which the test compound was compared to a control. The efficacies of test compounds were determined by the improvement in symptoms of skin erythema, edema, excoriations, dryness, and scratching behavior. Other parameters measured depended on the trial and included plasma Ig levels, cytokines and chemokine profiles, and evaluation of skin biopsies. All of these studies had positive outcomes based on the design parameters and were recommended by their research teams for use in human clinical trials.

Rumex Japonicus Houtt

Rumex is an herb used in the traditional medical systems originating from Eastern Asian countries (Japan, Korea, China) for the treatment of various skin diseases including AD (H. S. Lee *et al.*, 2006). Previous studies have shown that it contains components with anti-oxidant and antibacterial properties (Elzaawely *et al.*, 2005). Identified Bioactive compounds include anthraquinone derivatives: emodin, chrysophanol, physcion. These compounds studied from other natural sources are reported to have antibacterial, antifungal, anti-inflammatory, immunosuppressive and antiviral properties (H. S. Lee *et al.*, 2006) After 42 days, mice treated with the test compound were found to have significant decreases in the severity of all symptoms when compared to the control, particularly the scratching behavior, which is the most distressing symptom of AD. There was a decrease in plasma IgE and IL4 (which mediate type I hypersensitivity) and noticeable decrease of inflammatory changes in the skin biopsies. The results were more pronounced in the higher concentration groups indicating this compound causes a dose response (H. S. Lee *et al.*, 2006).

PG 102 – Actinidia Arguta

Actinidia Argurta, commonly known as Hardy Kiwi, is a fruit native to Korea, Northern China and Siberia. Compound PG102 and isolated from this fruit by Park *et al.* in 2005 and found to have oral immune modulating effects in mice (Park *et al.*, 2005). A follow up study conducted to determine the effect on the NC/Nga mice model (Park *et al.*, 2007), found that after 9 weeks, PG102 showed statistically significant beneficial effect on AD symptoms and scratching behavior, while noted immunomolecular effects showed a decrease in IgE, IgG, IL4 while IL12 was increased. Other reported effects including the prevention of eosinophilia, decreased levels of eotaxin and TARC, inhibiting the infiltration of inflammatory cells into the dermis, preventing the thickening of the epidermis and dermis and reduced expression of Th2 mediated cytokines and chemokines (Park et al., 2007). All of these effects are beneficial in attenuating the pathophysiological changes seen in Atopic dermatitis. Kim *et al.* tested the extract for efficacy compared to dexamethasone (corticosteriod) and tacrolimus and found PG102 attenuated the physical symptoms of AD similar to dexamethasone and more efficiently than tacrolimus. It also had positive effects on the molecular inflammatory markers as well (ex. IgE, IL4, INFY and others). However, all three compounds affected the physical changes in the dermis in a similar manner (Kim *et al.*, 2009). The initial results indicated this compound shows a promising potential for future use as an oral dietary supplement for the long term treatment of AD.

Saururus Chinensis Baill

Saururus is a perennial herbaceous plant used in Korean folk medicine for the treatment of various conditions such as edema, jaundice, gonorrhea and used has been employed as an antipyretic, diuretic, and anti-inflammatory agent (Choi *et al.*, 2008). It has been shown to have anti-oxidant activity (Y. S. Lee *et al.*, 2004) and has been used in the management of various skin diseases including AD in Eastern countries. It contains flavonoids (quercetin, quercitrin, isoquercitrin, rutin) as active components which are reported as possessing number of biological effects: antiallergic, anti-inflammatory, antiviral, antiproliferative, anticarcinogenic (Scalbert & Williamson, 2000). After 63 days this compound was found to significantly improve skin severity scores and improved itching behavior, with the higher concentration preforming better. Molecular evaluation found a decrease in IgE but no changes in IL4.

Lyophyllum Decastes

Lyophyllum is an edible mushroom cultivated in Japan that is commonly known as 'Fried Chicken Mushroom'. In a previous study, 11 polysaccharide extracts were found to have anti-tumour activity (Ukawa *et al.*, 2000) particularly (1-3)B-D-Glucan and (1-6)B-D-Glucan. In 2006, it was examined for its potential effect on the AD mice model (Ukawa *et al.*, 2007) using a 6 week feeding study. At the end of the study the treatment group had significant decreases in skin severity scores, as well as decreases in serum IgE, Histamine, and IL-4.

Persimmon Leaf Extract

Persimmon is the edible fruit of the Diospyros kaki Thunberg (Ebenanceae) tree which grows in China, Korea and Japan (Matsumoto *et al.*, 2002). Kaempferol, a flavonoid contained in the leaf, was found to inhibit antigen and calcium ionophore A23187 induced histamine release. Kaempferol-3-glucoside (astraglandin) has been shown to have anti-pruritic effects(Ishiguro & Oku, 1997). Kotani *et al.* found the leaf extract inhibited the release of histamine from human basophilic cell line KU812 (M Kotani, 1999) promoting them to study the effect on NC/Nga model (Kotani *et al.*, 2000). A 14 week oral feeding study using both Persimmon Leaf extract and Astraglandin alone found both were effective in decreasing the severity of skin scores, inhibiting IgE, IL4, IL13 and Histamine release (Kotani *et al.*, 2000). A similar follow up study was conducted confirming these earlier results and included measurement of Transepidermal water loss (TEWL) (Major pathology in AD due to dermal barrier dysfunction) and was found to be improved by the extract (Matsumoto *et al.*, 2002).

Konjac Glucomannan

Konjac is a plant found in eastern Asia and is very popular in Japan as cooking supplement. Two compounds of interest have been isolated from this product and tested as possible treatments: Konjac glucomannan which has been tested in mice and Konjac ceramide which entered human trials (see section 4.2.4). Glucomannan, a dietary fiber isolated from the tubers of *Amorphophallus konjac,* is a highly viscous polysaccharide composed of glucose and mannose residues (Onishi *et al.*, 2005). During the 1970's dietary fibers were investigated as part of the epidemiology of colon cancer (Burkitt, 1971a, 1971b). During mice feeding studies it was observed that serum IgE levels decreased and IgA and IgG increased(Lim *et al.*, 1997) indicating dietary fibers indirectly influenced immunoglobulin production. This theory was investigated in NC/Nga mouse model during an 8 week controlled feeding trial. Skin severity symptoms were significantly improved and scratching events were decreased to 1/3 to 1/6 of controls. Serologically it almost totally suppressed IgE levels and decreased the total Immunoglobulin, with a noted decreased in IL-4 and INFY. Since the compound suppressed both Th1 and Th2 related cytokines it's mechanism of action cannot be attributed to Th1/Th2 polarization (Onishi *et al.*, 2004, 2005). Follow up studies found that it decreased scratching behvaiour in a dose dependent manner (OnishiKawamotoSuzuki *et al.*, 2007), and prevented IgE class switching in Balb/c mice following injection of keratinocyte extract (Oomizu *et al.*, 2006). It was also found to suppress allergic rhinitis like inflammation following nasal challenge with ovalabumin (OnishiKawamotoUeda *et al.*, 2007).

Gyokuheifusan

This is a traditional Chinese Medicine formulation that has been used for the treatment of allergic and respiratory disease (ex. infections, allergic rhinitis, asthma, and others) (Fang *et al.*, 2005).This preparation contains three herbal medications: *Astragalus membranaceus, Atractylodes ovata, Saposhinkovia divaricate*. In a study on the immunomodulatory effects of the formulation on allergic asthma, it was found to reduce the severity of asthma through normalization of INFΥ/IL4 ratio (Th1/Th2 balance) (Fang *et al.*, 2005). These results were hypothesized to extent to AD, after a 4 week oral feeding treatment placebo control study it was found that dermatitis severity scores were improved significantly, as well as IgE and the IFNΥ/IL4 balance (Nakatsukasa *et al.*, 2009).

COMPOUND	PARAMETER IMPROVEMENT	MOLECULAR IMPROVEMENTS
Rumex Japonicus Houtt	Skin Severity Scores, Scratching Behaviour, Skin inflammatory Changes	Decrease IgE, IL4
PG102 – *Actinidia Arguta*	Skin Severity Scores, Scratching Behaviour; Prevented eosinophilia, inflammatory cells entering dermis	Decrease IgE, IgG, IL4, TARC, Eotaxin; Increase IL12; Reduce expression of Th2 mediated cytokines
Saururis Chinensis Baill	Skin Severity Scores, Scratching Behaviour	Decrease IgE
Lyophyllum Decastes	Skin Severity Scores, Scratching Behaviour	Decrease IgE, IL4, Histamine
Persimmon Leaf Extract	Skin Severity Scores, Transepidermal Water Loss	Decrease IgE, IL4, IL13, Histamine,
Konjac Glucomannan	Skin Severity Scores, Scratching Behaviour	Decrease IgE, Ig, IL4, INFΥ
Gyokuheifusan	Skin Severity Scores	Decrease IgE, IFNΥ/IL4 balance

Table 4. Summary of Treatments Tested in Animal Models

4.2.3 Human clinical trials

When clinical trials are conducted for Atopic Dermatitis subjective symptoms such as erythema and pruritus, must be converted to objective and uniform results so that they may be compared with other studies. The following are some of the most commonly used systems and those employed in the following studies:

Transepidermal Water Loss (TEWL) (Pinnagoda et al., 1990): This is a measure of integrity of stratum corneum's water barrier function; it provides information about the integrity of the skin, which becomes compromised in AD and may be influenced and improved with treatment. It is measured using tewameter, with units expressed as $g/m^2/h$; with improvement indicated by a lower value.

Blood flow volume (BFV) :Measured as a parameter of inflammation using Laser Blood Flow Monitor; Arbitrary unit with improvement indicated by lower values.

Skin Color (a* Value): Erythema quantified by skin color reflectance it is measured using colorimeter

Visual Scoring – Visual judgment made by clinical investigator, scored 0-5

SCORAD (SCORing Atopic Dermatitis) (SCORAD, 1993): Standardized method for reporting dermatitis severity first published in 1993 by the European Task Force on Atopic Dermatitis, allows dermatitis severity to be reported numerically ranging from 0-103.

$$\text{SCORAD Calculation} = A/5 + 7 \, (B/2) + C$$

PARAMETER	TOTAL SCORE
A *SPREAD/BODY SURFACE AREA*	100
Judge based on rule of 9 for body surface area	
B *INTENSITY*	18
Erythema (1-3)	
Edema (1-3)	
Oozing/Crusting (1-3)	
Excoriation (1-3)	
Lichenification (1-3)	
C *SUBJECTIVE SYMPTOMS*	20
Pruritus (1-10)	
Insomnia (1-10)	

Table 5. Parameters for SCORAD Calculation

4.2.4 Human clinical of trials of natural products

WBI-1001 (IPBD: 2-isopropyl-5-[(E)-2-phenylethenyl] benzene-1,3-diol)

This compound is derived from a metabolite of a unique group of bacterial symbiots of entomopathogenic nematodes. It was found to inhibit inflammatory cytokine secretion by activated T cells including: TNFα, INF Y as well as inhibit allergic contact dermatitis in a mouse edema model (Bissonnette *et al.*, 2010). A phase 2A, double blind, vehicle controlled study resulted in statistically significant improvement in SCORAD, pruritus, and the amount of affected body surface area. These improvements were reached after 3-5 weeks of treatment. A 12 week Phase IIb trial was conducted (NCT01098734) as of June 9th 2011, the results are still pending publication.

Konjac Ceramide

Konjac ceramide is the second compound of interest isolated from konjac. Ceramides are a normal component of the lipid membrane, and their deficiency has been suggested as one of the pathological factors resulting in skin barrier disruption (Imokawa *et al.*, 1991), having being previously studied in the treatment of dermatitis (Berardesca *et al.*, 2001). Glucosylceramides are isolated, purified and produced as a nutritional supplement (Kimata, 2006) and oral intake has been found to decrease transepidermal water loss in normal adults (Miyanishi *et al.*, 2005). Konjac due to its high concentration of ceramide was studied for its effect on AD as an oral supplement. Following a 4 week oral feeding trial in 50 children, the SCORAD index was significantly improved when compared to the control group. INFY and IL-12 were significantly increased while IL-4 and IL-13 were decreased indicating a skewing of the cytokine pattern towards a Th1 type. Interestingly in this study, ceramide was found to attenuate allergen specific response to HDM (house dust mite) and JCP (Japanese cedar pollen) by improving skin symptoms and wheal response but had no effect following dermal challenge of Egg white, histamine or buckwheat (Kimata, 2006).

Borage Oil: Gamma-Linolenic Acid

In patients with AD, an abnormality in metabolism of polysaturated fatty acids (PUFA) is commonly observed (Wright, 1991). PUFA are structural components of cell membrane phospholipids which are important in maintaining membrane fluidity (Wright, 1991), as well as being important as precursors for pharmacologically active immunological agents (ie Eicosanoids) (R. Finkel *et al.*, 2009). Borage oil contains a high content (24%) of Υ-linolenic acid (GLA) which is a metabolite of linoleic acid, one of the essential fatty acids. It is postulated an abnormality in essential fatty acid metabolism affects production of GLA and its incorporation into membranes, occurs in AD (Horrobin, 2000; Wright, 1991). Previous studies have shown GLA supplementation lead to improvements in multiple diseases including seborrheic dermatitis in children (Tollesson & Frithz, 1993). In a small Japanese study in a pediatric population, undershirts coated with Borage oil were given to 32 children in a double-blind, placebo controlled study (Kanehara *et al.*, 2007) . After 2 weeks it was found that there was a statistically significant improvement in symptoms of itch and erythema, but no improvement papules, erosions, and trans-epidermal water loss (Kanehara *et al.*, 2007). In a literature review of 12 trials (oral and topical) on the efficacy of Borage Oil in the treatment of AD by Foster *et al.* in 2010 found that 5 studies show statistically significant improvement, while 5 showed borage oil to be ineffective and 2 studies were shown only to have partial response (Foster *et al.*, 2010). The efficacy of borage oil in the treatment of AD remains questionable, a previous product EpoGam used for treatment of AD was removed from market in 2002 in the UK when it was found to be ineffective. This product contained primrose oil which contains lower concentration of GLA then borage oil but was based on the same pathophysiologic principle(H. Williams, 2003). Borage oil while providing some benefit in some studies requires future study to determine its efficacy and it remains to be determine if it will be steroid sparing.

Emollient Therapy

Emollient therapy is a mainstay in the management of the symptoms of AD (Szczepanowska *et al.*, 2008). While studies into the prevention of AD are less common, Simpson *et al.* proposed that 'skin barrier protection from birth using bland emollients is a safe and feasible strategy for AD prevention' (Simpson *et al.*, 2010). This was based on the results from previous studies that found use of petrolatum early in life may be protective against AD development, there was trend towards increased TEWL and skin hydration before development of AD, use of emollients in premature infants protects against skin inflammation and emollients are effective at preventing flares in established AD (Simpson *et al.*, 2010). In 20 high risk infants (based on the ISSAC criteria (Asher *et al.*, 2006)) emollient therapy was initiated in the first week of life in order to maintain intact skin barrier. After 2 years it was found that only 15% of subject developed AD when conservative estimates of high risk infants would be positive for AD in the range of 30-50% suggesting this treatment could have both a protective and preventative effect (Simpson *et al.*, 2010).

Probiotics

Living or inactivated organisms that are claimed to exert beneficial effects on health when ingested are referred to as Probiotics (Schrezenmeir & de Vrese, 2001). The use of probiotic and prebiotics in the field of allergology is a controversial subject, with the results of prenatal and postnatal supplementation for the prevention of atopic dermatitis having mixed results (J. Lee *et al.*, 2008). Probiotic intestinal colonization is theorized to affect the Th1/Th2 immunological maturation prior to the establishment of atopic dermatitis (Gruber *et al.*, 2010). Physiologically the normal gut milieu has an immune system that is balance between protective mucosal immunity and systemic tolerance. In food allergies the balance is impaired and oral tolerance of dietary antigens is not achieved. Risk Factors for the development of food allergy include immature gut barrier and type II Th2 cell skewed cytokine profile are present in early infancy. This may lead to atopic sensitization as antigen uptake is aberrant and Th2 cells further produce IL4 a cytokine essential for B cell differentiation into IgE producing cells and IL5 which is important for eosinophils . Normal bacterial flora at birth is shown to counterbalance the Th2 activity and promote oral tolerance. The predilection of bacteria to promote the differentiation of Th1 cell lineage may be due to specific CpG motif characteristics of bacterial DNA which has been show to induce polycolonal B-cell activation and secretion of Th1 Cytokines IL6, IL12 and interferon Y (Passeron *et al.*, 2006).The guts of infants born in poor areas of developing countries where allergy prevalence is lower, are colonized earlier by enterobacteria, enterococcim lactobacilli, and eubacteria and displays a higher turnover of different E. coli strains in the intestinal microflora ((Matricardi *et al.*, 2003). In a meta-analysis of 21 studies (1997-2007) by Lee *et al.* (2007) containing 1898 subjects looking at Probiotics in the prevention of atopic dermatitis found a risk reduction of 61% in the development of atopic dermatitis in high risk infants (J. Lee *et al.*, 2008). Newer studies have found conflicting results (Boyle *et al.*, 2011) so its use remains controversial. Strains of bacteria that have been investigated include *Lactobacillus rhamnosus GG* (Gruber *et al.*, 2007), *Bifidobacterium lactis (Kukkonen et al., 2007), Mycobacterium vaccae* and others (Matricardi *et al.*, 2003). In studies of the use of the Probiotics following the establishment of AD has been met with mixed results. In one study it was found that while probiotics did improve SCORAD results they were not statistically significant when compared to placebo (Viljanen *et al.*, 2005) . Other studies have shown the probiotics following established AD in children did improve SCORAD (Passeron *et al.*, 2006) .

St. John's Wort Cream

St. John Wort is a family of plants with worldwide distribution accounting for about 370 species. It has been use as a herbal treatment for depression (Rapaport *et al.*, 2011), ADHD (Chan, 2008) and other psychological condition, however without proven clinical effects. It has been traditionally used for the topical treatment of wounds, burns, nerve lesions and has used as a remedy for eczematous skin conditions (Schempp *et al.*, 2000). Hypericin is a major component of St. John wort and has been found to have bioactive properties exhibiting dose dependent photosensitizing activity (Schempp *et al.*, 2000). Hyperforin, a second compound, was found to have anti-bacterial activity (Gurevich *et al.*, 1971). After a 7 day topical trial, the treatment compound was found to significantly improved SCORAD scores. Colony forming units of *S. aureus* were measured, and found to be decreased by the treatment compound when compared to control, however not significantly. No molecular markers of inflammation were measure in this study.

Herbal Preparations – Traditional Chinese Medicine

Multiple trials have been conducted using formulas of traditional Chinese medicine. These formulas have a long history of use and documentation within their medical systems. The difficulty in investigating these compounds are due to the manner of preparation and individuality of the treatment. In a 2007 study by Hon *et al.* of a five herb formulation (*Flos lonicerae, Herba menthae, Cortex moutan, Rhizoma atractylodis, Cortex phellodendri*) in a placebo controlled 12 week oral feeding trial found that while the treatment group and placebo group both improved symptoms there was no statistically significance between the two. However in the treatment group, the number of days of corticosteroids use during the month was significantly decreased, improving the quality of life of the subject (Hon *et al.*, 2007). In a follow up study it was found the formulation suppressed brain-derived neurotrophic factor (BDNF), Thymus and activation regulated chemokine (TARC), INF-Υ, and TNFα (Leung *et al.*, 2008).

COMPOUND	PARAMETER IMPROVEMENT	MOLECULAR IMPROVEMENTS
WBI-1001	SCORAD, Pruritus, Body Surface Area	Inhibited TNFα, Increased INF Υ
Konjac Ceramide	SCORAD, Transepidermal Water loss, Allergen specific response	Increased INFΥ, IL12; Decreased IL4, IL13
Borage Oil	SCORAD?, Itch, Erythema	Metabolism of PUFA
Emollient Therapy	Prevention of AD	
Probiotics		
St. John's Wort Cream	SCORAD, Decreased *Staph. Aureus* CFUs	
TCM		

Table 6. Summary of Treatments Tested in Human Clinical Trials

4.2.5 Approved compounds

The calcineurin inhibitors are among the most recent example of natural products that had been identified having potential biological activity, then successfully proceeded through the clinical trial phase and have been approved for use in the treatment of AD and other dermatological hypersensitivity conditions. The following natural product concoction is the most recent treatment approved for use in AD by the FDA. Using an understanding of the pathophysiology of AD, compounds were selected that targeted different facets of the pathology to work in concert in the treatment of AD.

Atopiclair MAS063D (Atopiclair)

Hydrolipidic cream developed for the management of Atopic dermatitis, containing moisturizing elements and natural products (Belloni *et al.*, 2005): The agent contains a combination of the bioactive compounds from *Vitis vinifera*, glycyrrhetinic acid and Hyaluronic acid. Hyaluronic acid is barrier forming and hydrating agent, traditionally used as lubricant in surgery (Manuskiatti & Maibach, 1996). It is a naturally occurring glycosaminoglycan in the body found in healthy connective tissue and induces tissue hydration (traditionally used as lubricant in other areas of medicine – ocular surgery, orthopedic surgery). Telmesterine and extracts from *vitis viniferia* have been found to have anti protease activities, (inhibiting harmful enzymes that exuded by damaged skin; and antioxidant effects protecting against free radicals (Belloni *et al.*, 2005). Procyanidins found in *vitis viniferia* have been examined at the vascular endothelium, where they help to prevent oxidative damage, they also form a barrier to protect against elastase, collagenase, hyaluronidase, and B-glucuronidase. Glycyrrhetinic acid is a compound found to have anti-inflammatory activity (Teelucksingh *et al.*, 1990) In 2003, the first vehicle controlled, double blind study of Atopiclair was conducted in a study group of 20 subjects with contact dermatitis. Subjects applied vehicle to one arm and treatment compound to the other and were measured at 24, 48 and 72 hours. Results from this compound were promising, with significant improvements in Transepidermal water loss (by 50%), Blood flow volume, Skin color, Visual Scoring. Only itch magnitude results fell below significance but showed improvement (Hongbo Zhai, 2003). In a follow up study in 2004, Atopiclair was tested in patients with Atopic Dermatitis and found significant improvement in all patients after 22 days. Statistically significant improvements were measure in total body surface area affected, Itch score, SCORAD value, and Quality of sleep. In an informal survery following the study 93% of subjects responded positively to the product (Belloni et al., 2005). Following this study Atopiclair was approved by the FDA for the use in the treatment of atopic dermatitis (Abramovitis & Perlmutter, 2007).

5. Conclusions

Natural Products have been identified as potential sources of bioactive compounds used in the treatment of immune disorders. Historically some of the major and most important pharmaceutical compounds have their origin as natural products (Newman & Cragg, 2007). Penicillin, discovered as a metabolite of mold in a petri dish, revolutionized the manner in which medicine has been practiced since wide spread implementation following World War II (R. Finkel et al., 2009). Many of the classes of treatment compounds currently being used in immunology and dermatology have originated from natural products. It might hold true that the next revolutionary treatment might likewise have its origin from the natural world, potentially being already explored by patients looking into CAMs.

It is inevitable that nature will continue to provide pharmaceutical active compounds that will be used in all practices and disciplines of medicine. It is those conducting the exploration for these compounds to keep an open mind to the possibility that an already employed alternative medicine might provide the next clue or even a source unknown.

6. References

Abramovitis, W, & Perlmutter, A. (2007). Atopiclair: its position within a topical paradigm for the treatment of atopic dermatitis. *Expert Rev. Dermatol, 2*(2), 115-119.

Allan, K., & Devereux, G. (2011). Diet and asthma: nutrition implications from prevention to treatment. *J Am Diet Assoc, 111*(2), 258-268.

Asher, M. I., Montefort, S., Bjorksten, B., Lai, C. K., Strachan, D. P., Weiland, S. K., et al. (2006). Worldwide time trends in the prevalence of symptoms of asthma, allergic rhinoconjunctivitis, and eczema in childhood: ISAAC Phases One and Three repeat multicountry cross-sectional surveys. *Lancet, 368*(9537), 733-743.

Assmann, T., Homey, B., & Ruzicka, T. (2000). Applications of tacrolimus for the treatment of skin disorders. *Immunopharmacology, 47*(2-3), 203-213.

Barnes, P.M., Bloom, B., & Nahin, R.L. (2008). Complementary and alternative medicine use among adults and children: United States, 2007. *Natl Health Stat Report*(12), 1-23.

Barnes, P.M., Powell-Griner, E., McFann, K., & Nahin, R.L. (2004). Complementary and alternative medicine use among adults: United States, 2002. *Adv Data*(343), 1-19.

Belloni, G., Pinelli, S., & Veraldi, S. (2005). A randomised, double-blind, vehicle-controlled study to evaluate the efficacy and safety of MAS063D (Atopiclair) in the treatment of mild to moderate atopic dermatitis. *Eur J Dermatol, 15*(1), 31-36.

Berardesca, E., Barbareschi, M., Veraldi, S., & Pimpinelli, N. (2001). Evaluation of efficacy of a skin lipid mixture in patients with irritant contact dermatitis, allergic contact dermatitis or atopic dermatitis: a multicenter study. *Contact Dermatitis, 45*(5), 280-285.

Bissonnette, R., Chen, G., Bolduc, C., Maari, C., Lyle, M., Tang, L., et al. (2010). Efficacy and safety of topical WBI-1001 in the treatment of atopic dermatitis: results from a phase 2A, randomized, placebo-controlled clinical trial. *Arch Dermatol, 146*(4), 446-449.

Bolognia, Jean, Jorizzo, Joseph L., & Rapini, Ronald P. (2008). *Dermatology* (2nd ed. / edited by Jean L. Bolognia, Joseph L. Jorizzo, Ronald P. Rapini ; associate and artwork editor, Julie V. Schaffer. ed.). St. Louis, Mo. ; London: Mosby Elsevier.

Boyle, R. J., Ismail, I. H., Kivivuori, S., Licciardi, P. V., Robins-Browne, R. M., Mah, L. J., et al. (2011). Lactobacillus GG treatment during pregnancy for the prevention of eczema: a randomized controlled trial. *Allergy, 66*(4), 509-516.

Brems, C., Johnson, M. E., Warner, T. D., & Roberts, L. W. (2006). Patient requests and provider suggestions for alternative treatments as reported by rural and urban care providers. *Complement Ther Med, 14*(1), 10-19.

Burkitt, D. P. (1971a). Epidemiology of cancer of the colon and rectum. *Cancer, 28*(1), 3-13.

Burkitt, D. P. (1971b). Possible relationships between bowel cancer and dietary habits. *Proc R Soc Med, 64*(9), 964-965.

Chan, E. (2008). St. John's Wort does not show benefit for ADHD in short trial. *J Pediatr, 153*(5), 724.

Chang, H. H., Chen, C. S., & Lin, J. Y. (2009). High dose vitamin C supplementation increases the Th1/Th2 cytokine secretion ratio, but decreases eosinophilic infiltration in bronchoalveolar lavage fluid of ovalbumin-sensitized and challenged mice. *J Agric Food Chem, 57*(21), 10471-10476.

Chida, Y., Steptoe, A., Hirakawa, N., Sudo, N., & Kubo, C. (2007). The effects of psychological intervention on atopic dermatitis. A systematic review and meta-analysis. *Int Arch Allergy Immunol, 144*(1), 1-9.

Choi, M. S., Kim, E. C., Lee, H. S., Kim, S. K., Choi, H. M., Park, J. H., et al. (2008). Inhibitory effects of Saururus chinensis (LOUR.) BAILL on the development of atopic dermatitis-like skin lesions in NC/Nga mice. *Biol Pharm Bull, 31*(1), 51-56.

Cohen, J. S. (2006). Risks of troglitazone apparent before approval in USA. *Diabetologia, 49*(6), 1454-1455.

Corbin Winslow, L., & Shapiro, H. (2002). Physicians want education about complementary and alternative medicine to enhance communication with their patients. *Arch Intern Med, 162*(10), 1176-1181.

Corin, R. E. (2000). Nedocromil sodium: a review of the evidence for a dual mechanism of action. *Clin Exp Allergy, 30*(4), 461-468.

Custovic, A., Simpson, A., Chapman, M. D., & Woodcock, A. (1998). Allergen avoidance in the treatment of asthma and atopic disorders. *Thorax, 53*(1), 63-72.

D'Acquisto, F., May, M. J., & Ghosh, S. (2002). Inhibition of nuclear factor kappa B (NF-B): an emerging theme in anti-inflammatory therapies. *Mol Interv, 2*(1), 22-35.

David, M., Hodak, E., & Lowe, N. J. (1988). Adverse effects of retinoids. *Med Toxicol Adverse Drug Exp, 3*(4), 273-288.

Del Rosso, J., & Friedlander, S. F. (2005). Corticosteroids: options in the era of steroid-sparing therapy. *J Am Acad Dermatol, 53*(1 Suppl 1), S50-58.

Devereaux, P. J., & Yusuf, S. (2003). The evolution of the randomized controlled trial and its role in evidence-based decision making. *J Intern Med, 254*(2), 105-113.

DiMasi, J. A., Hansen, R. W., & Grabowski, H. G. (2003). The price of innovation: new estimates of drug development costs. *J Health Econ, 22*(2), 151-185.

Dixon, Anna, Riesberg, Annette, Weinbrenner, Susanne, Saka, Omer, Grand, Julian Le, & Busse, Reinhard. (2003). Complementary and Alternative Medicine in the UK and Germany: *Research and Evidence on Supply and Demand* (pp. 128). London: Anglo-German Foundation for the Study of Industrial Society

Eisenberg, D. M., Davis, R. B., Ettner, S. L., Appel, S., Wilkey, S., Van Rompay, M., et al. (1998). Trends in alternative medicine use in the United States, 1990-1997: results of a follow-up national survey. *JAMA, 280*(18), 1569-1575.

Elzaawely, A. A., Xuan, T. D., & Tawata, S. (2005). Antioxidant and antibacterial activities of Rumex japonicus HOUTT. Aerial parts. *Biol Pharm Bull, 28*(12), 2225-2230.

Ernst, E. (2000). The usage of complementary therapies by dermatological patients: a systematic review. *Br J Dermatol, 142*(5), 857-861.

Fang, S. P., Tanaka, T., Tago, F., Okamoto, T., & Kojima, S. (2005). Immunomodulatory effects of gyokuheifusan on INF-gamma/IL-4 (Th1/Th2) balance in ovalbumin (OVA)-induced asthma model mice. *Biol Pharm Bull, 28*(5), 829-833.

Finch, J., Munhutu, M. N., & Whitaker-Worth, D. L. (2010). Atopic dermatitis and nutrition. *Clin Dermatol, 28*(6), 605-614.

Finkel, R., Clark, M., & Cubeddu, L. (2009). *Pharmacology* (4th ed.). Philadelphia: Lippincott Williams & Wilkins.

Finkel, Richard. (2009). *Pharmacology* (4th ed.). Baltimore: Lippincott Williams & Wilkins.

Fisher, P., & Ward, A. (1994). Complementary medicine in Europe. *BMJ, 309*(6947), 107-111.

Foster, R. H., Hardy, G., & Alany, R. G. (2010). Borage oil in the treatment of atopic dermatitis. *Nutrition, 26*(7-8), 708-718.

Gale, E. A. (2006). Troglitazone: the lesson that nobody learned? *Diabetologia, 49*(1), 1-6.

Gavin, J. A., & Boon, H. (2005). CAM in Canada: places, practices, research. *Complement Ther Clin Pract, 11*(1), 21-27.

Grassberger, M., Baumruker, T., Enz, A., Hiestand, P., Hultsch, T., Kalthoff, F., et al. (1999). A novel anti-inflammatory drug, SDZ ASM 981, for the treatment of skin diseases: in vitro pharmacology. *Br J Dermatol, 141*(2), 264-273.

Grassberger, M., Steinhoff, M., Schneider, D., & Luger, T. A. (2004). Pimecrolimus -- an anti-inflammatory drug targeting the skin. *Exp Dermatol, 13*(12), 721-730.

Gruber, C., van Stuijvenberg, M., Mosca, F., Moro, G., Chirico, G., Braegger, C. P., et al. (2010). Reduced occurrence of early atopic dermatitis because of immunoactive prebiotics among low-atopy-risk infants. *J Allergy Clin Immunol, 126*(4), 791-797.

Gruber, C., Wendt, M., Sulser, C., Lau, S., Kulig, M., Wahn, U., et al. (2007). Randomized, placebo-controlled trial of Lactobacillus rhamnosus GG as treatment of atopic dermatitis in infancy. *Allergy, 62*(11), 1270-1276.

Gurevich, A. I., Dobrynin, V. N., Kolosov, M. N., Popravko, S. A., & Riabova, I. D. (1971). [Antibiotic hyperforin from Hypericum perforatum L]. *Antibiotiki, 16*(6), 510-513.

Hanifin, J. M., & Rajka, G. (1980). Diagnositic features of atopic dermatitis. *Acta Derm Venereol (Stockh), Suppl 92*, 44-47.

Hanifin, J. M., Schneider, L. C., Leung, D. Y., Ellis, C. N., Jaffe, H. S., Izu, A. E., et al. (1993). Recombinant interferon gamma therapy for atopic dermatitis. *J Am Acad Dermatol, 28*(2 Pt 1), 189-197.

Harris, P., & Rees, R. (2000). The prevalence of complementary and alternative medicine use among the general population: a systematic review of the literature. *Complement Ther Med, 8*(2), 88-96.

Herman, S. M., & Vender, R. B. (2003). Antihistamines in the treatment of dermatitis. *J Cutan Med Surg, 7*(6), 467-473.

Hon, K. L., Leung, T. F., Ng, P. C., Lam, M. C., Kam, W. Y., Wong, K. Y., et al. (2007). Efficacy and tolerability of a Chinese herbal medicine concoction for treatment of atopic dermatitis: a randomized, double-blind, placebo-controlled study. *Br J Dermatol, 157*(2), 357-363.

Hongbo Zhai, Clarissa D Villarama, Zeba Hasan Hafeez, Howard I Maiback. (2003). Efficacy of a Topical Agent, MAS063D ('Atopiclair'), in the Treatment of Sodium Lauryl Sulphate-Induced Irritant Contact Dermatitis. *Exog Dermatol, 2*, 301-305.

Horrobin, D. F. (2000). Essential fatty acid metabolism and its modification in atopic eczema. *Am J Clin Nutr, 71*(1 Suppl), 367S-372S.

Imokawa, G., Abe, A., Jin, K., Higaki, Y., Kawashima, M., & Hidano, A. (1991). Decreased level of ceramides in stratum corneum of atopic dermatitis: an etiologic factor in atopic dry skin? *J Invest Dermatol, 96*(4), 523-526.

Ishiguro, K., & Oku, H. (1997). Antipruritic Effect of Flavonol and 1,4-Naphthoquinone Derivatives form *Impatiens balsamina* L. *Phytotherapy Research, 11*, 343-347.

Jauregui, I., Ferrer, M., Montoro, J., Davila, I., Bartra, J., del Cuvillo, A., et al. (2007). Antihistamines in the treatment of chronic urticaria. *J Investig Allergol Clin Immunol, 17 Suppl 2*, 41-52.

Kaitin, K. I., & DiMasi, J. A. (2011). Pharmaceutical innovation in the 21st century: new drug approvals in the first decade, 2000-2009. *Clin Pharmacol Ther, 89*(2), 183-188.

Kanehara, S., Ohtani, T., Uede, K., & Furukawa, F. (2007). Clinical effects of undershirts coated with borage oil on children with atopic dermatitis: a double-blind, placebo-controlled clinical trial. *J Dermatol, 34*(12), 811-815.

Karha, J., & Topol, E. J. (2004). The sad story of Vioxx, and what we should learn from it. *Cleve Clin J Med, 71*(12), 933-934, 936, 938-939.

Kiebert, G., Sorensen, S. V., Revicki, D., Fagan, S. C., Doyle, J. J., Cohen, J., et al. (2002). Atopic dermatitis is associated with a decrement in health-related quality of life. *Int J Dermatol, 41*(3), 151-158.

Kim, J. Y., Lee, I. K., Son, M. W., & Kim, K. H. (2009). Effects of orally administered Actinidia arguta (Hardy Kiwi) fruit extract on 2-chloro-1,3,5-trinitrobenzene-induced atopic dermatitis-like skin lesions in NC/Nga mice. *J Med Food, 12*(5), 1004-1015.

Kimata, H. (2006). Improvement of atopic dermatitis and reduction of skin allergic responses by oral intake of konjac ceramide. *Pediatr Dermatol, 23*(4), 386-389.

Kotani, M., Matsumoto, M., Fujita, A., Higa, S., Wang, W., Suemura, M., et al. (2000). Persimmon leaf extract and astragalin inhibit development of dermatitis and IgE elevation in NC/Nga mice. *J Allergy Clin Immunol, 106*(1 Pt 1), 159-166.

Kukkonen, K., Savilahti, E., Haahtela, T., Juntunen-Backman, K., Korpela, R., Poussa, T., et al. (2007). Probiotics and prebiotic galacto-oligosaccharides in the prevention of allergic diseases: a randomized, double-blind, placebo-controlled trial. *J Allergy Clin Immunol, 119*(1), 192-198.

Kurtz, M. E., Nolan, R. B., & Rittinger, W. J. (2003). Primary care physicians' attitudes and practices regarding complementary and alternative medicine. *J Am Osteopath Assoc, 103*(12), 597-602.

Lane, J. E., Cheyney, J. M., Lane, T. N., Kent, D. E., & Cohen, D. J. (2006). Treatment of recalcitrant atopic dermatitis with omalizumab. *J Am Acad Dermatol, 54*(1), 68-72.

Lee, H. S., Kim, S. K., Han, J. B., Choi, H. M., Park, J. H., Kim, E. C., et al. (2006). Inhibitory effects of Rumex japonicus Houtt. on the development of atopic dermatitis-like skin lesions in NC/Nga mice. *Br J Dermatol, 155*(1), 33-38.

Lee, J., Seto, D., & Bielory, L. (2008). Meta-analysis of clinical trials of probiotics for prevention and treatment of pediatric atopic dermatitis. *J Allergy Clin Immunol, 121*(1), 116-121 e111.

Lee, Y.S., Baek, Y.I., Kim, J.R., Cho, H.K., Sok, D.E., & Jeong, H.S. (2004). Antioxidant activities of a new lignan and a neolignan from *Saururus chinensisis. Bioorganic & Medicinal Chemistry Letters, 14*, 5623-5628.

Leung, T. F., Wong, K. Y., Wong, C. K., Fung, K. P., Lam, C. W., Fok, T. F., et al. (2008). In vitro and clinical immunomodulatory effects of a novel Pentaherbs concoction for atopic dermatitis. *Br J Dermatol, 158*(6), 1216-1223.

Levine, S. M., Weber-Levine, M. L., & Mayberry, R. M. (2003). Complementary and alternative medical practices: training, experience, and attitudes of a primary care medical school faculty. *J Am Board Fam Pract, 16*(4), 318-326.

Li, J. T. (2002). Allergy testing. *Am Fam Physician, 66*(4), 621-624.

Lim, B., Yamada, K., Nonaka, M., Kuramoto, Y., Hung, P., & Sugano, M. (1997). Dietary fibers modulate indices of intestinal immune function in rats. *J Nutr, 127*(5), 663-667.

M Kotani, A Fujita, T Tanaka. (1999). Inhibitory effects of persimmon leaf extract on allergic reaction in human basophilic leukemic cells and mice. *J Jpn Soc Nutr Food Sci, 52*, 147-151.

Manuskiatti, W., & Maibach, H. I. (1996). Hyaluronic acid and skin: wound healing and aging. *Int J Dermatol, 35*(8), 539-544.

Matricardi, P., Bjorksten, B., Bonini, S., Bousquet, J., Djukanovic, R., Dreborg, S., et al. (2003). Microbial products in allergy prevention and therapy. *Allergy, 58*(6), 461-471.

Matsuda, H., Watanabe, N., Geba, G. P., Sperl, J., Tsudzuki, M., Hiroi, J., et al. (1997). Development of atopic dermatitis-like skin lesion with IgE hyperproduction in NC/Nga mice. *Int Immunol, 9*(3), 461-466.

Matsumoto, M., Kotani, M., Fujita, A., Higa, S., Kishimoto, T., Suemura, M., et al. (2002). Oral administration of persimmon leaf extract ameliorates skin symptoms and transepidermal water loss in atopic dermatitis model mice, NC/Nga. *Br J Dermatol, 146*(2), 221-227.

Metcalfe, A., Williams, J., McChesney, J., Patten, S. B., & Jette, N. (2010). Use of complementary and alternative medicine by those with a chronic disease and the general population--results of a national population based survey. *BMC Complement Altern Med, 10*, 58.

Milden, S. P., & Stokols, D. (2004). Physicians' attitudes and practices regarding complementary and alternative medicine. *Behav Med, 30*(2), 73-82.

Miller, Alicia D, & Eichenfield, Lawrence F. (2006). Evolving management of atopic dermatitis. *Expert Review of Dermatology, 1*(1), 31-41.

Miyanishi, K., Shiono, N., Shirai, H., Dombo, M., & Kimata, H. (2005). Reduction of transepidermal water loss by oral intake of glucosylceramides in patients with atopic eczema. *Allergy, 60*(11), 1454-1455.

Molassiotis, A., Fernadez-Ortega, P., Pud, D., Ozden, G., Scott, J. A., Panteli, V., et al. (2005). Use of complementary and alternative medicine in cancer patients: a European survey. *Ann Oncol, 16*(4), 655-663.

Montoro, J., Sastre, J., Jauregui, I., Bartra, J., Davila, I., del Cuvillo, A., et al. (2007). Allergic rhinitis: continuous or on demand antihistamine therapy? *J Investig Allergol Clin Immunol, 17 Suppl 2*, 21-27.

Nakatsukasa, Hiroko, Tago, Fumitoshi, Okamoto, Takuya, Tsukimoto, Mitsutoshi, & Kojima, Shuji. (2009). Therapeutic Effects of Gyokuheifusan on NC/Nga Mouse Model of Allergic Dermatitis. *Journal of Health Science, 55*(4), 516-524.

NCCAM. (2011). *Exploring the science of complementary and alternative medicine : third strategic plan, 2011-2015.* Bethesda, Md.: U.S. Dept. of Health and Human Services, National Institutes of Health.

Newman, D. J., & Cragg, G. M. (2007). Natural products as sources of new drugs over the last 25 years. *J Nat Prod, 70*(3), 461-477.

Onishi, N., Kawamoto, S., Nishimura, M., Nakano, T., Aki, T., Shigeta, S., et al. (2004). The ability of konjac-glucomannan to suppress spontaneously occurring dermatitis in NC/Nga mice depends upon the particle size. *Biofactors, 21*(1-4), 163-166.

Onishi, N., Kawamoto, S., Nishimura, M., Nakano, T., Aki, T., Shigeta, S., et al. (2005). A new immunomodulatory function of low-viscous konjac glucomannan with a small particle size: its oral intake suppresses spontaneously occurring dermatitis in NC/Nga mice. *Int Arch Allergy Immunol, 136*(3), 258-265.

Onishi, N., Kawamoto, S., Suzuki, H., Santo, H., Aki, T., Shigeta, S., et al. (2007). Dietary pulverized konjac glucomannan suppresses scratching behavior and skin inflammatory immune responses in NC/Nga mice. *Int Arch Allergy Immunol, 144*(2), 95-104.

Onishi, N., Kawamoto, S., Ueda, K., Yamanaka, Y., Katayama, A., Suzuki, H., et al. (2007). Dietary pulverized konjac glucomannan prevents the development of allergic rhinitis-like symptoms and IgE response in mice. *Biosci Biotechnol Biochem, 71*(10), 2551-2556.

Oomizu, S., Onishi, N., Suzuki, H., Ueda, K., Mochizuki, M., Morimoto, K., et al. (2006). Oral administration of pulverized Konjac glucomannan prevents the increase of plasma immunoglobulin E and immunoglobulin G levels induced by the injection of syngeneic keratinocyte extracts in BALB/c mice. *Clin Exp Allergy, 36*(1), 102-110.

Pagan, J. A., & Pauly, M. V. (2005). Access to conventional medical care and the use of complementary and alternative medicine. *Health Aff (Millwood), 24*(1), 255-262.

Park, E. J., Kim, B., Eo, H., Park, K., Kim, Y., Lee, H. J., et al. (2005). Control of IgE and selective T(H)1 and T(H)2 cytokines by PG102 isolated from Actinidia arguta. *J Allergy Clin Immunol, 116*(5), 1151-1157.

Park, E. J., Park, K. C., Eo, H., Seo, J., Son, M., Kim, K. H., et al. (2007). Suppression of spontaneous dermatitis in NC/Nga murine model by PG102 isolated from Actinidia arguta. *J Invest Dermatol, 127*(5), 1154-1160.

Passeron, T., Lacour, J. P., Fontas, E., & Ortonne, J. P. (2006). Prebiotics and synbiotics: two promising approaches for the treatment of atopic dermatitis in children above 2 years. *Allergy, 61*(4), 431-437.

Peroni, D. G., Piacentini, G. L., Bodini, A., Rigotti, E., Pigozzi, R., & Boner, A. L. (2008). Prevalence and risk factors for atopic dermatitis in preschool children. *Br J Dermatol, 158*(3), 539-543.

Pinnagoda, J., Tupker, R. A., Agner, T., & Serup, J. (1990). Guidelines for transepidermal water loss (TEWL) measurement. A report from the Standardization Group of the European Society of Contact Dermatitis. *Contact Dermatitis, 22*(3), 164-178.

Presta, L. G., Lahr, S. J., Shields, R. L., Porter, J. P., Gorman, C. M., Fendly, B. M., et al. (1993). Humanization of an antibody directed against IgE. *J Immunol, 151*(5), 2623-2632.

Rapaport, M. H., Nierenberg, A. A., Howland, R., Dording, C., Schettler, P. J., & Mischoulon, D. (2011). The treatment of minor depression with St. John's Wort or citalopram: Failure to show benefit over placebo. *J Psychiatr Res, 45*(7), 931-941.

Rawson, N. S. (2000). Time required for approval of new drugs in Canada, Australia, Sweden, the United Kingdom and the United States in 1996-1998. *CMAJ, 162*(4), 501-504.

Sakuma, S., Higashi, Y., Sato, N., Sasakawa, T., Sengoku, T., Ohkubo, Y., et al. (2001). Tacrolimus suppressed the production of cytokines involved in atopic dermatitis by direct stimulation of human PBMC system. (Comparison with steroids). *Int Immunopharmacol, 1*(6), 1219-1226.

Salameh, F., Perla, D., Solomon, M., Gamus, D., Barzilai, A., Greenberger, S., et al. (2008). The effectiveness of combined Chinese herbal medicine and acupuncture in the treatment of atopic dermatitis. *J Altern Complement Med, 14*(8), 1043-1048.

Scalbert, A., & Williamson, G. (2000). Dietary intake and bioavailability of polyphenols. *J Nutr, 130*(8S Suppl), 2073S-2085S.

Schachner, L., Field, T., Hernandez-Reif, M., Duarte, A. M., & Krasnegor, J. (1998). Atopic dermatitis symptoms decreased in children following massage therapy. *Pediatr Dermatol, 15*(5), 390-395.

Schafer, T. (2004). Epidemiology of complementary alternative medicine for asthma and allergy in Europe and Germany. *Ann Allergy Asthma Immunol, 93*(2 Suppl 1), S5-10.

Schafer, T., Riehle, A., Wichmann, H. E., & Ring, J. (2002). Alternative medicine in allergies - prevalence, patterns of use, and costs. *Allergy, 57*(8), 694-700.

Schempp, C. M., Ludtke, R., Winghofer, B., & Simon, J. C. (2000). Effect of topical application of Hypericum perforatum extract (St. John's wort) on skin sensitivity to solar simulated radiation. *Photodermatol Photoimmunol Photomed, 16*(3), 125-128.

Schmitt, J., Meurer, M., Schwanebeck, U., Grahlert, X., & Schakel, K. (2008). Treatment following an evidence-based algorithm versus individualised symptom-oriented treatment for atopic eczema. A randomised controlled trial. *Dermatology, 217*(4), 299-308.

Schrezenmeir, J., & de Vrese, M. (2001). Probiotics, prebiotics, and synbiotics--approaching a definition. *Am J Clin Nutr, 73*(2 Suppl), 361S-364S.

SCORAD. (1993). Severity scoring of atopic dermatitis: the SCORAD index. Consensus Report of the European Task Force on Atopic Dermatitis. *Dermatology, 186*(1), 23-31.

Sewitch, M. J., & Rajput, Y. (2010). A literature review of complementary and alternative medicine use by colorectal cancer patients. *Complement Ther Clin Pract, 16*(1), 52-56.

Simpson, E. L., Berry, T. M., Brown, P. A., & Hanifin, J. M. (2010). A pilot study of emollient therapy for the primary prevention of atopic dermatitis. *J Am Acad Dermatol, 63*(4), 587-593.

Sirois, F. M., & Gick, M. L. (2002). An investigation of the health beliefs and motivations of complementary medicine clients. *Soc Sci Med, 55*(6), 1025-1037.

Spergel, J. M., & Leung, D. Y. (2006). Safety of topical calcineurin inhibitors in atopic dermatitis: evaluation of the evidence. *Curr Allergy Asthma Rep, 6*(4), 270-274.

Stevens, S. R., Hanifin, J. M., Hamilton, T., Tofte, S. J., & Cooper, K. D. (1998). Long-term effectiveness and safety of recombinant human interferon gamma therapy for atopic dermatitis despite unchanged serum IgE levels. *Arch Dermatol, 134*(7), 799-804.

Streiner, DL , & Normam, GL. (2009). Drug Trial Phases. *Community Oncology, 6*(1), 36-40.

Strunk, R. C., & Bloomberg, G. R. (2006). Omalizumab for asthma. *N Engl J Med, 354*(25), 2689-2695.

Su, D., & Li, L. (2011). Trends in the use of complementary and alternative medicine in the United States: 2002-2007. *J Health Care Poor Underserved, 22*(1), 296-310.

Suto, H., Matsuda, H., Mitsuishi, K., Hira, K., Uchida, T., Unno, T., et al. (1999). NC/Nga mice: a mouse model for atopic dermatitis. *Int Arch Allergy Immunol, 120 Suppl 1*, 70-75.

Szczepanowska, J., Reich, A., & Szepietowski, J. C. (2008). Emollients improve treatment results with topical corticosteroids in childhood atopic dermatitis: a randomized comparative study. *Pediatr Allergy Immunol, 19*(7), 614-618.

Teelucksingh, S., Mackie, A. D., Burt, D., McIntyre, M. A., Brett, L., & Edwards, C. R. (1990). Potentiation of hydrocortisone activity in skin by glycyrrhetinic acid. *Lancet, 335*(8697), 1060-1063.

Tollesson, A., & Frithz, A. (1993). Borage oil, an effective new treatment for infantile seborrhoeic dermatitis. *Br J Dermatol, 129*(1), 95.

Ukawa, Y., Ito, H., & Hisamatsu, M. (2000). Antitumor effects of (1-->3)-beta-D-glucan and (1-->6)-beta-D-glucan purified from newly cultivated mushroom, Hatakeshimeji (Lyophyllum decastes Sing.). *J Biosci Bioeng, 90*(1), 98-104.

Ukawa, Y., Izumi, Y., Ohbuchi, T., Takahashi, T., Ikemizu, S., & Kojima, Y. (2007). Oral administration of the extract from Hatakeshimeji (Lyophyllum decastes sing.) mushroom inhibits the development of atopic dermatitis-like skin lesions in NC/Nga mice. *J Nutr Sci Vitaminol (Tokyo), 53*(3), 293-296.

Υσηα Ρανι, ΜΥΡ Ναιδι. (2009). Phase 0 - Microdosing strategy in clinical trials. *Indian Journal of Pharmacology, 40*(6), 240-242.

Vestergaard, C., Yoneyama, H., Murai, M., Nakamura, K., Tamaki, K., Terashima, Y., et al. (1999). Overproduction of Th2-specific chemokines in NC/Nga mice exhibiting atopic dermatitis-like lesions. *J Clin Invest, 104*(8), 1097-1105.

Viljanen, M., Savilahti, E., Haahtela, T., Juntunen-Backman, K., Korpela, R., Poussa, T., et al. (2005). Probiotics in the treatment of atopic eczema/dermatitis syndrome in infants: a double-blind placebo-controlled trial. *Allergy, 60*(4), 494-500.

Wallach, D., Coste, J., Tilles, G., & Taieb, A. (2005). The first images of atopic dermatitis: an attempt at retrospective diagnosis in dermatology. *J Am Acad Dermatol, 53*(4), 684-689.

WHO. (2005). *National policy on traditional medicine and regulation of herbal medicines : report of a WHO global survey*. Geneva: World Health Organization.

Wichers, H. (2009). Immunomodulation by food: promising concept for mitigating allergic disease? *Anal Bioanal Chem, 395*(1), 37-45.

Wiles, J., & Rosenberg, M. W. (2001). 'Gentle caring experience'. Seeking alternative health care in Canada. *Health Place, 7*(3), 209-224.

Williams, H. (1992). Is the prevalence of atopic dermatitis increasing? *Clin Exp Dermatol, 17*(6), 385-391.

Williams, H. . (2003). Evening primrose oil for atopic dermatitis. *BMJ, 327*(7428), 1358-1359.

Wise, F., & Sulzberger, MG. (1933). *In Year Book of Dermatology and Syphiolology*.

World Health Organization. (2009). *Report of the WHO Interregional Workshop on the Use of Traditional Medicine in Primary Health Care : Ulaanbaatar, Mongolia, 23-26 August 2007*. Geneva: World Health Organization.

Wright, S. (1991). Essential fatty acids and the skin. *Br J Dermatol, 125*(6), 503-515.

7

Specific Immunotherapy and Central Immune System

Celso Pereira, Graça Loureiro, Beatriz Tavares and Filomena Botelho
Immunoallergology Department, Coimbra University Hospital,
Portugal

1. Introduction

Despite the current knowledge, the mechanisms by which the specific immunotherapy (SIT) achieves clinical improvement remains unclear. However, it is now clear that the immune tolerance is one of the major targets of this kind of treatment. Immune tolerance depends on different mechanisms, including T-cell anergy, T-cell depletion by apoptosis, and active immune suppression (Akdis & Akdis, 2011). One of the goals of SIT is the induction of tolerance to allergens to which the patient is sensitized. IL-10 is probably a relevant cytokine induced by this treatment and is associated to regulatory T cells (T-regs) that actively control or suppress the function of other cells, generally in an inhibitory pattern (Frew, 2010).

The changes in microenvironment due to the decrease in histamine and PGE2 release by mast cell, and the IL-10 and TGF-β release by dendritic cells (DC) could switch the T-cell population into T-regs. These alterations will then lead to tolerance (Schmidt-Weber & Blaser 2005).

Much of the knowledge about SIT has been based on studies using subcutaneous route of administration (SCIT), but increasing data is now available based on studies using sublingual immunotherapy (SLIT).

The sublingual mucosa, where the deposition of the extract occurs, has very particular characteristics, quite different from the cellular subcutaneous tissue. The dendritic cells present in the buccal region are distinct from the Langerhans cells present in the skin. These cells present, constitutively, receptors with high affinity for IgE, FcεRI+, MHC class I and II molecules, as well as co-stimulation molecules, namely CD40, CD80/B7.1 and CD86/B7.2 (Allam et al., 2006). There is also expression of CD14, a lipopolysaccharide (LPS) receptor, which is relevant for the modulation of Th2 and Th1.

In SLIT, the allergen is captured by the DC cell by *C-lectin* endocytosis receptors and/or by ligation to the IgE on the surface. After the internalization, the migration to the regional lymphoid nodules occurs, and it is then presented to the T cells (Geijtenbeek, 2006). A study that compares the DC population in the oral and nasal mucosa was able to demonstrate that only the DC myeloid type is profusely present in the oral region, in contrast with the nasal mucosa where both populations are present (Allam et al., 2006). Another very important difference is the high expression levels of FcεRI in the oral mucosa, which is almost absent in the skin's Langerhans cells (Allam et al., 2003). Furthermore, the expression levels of MHC class I and II molecules, CD40, CD80 and CD86 is significantly higher in oral DC than in the skin.

The integrity of the lamina propria in the oral mucosa, along with the highly reduced population of mast cells, eosinophils and basophils, are the factors that limit the contact of the allergen with submucosal areas or with circulating blood cells. All of these together constitute the excellent security profile characteristic of the SLIT (Moingeon et al., 2006). The DC seems to be crucial in the induction of the tolerance profile due to the production of IL-10 and TGF-β after activation, as well as an increase in indoleamine dioxygenase type 2 (IDO), necessary to the decrease in T cells proliferation.

The allergen absorption through the intact mucosa and the interaction with local dendritic cells could switch on the process leading to immune-tolerance. In addition to the local effect, the swallowed allergen could induce a supplementary outcome based on a GALT-related mechanism (Akdis et al., 2001). In fact, the first method of sublingual administration of SIT, in which the allergen was spat out, was significantly less effective. Most of the immunological changes and mechanisms that occur with sublingual administration of high allergen dosage have been recently demonstrated (Moingeon et al., 2006).

The aqueous extracts are highly effective, but induce more side-effects (local and systemic) than depot and modified vaccines (Larché et al., 2006). These have been developed in an attempt to reduce or remove allergenicity, while preserving or increasing the immunogenicity (Casanovas et al., 2005). Aqueous subcutaneous SIT is now the gold standard treatment for hymenoptera venom allergy and depot aeroallergen extracts for respiratory allergy (Wheeler & Woroniecki, 2004). The use of chemically modified allergens is not consensual. Although recent papers demonstrate a clinical benefit with allergoid therapy (Ibarrola et al., 2004), double blind placebo controlled studies comparing both extracts are still missing. On the other hand, the sublingual-swallowed administration of SIT in higher dosages had a clinical efficacy entirely demonstrated with similar immunological effects, namely the increase in allergen-blocking IgG, the induction of IgE-modulating CD8[+] T cells, the reduction of mast cells and eosinophils on the target mucosa, the decrease in inflammatory mediators, and a modulation on the inflammatory trafficking cells by reduced expression of adhesion molecules (Bousquet, 2006).

2. Kinetics of immunotherapy mechanism

The studies on the dynamics of SIT are of extreme relevance, because they represent the only approach available to define, on a biological point of view, the mechanism by which the therapeutics works. Despite the current advances contributing to the wide knowledge of the modulator effect, these studies are extremely rare, as a result of several ethical, technical and economical boundaries. Furthermore, there are also several difficulties in transposing the results from experimental studies using laboratory animals to Humans.

In a study using mice, the systemic activity of a modified aeroallergen, an allergoid administered sublingually, was shown (Mistrello, 1994). However, before the study of an Italian group from Genoa in 1997, the kinetics and dynamics of the allergen in Humans was not known (Bagnasco, 1997). This study had the merit of assessing the response of the sublingual administration of a radioactively labeled allergen in a group of 9 healthy individuals (Bagnasco, 1997). *Par j* 1, the major *Parietaria judaica* allergen, was labeled with [123]I. In respect to the sublingual route, the application and deposition of the labeled allergen in 3 individuals was monitored for a period of 30 minutes before deglutition, by the acquisition of static images in the following 1, 2, 3, 5, 24 and 48 hours. In parallel, blood draws were collected for the determination of the radioactive counts at 5, 10, 20, 30 and 60 minutes, and then at 2, 3, 5 and 24 hours after the administration. A quantification of the same parameters in the urine was also performed. This study was able to demonstrate that the allergen was not degraded by the saliva and interestingly that there was no absorption by the sublingual mucosa.

The plasma radioactive activity only occurs after the deglutition of the allergen. Another surprising fact is that an enormous radioactive activity of the labeled allergen in the sublingual region is still detected, even after 48hours and despite the deglutition. Furthermore, the study also compared the same methodology either with nasal and oral (immediate deglutition) administration. The results from the application of the allergen in a nasal pulverization demonstrated activity in the superior region of the pharynx and proximal esophagus, and persistence of the labeled allergen until 36hours, with no bronchial deposition, but having activity in the plasma since the beginning. The oral route is simultaneous to the detection of immediate activity in the plasma, characterized by a pick at 2hours, followed by a decline, but with no identification of the labeled allergen. Probably there is protein degradation and only small peptides are absorbed at the level on the intestinal mucosa.

These results, done afterwards by the same group and obtained from healthy individuals, were crucial for the evaluation of the kinetics and dynamics of the allergen administration in 9 allergic patients with rhinitis (Bagnasco, 2001). The study compared the different alternatives of sublingual administration of the *Par j* 1 allergen labeled with [123]I. Namely non-modified allergen solution (drops), non-modified allergen in pills and modified allergen (allergoid) also in pills. The patients were monitored with dynamic acquisition in the first 20 minutes and static acquisitions of 5 minutes every hour until the 16th hour. Serial blood draws were also collected in order to quantify the radioactive plasmatic activity. The results confirmed persistent radioactive activity at the local of the administration of the allergen. For all the extracts, the plasmatic activity only occurs after deglutition. With the allergoid, the activity is higher, probably dependent of a lower enzymatic degradation and consequent lower possibility of intestinal absorption. The acquisitions in a gamma-rays camera only visualizes the activity after deglutition (1-5 minutes later), in the pharyngeal and esophagic region.

The same group of investigators studied the kinetics of the intranasal administration of *Par j* 1 labeled with ^{123}I in a group of 3 patients with allergic rhinitis, using a similar methodology although with distinct time points (Passalacqua, 2005). The radioactive activity in the nasal region disappears rapidly in allergic patients when compared to healthy individuals. The clinic inflammation controlled by the administration of the therapeutic allergen in these patients may condition an increase in the depuration or clearance of the mucosa. Plasmatic activity is also observed after an effective deglutition of the allergen. Despite the reduced number of patients used to conducted this study, the results are significantly distinct from the results observed when using the sublingual route, in which the radioactive activity persist at the local of administration, long after the deglutition of the therapeutic extract (Bagnasco, 2001).

The same Italian group responsible for the study with allergens administered by non-injectable routes prompt the question of whether the results obtained up until that moment were restricted to specific characteristics of *Parietaria judaica*. Following this, the group published another study using a major allergen from *Dermatophagoides pteronyssinus*, the *Der p* 2 (Bagnasco, 2005). For the 7 patients with allergic rhinitis, the results were analogous to the ones mentioned above. This lead to the conclusion that the persistence of the radioactive activity at the local of administration of the allergen and the systemic absorption after the deglutition is independent of the allergen used in the treatment and the chemical modification used.

The studies regarding the kinetics and dynamics of immune-therapy administrated by non-injectable routes were pioneer, even though its implementation was substantially more recent than conventional route, and interestingly they included the nasal route, which had no scientific validation for its efficacy (Bousquet, 1998; Alvarez-Cuesta, 2006). In respect to the subcutaneous route, our group has published in 2004 the first *in vivo* results regarding the dynamics of SIT in patients with allergic disease (Pereira, 2004).

3. Dynamics of the immunotherapy mechanism

The radioactive labeling of an allergen from the therapeutic extract is possible, but it would be restricted, exclusively, to one protein only. This could have been a strategy to evaluate the dynamics of the biological response to SIT. However, for patients under a maintenance treatment, the exclusion of some allergenic epitopes present in the therapeutic extracts would condition the interpretation of the results. Furthermore, it could, eventually, change the immunogenic structure of that epitope and as a consequence, the immune response that was induced. In these studies, the administration of the allergen extract, according to the maintenance scheme in place for each patient, would occur simultaneously with the reinjection of leucocytes labeled with ^{99m}Tc-HMPAO. The labeling of leucocytes with ^{99m}Tc-HMPAO is a technique that, on the theoretical level, has affinity for all the cellular elements of the white series (mononuclear and polymorphonuclear) and all of these have a specific contribution in the inflammatory process (Kumar, 2005; Peters, 1986).

The therapeutic allergenic extract injections always induce an inflammatory reaction at the local of the administration, detectable clinically by the presence of typical local signals. In the maintenance treatment, these symptoms have variable intensity and depend not only on the type of extract but also on the severity of the basal clinical features (Alvarez-Cuesta et al., 2006). The modified extracts and the extracts administrated sublingually are the ones that induce minor local secondary effects, as mentioned before. Therefore, although in a limited and controlled way, the SIT leads to an effective inflammatory allergic reaction in the area where the extract is applied, despite all the relevant immune-modulator mechanisms, which at the moment are well established for this therapeutic.

This local inflammatory allergic reaction will be, presumably, responsible by the dynamics of a response highly similar to the one observed in the allergic response in general (Pereira, 2009). Therefore, it can be admitted that the autologous reinjection of leucocytes will have a migration at that level by mechanisms dependent on the IgE-mediated mast cells activation (Bousquet, 1998; Alvarez-Cuesta et al., 2006).

3.1 Patients studied

Seventeen adult volunteer allergic patients were selected, 15 of them under maintenance therapeutic with specific immunotherapy. All were under a regular and programmed follow-up at the Immunoallergology department for the treatment of allergic pathology: respiratory allergy (bronchial asthma and rhinitis) and anaphylaxis (latex or hymenoptera venom). Until the date of selection of the patients, this treatment scheme has demonstrated clinical efficacy, translated by the complete remission of the symptoms, absent regular and preventive anti-allergic medication, no need of symptomatic medication in periods of worsening of the symptoms. Along with these criteria, it was also taken into account the favorable evolution of the laboratory parameters, namely reduction of the cutaneous reactivity to the responsible allergen by allergic diathesis in cutaneous prick tests using standardized extracts, and the reduction in the levels of the serum specific IgE, relatively to the beginning of the treatment. For the study of the dynamics of this therapeutic, samples from patients using different routes of administration of SIT and different allergenic extracts were also included. Patients were selected according to the type of allergen extract and route of administration of the SIT (Table 1).

Subcutaneous Administration Route
Aqueous subcutaneous extract (anaphylaxis)
4 patients: latex extract
2 patients: Apis mellifera extract
Subcutaneous depot extract (respiratory allergy)
2 patients: D pteronyssinus extract
2 patients: pollen from Poaceae extract
Subcutaneous modified allergen extract (respiratory allergy)
1 patient: pollen from Poaceae extract
1 patient: pollen from Parietaria judaica extract
Sublingual Administration Route (respiratory allergy)
2 patients: D pteronyssinus extract
1 patient: pollen from Parietaria judaica extract

Table 1. Patients under a specific immunotherapy treatment (extract, route of administration and allergic disease)

The control group included 2 patients allergic to *Dermatophagoides pteronyssinus*, with asthma and rhinitis, non-submitted to SIT and controlled with daily inhaled corticotherapy (fluticasone furoate). None of the selected patients presented any other concomitant pathology, namely inflammatory, which could interfere with the interpretation of the results. Furthermore, neither of the patients was under any other medication, besides the ones mentioned. All female patients were submitted to a quick urinary test to exclude pregnancy. All the studies were conducted under strict hospital vigilance, and the day of the immunotherapy administration was exactly the one previously defined in the maintenance therapeutic scheme. This study was, obviously, submitted for the approval of the Ethics Committee of the Institution, according to the "Declaration of Helsinki" of the World Medical Association (Helsinki 1964; Tokyo 1975; Venice 1983; Hong-Kong 1989).

3.2 Methodology for this study
A standard technique was used for the labeling of circulating leucocytes with ^{99m}Tc-HMPAO (Peters, 1986).
The allergen extracts used in the patients with subcutaneous immunotherapy (aqueous and depot) or submitted to sublingual *Dermatophagoides pteronyssinus* treatment were produced by the ALK-Abelló Laboratory (Madrid, Spain). For another patient in SLIT, the *Parietaria judaica* extract was provided by the Stallergenes Laboratory (Paris-France). In respect to the SCIT with modified extracts (allergoid), the glutaraldehyde-modified extract from pollens of

Poaceae was supplied by BIAL-Aristegui Laboratory (Bilbao, Spain) and the *Parietaria judaica* extract modified by depigmentation was provided by the Leti Laboratory (Madrid, Spain).

The maintenance dosage to which the patients were submitted on the day of the study corresponded to the one established on their treatment scheme, and was administrated on the pre-defined schedule. Two controls non-submitted to SIT with respiratory allergy to *Dermatophagoides pteronyssinus* were also studied. They were submitted, respectively, to:

-0,5cc of bacterial aqueous extract by the subcutaneous route, immune stimulant inductor of a IgG response (Ribomunyl ®, Pierre Fabre Médicament, France), containing ribosomal fractions of *Klebsiella pneumoniae*, *Streptococcus pneumoniae*, *Streptococcus pyogenes*, *Haemophilus influenzae* and membrane fractions of *Klebsiella pneumoniae*.

-0,5cc of phenolated aqueous solution administrated by the subcutaneous route, diluting the solution from the ALK-Abelló Laboratory (Madrid, Spain).

Patients were positioned in dorsal decubitus, under a gamma camera. The puncture of the cubital vein with a caliber 14 catheter allowed the reinjection of the autologous leucocytes labeled with a radio-labeled pharmaceutical compound in fast bolus, followed by a venous wash with physiological serum. Simultaneously, the allergenic extract was administrated subcutaneously, according to the usual technique (Bousquet et al., 1998) in the external surface of the arm contralateral to the administration of the labeled cells. Both injections occurred at the same time, simultaneously to the beginning of the scintigraphic acquisition.

The 3 allergic patients submitted to SLIT were placed in dorsal decubitus under a gamma-rays camera, and drops containing the allergenic extract were administrated at the same time that the reinjection of radio labeled leucocytes in the cubital vein was performed. Three minutes later the allergen was swallowed, according to the usual protocol.

For the control group, the subcutaneous administration of the saline solution and the bacterial extract were performed the same way as for the patients in the active group.

In all the studies, the residual activity of the syringe containing the autologous cells that were reinjected was assessed, in order to quantify the radioactive dosage effectively administrated. The scintigraphic studies were performed under a gamma rays camera (GE XR, Milwaukee, USA) using a low energy and parallel cavities collimator coupled to a Camstar acquisition unity and to a eNTEGRA processing unity. The dynamic acquisition was obtained in an anterior side view of the head and neck to 64x64 resolution matrixes during 60 minutes (120 images x 30 seconds), followed by a static study at 60, 120, 180, 240, 300 and 360 minutes after the administration of the allergen and leucocytes labeled with ^{99m}Tc-HMPAO, during 5 minutes for each acquisition (256 x 256 resolution elements). The static images were obtained in anterior and posterior side views for the following projections: head and neck, thorax and abdomen. During the acquisitions, patients were asked to remain at rest, despite the induction of nasal symptoms, in order to maintain the geometry of the projections, and at the same time minimizing the distance to the detector.

A qualitative evaluation of the images obtained in the dynamic acquisition was then performed, either by sequential analysis or using a video of 120 images. The moment in which the activity in the nasal region started was determined, as well as the local of the administration and the subsequent focalizations of the inflammatory activity that was induced. In the same way, a qualitative evaluation of the focalized inflammatory activity on defined timings for the static acquisition was performed. For the quantitative results, a different approach was chosen, in respect to the type of image in study. For the dynamic images obtained from the head and neck, the regions of interest were drawn (ROIs, *region of interest*) at the local of the administration of the allergen extract and /or controls, the *background* area (muscle) and also the following areas: oropharynx, cranial calotte and cervical lateral-external region of the neck. The dynamic acquisition was obtained in anterior view of the thorax and neck for matrixes with a resolution of 64 x 64 elements, during 60 minutes (120 images x 30 seconds), followed by a static study at 60, 120, 180, 240, 300 and 360 minutes for 5 minutes each acquisition (256 x 256 elements of resolution), after the administration of leucocytes labeled with ^{99m}Tc-HMPAO and the therapeutic allergen. The static images were obtained in anterior and posterior view for the thoracic projection and in anterior view for the abdominal projection.

A qualitative study of the images obtained in dynamic acquisition was then conducted by a sequential analysis or in a video of 120 images. The moment of the beginning of the activity at the local of the administration of the extract and in subsequent focalizations of the inflammatory activity that was induced was then determined. In the same way, a qualitative evaluation of the inflammatory activity focalized at defined timings for the static acquisition was performed. For the quantitative analysis a different approach was taken, regarding the type of image in study. For the dynamic thoracic images, ROIs were draw at the local of administration of the allergen and/or controls, as well as in the *background* area (muscle) and in possible focalizations (cervical, armpit and thoracic). For each ROI the total values, the average per pixel and the maximum values were determined. The uptake coefficient (UC, *uptake coefficient* ROI) was then calculated as the ratio between the maximum measurements of each ROI and the average value in the background area. For a best accuracy of the results it was also calculated the corrected uptake coefficient (UCC, *corrected uptake coefficient* ROI) by subtracting the uptake coefficient ROI in the background from the uptake coefficient ROI for each of the areas analyzed.

3.3 Results

The qualitative and quantitative results from patients submitted to specific treatment will be presented.

3.3.1 Qualitative results

All images from patients submitted to SIT were interpreted by analyzing the images with the same color scale, Figure 1. These crescent colors (from black to white) translate the inflammatory activity induced by the therapeutic action.

Fig. 1. Color scale from minimum activity (black) to maximum activity (white).

The studies regarding each type of SIT in analysis, namely regarding the type of extract and route of administration, are presented here (Figures 2 – 7). Besides the static images for the acquisitions of the thoracic and abdominal side view of each of the exemplified patients, an image from the dynamic sequence corresponding to the time point in which the beginning of the anti-inflammatory activity is observed at the site of administration of the extract will be presented. Furthermore, images obtained from two control patients will also be presented, namely with administration of a saline phenolated solution (SS) and a bacterial extract (BE). In all the studies the hepatosplenic region should be considered as an image of subtraction that should not be taken into account or interpreted. The spleen since it sequesters labeled erythrocytes, even though at residual levels, but always present in the pellet of isolated cells; the liver because it represents the preferential location for metabolization of the radio labeled pharmaceutical compound.

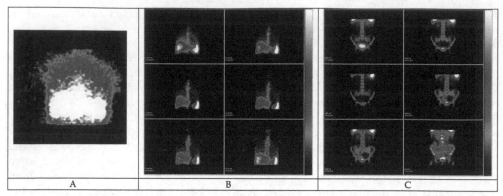

Fig. 2. Scintigraphic study of patient C1, control, with respiratory allergy to *Dermatophagoides pteronyssinus*, submitted to subcutaneous injection with bacterial extracts. Panel A shows the beginning of the activity at the external side of the arm after 45 minutes. Panels B and C show, respectively, thoracic and abdominal static acquisitions, in an anterior view.

For patient C1, submitted to subcutaneous injection with bacterial extract (BE), at 45 minutes we can observe inflammatory activity focalized at the site of administration. Furthermore, we observe focalizations, in the static studies, with inflammatory activity in bone structures (humeral head and iliac crest), as well as in the suprasternal region. The activity observed in the sternum and spinal cord (in anterior side view, not shown) should be interpreted with caution since there are superimposed structures with potential involvement. We do not observe intrapulmonary or intra-abdominal (intestinal) focalizations.

Regarding patient C2, submitted to subcutaneous injection of phenolate saline solution (SS) in the external face of the right arm, we notice minimum activity 50 minutes after the injection. For the static acquisitions we also observe activity localized to the structures described.

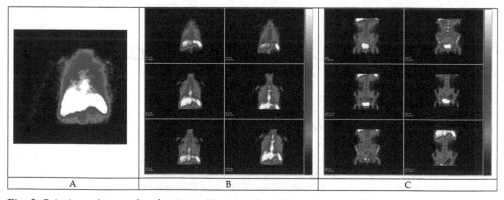

Fig. 3. Scintigraphic study of patient C2, control, with respiratory allergy to *Dermatophagoides pteronyssinus*, submitted to subcutaneous injection with phenolate saline solution. Panel A shows the beginning of the activity at the external side of the arm after 50 minutes. Panel Panels B and C show, respectively, thoracic and abdominal static acquisitions, in an anterior view.

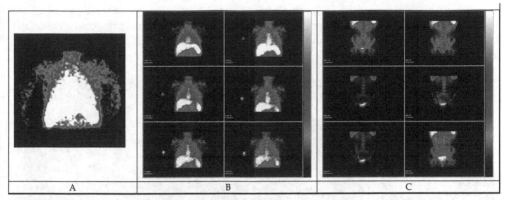

Fig. 4. Scintigraphic study of patient 6 (anaphylaxis to *Apis mellifera*), submitted to subcutaneous injection with aqueous extract. Panel A shows the beginning of the activity at the external side of the arm after 35 minutes. Panel Panels B and C show, respectively, thoracic and abdominal static acquisitions, in an anterior view.

For the patient (Figure 4), under treatment for anaphylaxis to hymenoptera venom, we observe inflammatory activity earlier at the local of administration of the therapeutic allergen extract, but the systemic involvement is also observed in all of the posterior scintigraphic images. Higher activity was detected in the bone structures, when compared to patient 3 with anaphylaxis to latex. We did not detect intra-abdominal (intestinal) focalizations in this patient. For these patients, as well as for all the other studies, the sternum bone structures and spinal cord will not be interpreted because of all the reasons already discussed.

For the patient allergic to pollens (Figure 5), the beginning of the inflammatory activity was detected at 35 minutes on the site of administration of the therapeutic extract. A systemic involvement in all the acquisitions was observed. In the armpit homolateral to the injection of the extract, we detect activity that persists throughout the study, similar to what happened in the cervical-lateral region of the neck. In the intestinal area we only observe focalizations at 60 and 120 minutes.

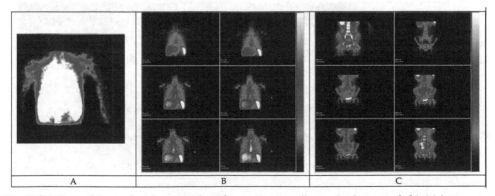

Fig. 5. Scintigraphic study of patient 8 with respiratory allergy (asthma and rhinitis) to grass pollen submitted to subcutaneous injection with depot extract. Panel A shows the beginning of the activity at the external side of the arm after 35 minutes. Panel Panels B and C show, respectively, thoracic and abdominal static acquisitions, in an anterior view.

For patient on figure 6, the inflammatory activity at the site of administration of the allergoid extract is highly reduced, when compared to the patients previously described. The systemic activity persists in all the structures considered, including the intra-abdominal area, from minute 60 to 120.

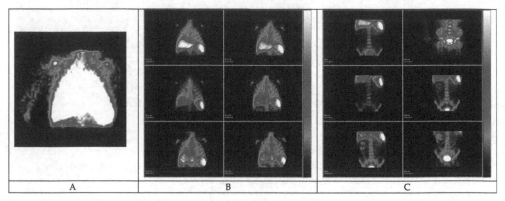

Fig. 6. Scintigraphic study of patient 11 with respiratory allergy (asthma and rhinitis) to grass pollens, submitted to subcutaneous injection of a glutaraldehyde modified extract. Panel A shows the beginning of the activity at the external side of the arm after 50 minutes. Panel Panels B and C show, respectively, thoracic and abdominal static acquisitions, in an anterior view.

The SLIT administration induced a very precocious beginning of activity when compared to the subcutaneous route. Patient from Figure 7, submitted to treatment with *D pt* extract, the inflammatory activity in the oropharynx occurred 3 minutes after the administration of the drop extract. We also observed a more relevant involvement of the cervical-lateral structures of the neck, which persisted throughout the trial. The systemic involvement was also present in this patient in different structures: intrapulmonary, bones and suprasternal region.

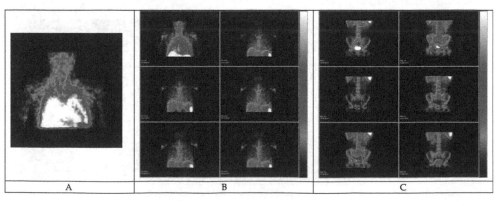

Fig. 7. Scintigraphic study of patient 13, with respiratory allergy (asthma and rhinitis) to *Dermatophagoides pteronyssinus*, submitted to sublingual administration. Panel A shows the beginning of the activity in the oral region after 3 minutes. Panel Panels B and C show, respectively, thoracic and abdominal static acquisitions, in an anterior view.

3.3.2 Quantitative analysis

All the scintigraphic studies were submitted to a quantitative evaluation in order to determine the corrected uptake coefficients. ROIs were draw in the areas with focalized activity, which included: local of administration of the allergenic extract, suprasternal region, humerus head and iliac crest. Besides this, every time intra-abdominal (intestinal) focalizations were present, the respective UCCs were calculated. Naturally, for each projection a ROI in the muscle area was draw, representing the background area.

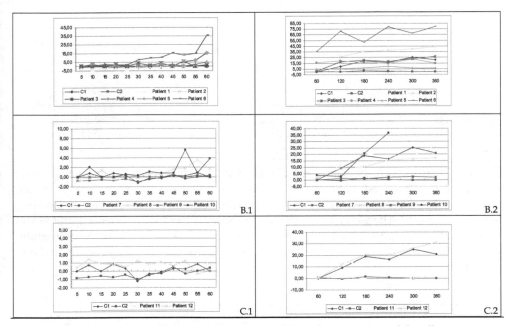

Fig. 8. Corrected uptake coefficients in the region of the administration of the allergenic therapeutic extract for the subcutaneous injectable treatments (1. Dynamic; 2. Static) throughout the study (expressed in minutes). A: aqueous extracts; B: depot extracts; C: chemically modified extracts (allergoid).

The beginning of the inflammatory activity for patients submitted to SCIT was different between the groups of patients in this study. The aqueous extracts for the treatment of anaphylaxis were the ones that induced higher UCCs, both in the dynamic and static evaluations. However, for the same type of extract, it seems that there are no relevant differences in respect to the type of allergen in the treatment, Figure 8.

Patients under treatment with the depot extracts showed intermediate levels between patients with aqueous extracts and allergoid. However, we should emphasize that a patient under depot extracts to dust mites showed a highly reduced UCC at the spot of the therapeutic injection, as well as a patient under treatment with pollinic extract modified with glutaraldehyde. The control patient submitted to BE, showed very significant UCCs at the local of administration in the evaluations made after the first 60 minutes. On the other side, for the patient submitted to SS, the quantification of the activity at the local of injection persisted always in much reduced levels.

For patients submitted to treatment with SLIT, the inflammatory activity is detected very early in the process, and persists throughout time at relatively constant levels, Figure 9. The patients allergic to dust mites showed higher levels when compared to the patient allergic to *Parietaria judaica*. However, for this patient, the study took place during the pollinic period, and therefore a reduced therapeutic dosage was administrated, which can justify, eventually, the results obtained.

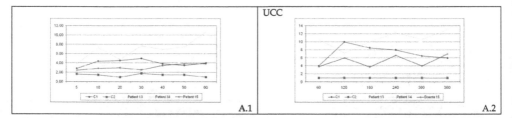

Fig. 9. Corrected uptake coefficients in the region of the administration of the sublingual allergenic therapeutic extract throughout the study (expressed in minutes). 1. Dynamic; 2. Static

The area located above the sternal furcula presented an early inflammatory activity, even during the dynamic studies. Since this region includes an extremely rich set of vascular structures, the effect of leukocyte recirculation maintained in the beginning of the study cannot be excluded. Therefore, it was decided to only evaluate the coefficients acquired with the static studies, Figure 10. Globally, the results are substantially higher than the control patient submitted to SS injection. Furthermore, it was also observed a slow increase during the experiment.

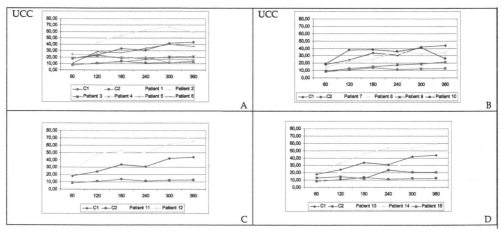

Fig. 10. Corrected uptake coefficients, taken at different time points during the experiment (minutes), obtained in the suprasternal region after the administration of the therapeutic extract. A: aqueous extracts; B: depot extracts; C: chemically modified extracts (allergoid); D: sublingual extracts

The evaluation of the UCCs in the bone structures localized in the humeral head and iliac crest was then performed, exclusively for static acquisitions, Figure 11.

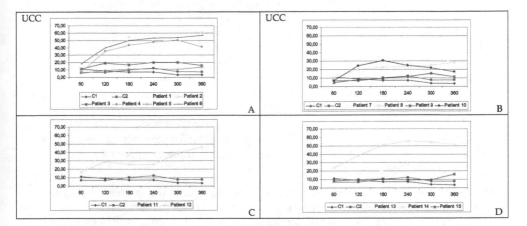

Fig. 11. Corrected uptake coefficients, taken at different time points during the experiment (minutes), obtained in the iliac crest after the administration of the therapeutic extract. A: aqueous extracts; B: depot extracts; C; chemically modified extracts (allergoid); D: sublingual extracts

The coefficients obtained in the two bone structures were similar and, globally, there was an apparent progressive increase throughout the experiment. However, regarding the type of extract and the method of administration, there wasn't a characteristic profile of the inflammatory activity in these structures. For the motives previously expressed, no other bone focalizations were considered.

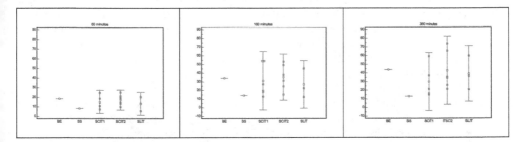

Fig. 12. Comparative results of the UCC obtained for the suprasternal of patients submitted to aqueous extracts (SCIT1) for the treatment of anaphylaxis; depot and allergoid extracts (SCIT2) for the treatment of respiratory allergy and sublingual aqueous extracts (SLIT), also for the treatment of respiratory allergy. The results obtained for control patients submitted to injection of bacterial extract (BE) or phenolated saline solution (SS). For all patients, samples were collected at 60, 180 and 360 minutes.

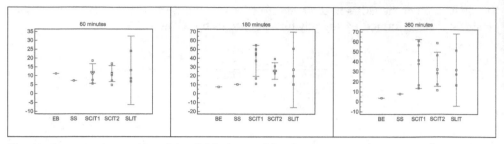

Fig. 13. Comparative results of the UCC obtained for the iliac crest of patients submitted to aqueous extracts (SCIT1) for the treatment of anaphylaxis; depot and alergoids extracts (SCIT2) for the treatment of respiratory allergy and sublingual aqueous extracts (SLIT), also for the treatment of respiratory allergy. The results obtained for control patients submitted to injection of bacterial extract (BE) or phenolated saline solution (SS). For all patients, samples were collected at 60, 180 and 360 minutes.

In the inflammatory focalization dependent of the ROI from the suprasternal region, no prevalence for a type of extract or method of administration of the treatment seems to exist, Figure 12. Similarly, it can be observed an increase in UCCs throughout the experiment. The same considerations can be applied to the inflammatory activity induced in the iliac crest, Figure 13.

3.4 Discussion

The administration of an allergenic therapeutical extract induces, always, an inflammatory reaction at the administration site that is characterized by the presence of clinically validated local symptoms. The modified extracts and the extracts delivered sublingually are the ones that induced lower secondary effects, as previously described. Although the main immunomodulator mechanism is already well established in SIT, it can dictate, in a limited and controlled approach, the effective inflammatory allergic reaction at the administration site. Therefore, we can admit that the autologous reinjection of leucocytes will have a migration dependent of the mast cell activation mediated by IgE (Togias, 2004; Kelly, 2007). This local inflammatory allergic reaction is, presumably, responsible for the dynamics of a response similar to allergy. Regarding the lymphocyte population, the circulatory migration to the tissue where the specific allergic reaction took place, is mediated by the expression of specific adhesion molecules that specify the type of cell implicated in the migration to the tissue (Togias, 2004). The migration of Th2 cells is associated to the expression of VCAM-1 and P-selectin, under effect of IL-4 and IL-13, that depends on the activation of lymphocyte transduction signals by transcription factors similar to STAT6 (Lukacs, 2000). On the other hand, the migration of Th1 cells seems to be dependent on the expression of STAT4, due to the effect of IL-12, and associated to the RANTES and ICAM-1 mechanism. In an interesting study with intradermal injection of allergenic peptides without the ability to induce an IgE response, it was possible to observe lymphocyte trafficking from the vascular department (Haselden, 1999). Also, the intervention of T-reg cell in the mechanisms of immunomodulation of SIT are well established either by inducing the population of Th1 cells or reducing the number of Th2 (Woodfolk, 2007; Francis, 2003).

Nevertheless, in these cells, it is not clear which is the specificity towards the allergen or what is the eligibility of the method of the induction (systemic or inhaled). Furthermore, it was also not clear what is the dosage required for induction or what type of regulatory cells are induced (natural T-reg produced by the thymus and with an effect dependent of cellular contact or adaptive T-reg cells induced on the periphery and with the effect dependent of IL-10 or TGF-β) (Woodfolk, 2007). At the same time, other lymphocytes, such as CD8+ e NKT cells, have the ability to respond to the allergen and represent other vectors involved in the SIT mechanisms (Woodfolk, 2007, Agea, 2005)).

As previously mentioned, DCs are considered central cells in inflammation and immune tolerance often reported in the SIT mechanisms. These cells represent the antigen presenting cells (APC) that, after migrating to the regional lymph node, induce an effective and differentiated immune response. Nevertheless, this is a very heterogeneous and diversified population, ubiquitously present, although in a reduced number when compared to other resident or circulation populations (von Bubnoff, 2002; Novak, 2004). Furthermore, it is known that myeloid DC cells can migrate from the blood to the tissues in order to capture antigens (Novak, 2004; Schmit-Weber, 2002, Allam, 2003). In specific situations, and under appropriated stimulus, the peripheral monocytes can differentiate into myeloid DC (von Bubnoff, 2002).

The skin and sublingual mucosa are, naturally, distinct. Therefore the mechanisms derived from the administration of the therapeutical allergenic extract should reflect this difference. The Langerhans cell (LC) is a DC myeloid cell (DC1) and are the most representative APCs in the skin. After a correct local stimulus, the monocyte chemotactic protein (MCP) determines the recruitment of LC progenitors from the bone marrow to the skin and the subsequent migration to the peripheral lymph nodes (Novak, 2004). The DC in the oral mucosa presents differences relatively to the skin, namely it expresses a higher number of MHCI and MCHII molecules, as well as the co-stimulation molecules CD40, CD80 and CD86 and also more FcγRIII (CD16), FcγRI (CD64) and FcεRI receptors (Allam, 2003). Several lymphoid structures are present in the oropharynx: tonsils, lymphatic ganglions and diffuse lymphoid tissue (Bienestock, 2005). It is well established that plasmacytoid DCs (DC2) are the APC most abundant in the Waldeyer's tonsillar ring and in the ganglion areas dependent on T cells, but that these cells are unable to effectively internalize the antigen (Novak, 2004). This is surely, a biologic characteristic of this region with consequences on the immune response on this area.

The subcutaneous tissue is, undoubtedly, composed by a population of resident cells that are biologically less active that the ones present in the oral mucosa. Nevertheless, the therapeutical administration of allergenic extracts by both ways has proven to be effective and able to induce an immunomodulator response in patients of IgE mediated allergy. This project did not intended to validate the efficacy of this therapy, broadly documented, but to study the dynamic of the resulting mechanism due to the administration of the therapeutical extract in patients maintained in the previously determined individual dosage. Theoretically, it would be extremely relevant to have monitored, under the same methodology, this treatment in different periods throughout the year, but the radioactive dosage accumulated would be ethically unacceptable.

In patients under subcutaneous injectable treatment, the anaphylaxis treatment with aqueous extracts induced the fastest signs of inflammatory activity in the administration site. The activity became visible 35 minutes after the administration, while with depot extracts, the activity was only visible between 40 and 45 minutes after the administration. In all patients, an increase in the intensity of the activities was observed throughout the observation period. The higher activity induced by the aqueous extracts did not translate into more exuberant clinical signs. The patients in SCIT to latex presented local clinical signs more pronounced than two patients allergic to *Apis*. In these two patients, the inflammatory activity was bigger and deeper, which can be explained by a higher amount of protein and the volume of extract administered.

In patients with respiratory allergy submitted to SCIT with depot extracts there were no evident differences connected to the extract composition, either mites or pollens.

Regarding the allergoid extracts, a reduced inflammatory activity was observed at the administration site, similarly to what was previously reported in the literature and demonstrated in daily clinical practice (Casanovas et al., 2005, 2007; Ariano et al., 1999). The modification of the allergenic with glutaraldehyde reduced the local inflammatory activity to levels similar to the ones observed in the control patients submitted to SS. In patient C1, asthmatic allergic to dust mites submitted to subcutaneous injection with BE, a local inflammatory activity was observed 45 minutes after the administration. This is an extract with immunomodulator activity, which induces the response of an IgG polyclonal antibody well documented in the literature (Clot, 1997). Although the local demonstration of activity was expected, the time necessary to observe activity was also extremely reduced.

The patient submitted to a phenolated solution presented a minimal local inflammatory activity only seen 60 minutes after the subcutaneous injection. Similarly to the patients studied in the previous chapter, it is considered that the irritation potential of this preservative can justify this result (Spiller et al., 1993).

In this study it was possible to assess and confirm the dynamics of the inflammation induced by the subcutaneous application of an allergenic extract. These results, although not surprising, were not unequivocally demonstrated, namely in terms of extension, depth of the adjacent region or evolution of the reaction along the course of the experiment. One advantage of the depot extracts when compared to the aqueous extracts, besides the safety profile, was the slower release of the allergenic protein (Wheeler & Woroniecki, 2004). In our patients we clearly observed a lower activity of these extracts, despite the fact that the patients with the aqueous extracts presented a worse level of basal allergic disease. The lymphocyte traffic seemed to be more intense and persistent with these extracts since the soluble allergenic is more readily available. In all patients submitted to SCIT, it is possible to observe systemic focalizations before the locally induced inflammatory activity. In the dynamic acquisition during the first 60 minutes, the anterior thoracic projection only permits to infer the potential activity in this view. In the intramedullary area of the humeral head is evident a significant intensity, surely dependent on the recirculation of cells representing all leukocyte cell populations.

In patients submitted to SCIT, the activity in bone structures and in thymic tissue presented a very intense activity that increased throughout the experiment. It should be noticed that these structures anatomically overlap to other organs from the central immune systems, but that in the peripheral immune lymphoid system, such as regional ganglion, and presumably in the region of the mediastinum, there is also evidence of activity. Furthermore, the mucosa immune system seems to be involved namely the pulmonary and less consistently the intestinal. The early involvement of the central lymphoid structures was an unexpected event, but was very consistent in all patients.

Obviously, with the methodology used it is not possible to determine the cell type and profile that is responsible by the activity induced by the migration from the circulation to a specific focalization. Nevertheless, given the actual knowledge regarding the mechanism that modulate this therapeutic, it is possible to admit that a diversified set of cells with different activation profiles and with divergent implications in the different structures.

The subcutaneous administration of the allergenic extract, particularly with aqueous extracts, defines an evident local inflammatory process. To this level, we admit that some conjunctive mast cells can be activated, although with limited intensity. As described in the literature, we also admit that the presence of conjunctive DCs, with IgE receptors, can favor this type of reaction. However, the most likely mechanism can depend on an effective presentation of the allergen to presenting cells and posterior migration to local-regional structures. This mechanism could explain the ganglion activity observed in the homolateral arm, with the involvement of other ganglion structures more distant, such as the ones present in the cervical lateral-external area.

On the other hand, we admit the influx from the circulation of DC or monocytes into the site of administration of the allergenic extract, since it is well known the ability of these cells to maturate into DCs or phagocytes. This dual mechanism, that simultaneously induce a biological defense from the aggression and favors an effective immune response, are probable local mechanisms. Therefore, the local administration of therapeutical allergens limits the local response that rapidly seems to have local-regional and systemic consequences. Probably, not only the biologic mediator produced *in situ*, as well as the following cell migration, presumably DCs, and the cellular limitations in venular structures in the proximity of the allergenic, allow the amplification of the systemic effect by mechanisms, possibly similar to the ones verified in the allergic reaction (Togias, 2004; Kelly, 2007).

The qualitative analysis of our SCIT patients corroborates, although indirectly, the complexity of the tolerance mechanisms, well described in the literature. The anatomic involvement of structures implicated with organs of the central immune system seems to sustain these effects. The activity observed in the bone marrow areas allow us to speculate that it could limit the modification of cellular profiles, namely lymphocyte, that has been documented in these patients (Denburg et al., 2000). Also, the demonstration of the contribution of regulatory cells can be sustained by our results given the involvement of the anatomic region reported to the thymic tissue, whose function persists throughout life (Arellano et al., 2006). Nevertheless, the pace of this process and the systemic involvement, evidenced by the focalization of the inflammatory activity, is clearly higher than expected, given the present knowledge. It should be noticed that this dynamic study evaluates, in a certain way, the biologic response in the whole organism. This contrasts with the usage of small biologic samples (such as tissues or humors), a procedure that is very common in most clinical and experimental studies.

We admit that the lungs are involved in the influx of leukocytes to the BALT, but it should be noticed that this is a preponderant location for the clinical symptoms that lead to treatment in patients with respiratory allergy.

In patients in SLIT, the beginning of the inflammatory activity in the site of administration was substantially earlier than the observed in patients in SCIT. In the two patients allergic to mites and in the patient allergic to *Parietaria judaica*, the activity was noticed 3 and 5 minutes after the respective induction. Despite this early onset of activity, no substantial differences were registered when the final results were compared, namely in the effects of regional or distant structures.

In fact, it seems evident that since the administration of the extract, a continuous increase of the local inflammatory activity as well as in cervical structures, particularly in the cervical lateral-external region. As described previously for SCIT patients, the venous recirculation at very early stages does not allow an effective validation of this effect, but the assessment in later periods, both in the dynamic or static acquisitions, there is an evident focalization in these cervical structures. For these patients, and with exception of the patient injected with extract modified with glutaraldehyde, and using the color scale, the intensity of the oropharynx is clearly inferior than the one verified in the injection site. Other clear difference, is the absence of a progressive increase of the inflammatory response focalized at the administration site verified in subsequent static evaluations. However, the systemic effect is very similar to the observed in patients under injectable treatment. We observe pulmonary focalizations as well as in regions reported to the organs from the immune central system. In these regions, the areas reported to the bones and in suprasternal, the images from the static studies support an increase of activity throughout the experiment.

In patients under SLIT, the extract was swallowed 3 minutes after the administration. It would be expected an intra-abdominal involvement, with intestinal focalizations. However, in none of these 3 patients that effect was observed. We admit that the extract can be completely degraded in the stomach, which would prevent an effect in the intestinal mucosa. Our results seem to corroborate the therapeutic inefficiency of the oral immunotherapy, which is not scientifically validated by the literature (Bousquet et al., 1998). It is not possible to define and characterize the migrating population that focalizes in the distinct structures in patients under SLIT. Despite this, the available scientific knowledge allows us to assume that the allergenic persistence in the sublingual mucosa, as previously demonstrated (Bagnasco et al., 2005), allows the induction of the following immune response. As previously described, abundant lymphoid structures with specific biologic characteristics are present in this mucosa. The DC permits a fast transport to the tonsils and lymphatic ganglions in a magnitude that cannot be compared to the subcutaneous tissue. However, it is well established that the majority of DCs present in the tonsils are DC-2. These cells do not have the capacity to effectively internalize the allergenic protein and efficiently present it to the T-cell. Therefore, and although in smaller numbers, the DC-1 cells probably have a preponderant function. As a result, we admit that there might be an influx from the circulation of DC and monocytes, and that these, once in the mucosa, will differentiate and maturate. The early start of the activity will, presumably, result from the presence and availability of a biologically more active and diversified resident population. The reduced population of mast cells in the oral mucosa limits the local inflammatory response when compared to the subcutaneous administration. Therefore, and in theory, we can predict that the resulting mechanism derives from the activation of DCs and the presentation to lymphocytes in structures in the oral mucosa and that are dependent from the immune system. Thus, the therapeutical extract produces a powerful stimulus that initiates a local and systemic immune response, surely by regulating biologic mediators of cytokines and chemokines, as well as by limiting the entry of circulating cells from the vascular-lymphoid structures present in the oral mucosa.

The systemic effects in areas of the central immune system, similarly to what was observed for the injectable extracts, can corroborate the tolerance and immunomodulation, presently well documented in the therapeutical intervention.

In patients under injectable therapy, the UCCs results obtained in the homolateral armpit are higher that was expected by the exclusive visualization of the scintigraphic images. We admit that the results obtained in this focalization are, eventually, due to the migration of lymphatic cells from the administration site of the therapeutical extract to the ganglion structures present in the armpit region that allow a therapeutical amplification with natural systemic effect. In fact, functional studies in melanoma using a radio-labeled pharmaceutical compound administered intradermally evidenced the high rate of lymphatic migration to distant ganglion structures (Alazraki et al., 2002). Since the most important ganglion structures of the subcutaneous cellular tissue of the arm are located in the armpit, that the effective presentation of the allergenic protein to the T-cell in the lymph node is mediated by the DC and that the intralymphatic migration is very fast, the UCCs obtained in our patients are, probably, justified.

The eventual lymphatic migration proportions, are in fact, an amplification of the immune mechanism with characteristics that clearly favors tolerance. Therefore, it could lead not only to an effective diffusion of the response throughout the immune-lymphoid system, as well as a recirculation of cells from the allergenic administration site to distant central structures and organs that can allow the synergistic effects that concur with the immunomodulation of this therapy.

Therefore, the presumed ascending drainage justifies the precocious and persistent UCCs induced by the subcutaneous administration of the allergen in other vascular-lymphatic structures, anatomically located in the lateral-external region of the neck. Eventually, this process allows an amplification of the response to cervical structures with high biological activity. To this level, we do not observe significant differences of UCCs due to usage of different injectable extracts.

Although we verify focalization in the pulmonary region throughout the dynamic acquisition, we only calculated the coefficients in the static acquisition. The intense venous recirculation of leukocytes after the reinjection could falsify the results. However, all our patients presented intrapulmonary activity. Particularly in patients undergoing treatment for respiratory allergy, the influx of these cells to the targeted organ is compatible to the methods sensitivity. This way, the recirculation of leukocytes between the vascular compartment and the mucosa of the different organs of the immune system allow the convenient organic homeostasis that justifies the reduced numbers of pulmonary UCCs verified in control patients.

Given the results obtained in the patient submitted to BE, we presume that the unspecific bacterial immunomodulators have, besides favoring an IgG polyclonal response, a more central and selective regulator effect than the one presumed until now, but for which the clinically efficacy has been shown (Bousquet & Fiocchi, 2006). Regarding the patient allergic to dust mites submitted to SS injection, the reduced UCCs values were consistent throughout the experiment, and we presume that are derived from the organic recirculation of leukocytes, and correspond to the basal function of this tissue

The activity observed in the bone structures was confirmed by the UCCs calculated in the two considered ROIs. There were no differences in the results obtained in the medullary area of the humeral head or the iliac crest.

Our results suggest that either the bone marrow or the functional thymic tissue, organs from the central immune system, are preferential targets of the induction mechanism of SCIT, regardless of the type of allergenic extract. It should be noticed that in patients treated with modified extracts, allergoid, the dosage of allergenic used was substantially higher than the dosages in the depot extracts, and that the UCCs obtained in the regions associated with bone marrow were also higher. However, the size of the sample does not allow us to conclude if this treatment is more selective or effective. Nevertheless, we presume that given the previously described mechanisms, the bone marrow may participate in the SIT mechanism since earlier stages, right after the injection of the extracts.

In the suprasternal region, the UCCs were very similar in the different groups under active treatment and significantly distinct from the ones obtained in the patient submitted to SS injection. This data corroborates the eventual physiological dynamic of the leukocytes, possibly dependent of the persistent limitation of the medulla, even in cells apparently mature that were collected from the venous compartment.

In the intra-abdominal region, the UCCs obtained in the intestinal focalizations, observed occasionally in the scintigraphic images, confirmed the involvement of this mucosa. The calculations were only performed in focalizations areas during the first 4 hours, in order to minimize interferences due to faecal elimination.

For the three patients under sublingual treatment we do not have a control that we can compare to. Despite this, the values obtained in the asthma and rhinitis patients allergic to dust mites submitted to BE or SS in the nasal region (see previous chapter), are similar to the type of response verified in SLIT patients.

The capture and the inflammatory activity on the site of the administration of the therapeutic extract evidenced a very precocious activity that subdue in relatively high values throughout the experiment. These results are consistent with previously described dynamic studies (Bagnasco et al., 2005). The quantitative analysis does not evidence an increase of the local activity as seen in the majority of patients submitted to injectable extracts. In this mucosa, the presence of mast cells is extremely reduced which, despite the persistence of the extract (even after it was swallowed), does not induce a broader influx of circulating leukocytes due to this mechanism. Therefore, we presume that the much more limited activity observed can be due to circulating DCs and mast cells that have a recognized ability to mature and differentiate in the offended tissues. The readily availability of immune-lymphoid tissue in this localization will allow a fast amplification and dissemination of cells with the ability to induce an immunomodulator mechanism.

In patient 15, submitted to sublingual treatment with *Parietaria judaica* extracts, the UCCs obtained throughout the observation period were the lowest in these three patients. In fact, since the test was conducted during the pollinic period, we established a reduction of the allergenic dosage during the pollination period of this herb. It is a clinical procedure well established in the therapeutic with injectable extracts, although not consensual in sublingual treatment (Bousquet, 2006; Bousquet et al., 1998). Despite this, and since this patient lives in a geographic area with high levels of aeropalinologics, it was decided to reduce the maintenance dosage to 2/3 (10:15 drops). Eventually, this procedure had implications in the type of response that was evidenced, not only in the local activity as well as in the distant focalizations.

In patients under SLIT treatment, the UCCs obtained in the structures localized in the lateral-external region of the neck confirmed the analytic results from the scintigraphic images. The apparent descendent drainage in these vascular-lymphatic systems corroborates our proposal, particularly in the intrapulmonary capture. In the anatomic regions reported to the organs of the central immune system we observed UCCs with similar behavior than those verified in the patients under injectable treatment. Therefore, we presume that in SLIT there is also an early participation of the bone marrow and the functional thymic tissue.

4. Involvement of the organs from the immune system

In SCIT, we admit that the APC migration to ganglion structures is determinant to obtain a systemic effect and to acquire an immunomodulator and/or tolerance state. In patients submitted to SLIT, the inflammatory activity was observed in the first minutes, much earlier but with clearly lower gradients throughout the experiment. As previously described, the morphological characteristics of the conjunctive subcutaneous tissue and the oral, in particular from the sublingual region, are completely distinct. Therefore, the local availability of the whole array of the adjacent immuno-lymphatic-ganglion structures allows the effectiveness of the early stages of the mechanism. Paradoxically, the characteristics of the DCs present in the oral mucosa, mainly from the plasmacytoid type, are responsible for a less effective response (Novak et al., 2004). Previous work evidenced the presence of the allergenic extract in the sublingual mucosa long after it was swallowed, but it was extremely reduced 24 hours after that administration (Bagnasco et al., 2005). This difference, relatively to the subcutaneous administration, has natural implications in the periodicity of the therapeutical application. The amplification of the systemic effect seems to result from a descending involvement of structures presumably vascular-lymphatic in the lateral-external of the neck by a mechanism similar to SCIT.

Given the differences between the two administration methods and the type of therapeutic extract, the results obtained suggest a potentially selective influx of cells from the mononuclear-phagocyte system to the deposition site, similarly to the allergic reaction, which was documented in an interesting study done in ten patients submitted to an inhaled aggression (Upham et al., 2002). Naturally, the mediators produced locally will have a potential modulator effect in the adjacent vascular endothelium, which allows a possible immunomodulator effect in circulating leukocytes that allows a systemic involvement.

The recirculation and following focalization of intrapulmonary leukocytes was observed in all patients. The presence of the bronchus-associated lymphoid tissue (BALT) supports these results, in particular since this mucosa is a potential target in patients undergoing treatment of respiratory allergy. However, regarding the involvement of the intestinal mucosa, where the gut associated lymphoid tissue (GALT) is located, focalization of the inflammatory activity was occasionally observed. The SLIT with allergenic deglutition three minutes after the deposition did not produced any additional gain. In fact, we admit that the protein degradation can occur as result of the gastric enzymatic degradation as proposed in the literature (Bousquet et al., 1998).

The lymphocyte cellular modulation from a mainly Th2 profile into a lymphocyte profile mostly Th1, as well as the induction of T-lymphocytes with regulatory characteristics, are the most studied and documented mechanisms in the literature (Larché et al., 2006; Till et al., 2004; Canonica & Passalacqua, 2003). The complexity of the processes involved allows a constant effect throughout the treatment, but its dynamic mechanism is not well established. The need to extend in time the specific treatment translates the need to promote an immunologic memory *status*. The patients studied in this project were well documented, both clinically and laboratorial, and all were in maintenance treatment. Although we know several mechanisms involved, it is not known the dynamics and the regions implicated after the administration of the extract, nor in the induction stages or in maintenance periods.

It seems obvious the involvement of organs from the central immune system in the SIT action mechanisms. It also appears, given the results obtained in allergic patients submitted to specific provocation, that the participation of these organs could have a dynamic and pace with similar magnitude. These results look as redundant or expectable, but we had no previous knowledge about the location and timing of the immunomodulation process that has been so well characterized in the laboratory.

The induction of medullar cellular clones with phenotypes that favor the secretion type Th1 or clones precursors of DCs with tolerogenic characteristics are events that sustain the activity of the bone marrow, and is present at an early stage in patients undergoing treatment (van Helvoort et al., 2004; Moingeon et al., 2006). The essential function of several regulatory T-cells, well placed and with central function in the SIT mechanism, is an element that supports not only the intervention of bone marrow as well as the thymic activity (Schmidt-Weber & Blaser, 2005; Moingeon et al., 2006). Despite the anatomic involution, the organic function persists in adulthood (Hakim et al., 2005; Harris et al., 2005; Arellano et al., 2006). In this regard, we should notice that in one patient we had the opportunity to acquire a scintigraphic 21 hours after the simultaneous administration of leukocytes labeled with ^{99m}Tc-HMPAO and allergenic aqueous latex extract. In this patient we observe the persistence of the inflammatory activity in both the suprasternal and bone medullar areas, Figure 14.

It should be noticed that the half-life of the radio-labeled compound is 6 hours, and therefore the acquisition occurred at a time well past its half life. Nevertheless, the activity persisted at the administration site, allowing the therapeutic effect to continue, as well as activity in intra-bone areas and in the suprasternal region, which we judge representative the functional thymic tissue.

The study in this patient was done occasionally and was, in fact, a surprise, revealing activity that we supposed it was not possible due the anatomic physical conditionings. We proceeded with the quantitative evaluation that unequivocally contributed the qualitative assessment done in this patient. In Figure 15 we show the UCCs obtained for this patient after 6 hours (last programmed observation that coincides with ^{99m}Tc half-life) and 21 hours. Although the UCCs are lower after 21 hours when compared to the values obtained after 6 hours, it is evident that, despite after nearly four half-lives, the activity reported is very significant. We should highlight that the UCC in the ROI draw in the homolateral armpit maintains constant values of activity, which supports a continuous involvement.

The study in this patient, since it is not likely a continuous recirculation of leukocytes without focalization and influx to this organ, allows us to deduce that we were able to obtain an image of the functional thymic tissue.

Our results support the research developed since 1985 by a Canadian group that sustains the involvement of the central immune system's organs, mainly bone marrow, in the pathophysiology of the allergic inflammation (Denburg et al., 1998). The results obtained in experimental models and in humans with allergy are essential, regarding the participation of hematopoietic mechanisms during the response to an allergenic (Denburg et al., 1998; Denburg & van Eeden, 2006, Sehmi et al., 1996; Cyr & Denburg, 2001).

In a comparative study with 153 patients with pollinic rhinoconjunctivitis, the effect of the administration of SIT either subcutaneously or intralymphatic was compared (Senti et al., 2008). In the later group, the administration of the pollinic allergen directly in a inguinal lymphatic ganglion using ultrasound as a control, with only three injections separated by 4 weeks, in the response to a specific nasal induction 4 months after the last administration, required a dosage ten times higher than the one required in patients under SCIT treatment for three years and with a cumulative dosage drastically higher and with multiple allergenic injections. In addition to the clinical efficacy, the adverse effects were neglectable and the lymphatic intraganglionic injection was very well tolerated. This promising and innovative study can induce a complete reversion on the treatment of IgE mediated allergy. It should be noted that these results were obtained with conventional allergens. However we consider that the future use of highly selective peptides directly administered in immune structures can induce an even more elective therapeutical effect.

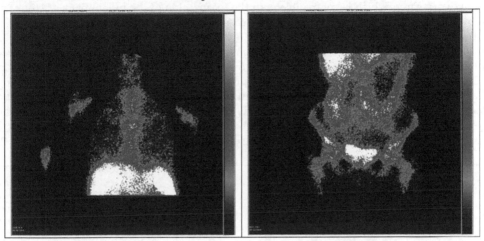

Fig. 14. Scintigraphic study in patient with anaphylaxis to latex, submitted to subcutaneous aqueous extract. Static acquisitions, anterior thoracic (A) and abdominal (B) views, 21 hours after the beginning of the study.

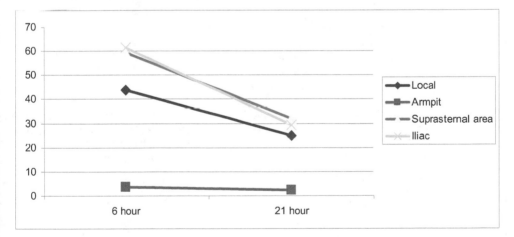

Fig. 15. Corrected uptake coefficient obtained in static acquisitions after 6 and 21 hours in different locations in patient with the diagnosis of latex anaphylaxis submitted to subcutaneous aqueous extract treatment.

5. Final remarks

SCIT limits the visualization of the inflammatory activity in systemic focalizations earlier than at the site of the extract administration. Generically, the local inflammatory activity evolves throughout time and is significantly broader than the one verified in the clinic, by the observation of the inflammatory signals. The pollinic extract modified with glutaraldehyde does not present nearly any inflammation at the injection site.

The involvement of the armpit's region homolateral to the administration of the extract occurs very early, which is compatible with the focalization of the inflammatory activity in immune ganglia structures. We admit an ascending drainage effect from the site of the extract's administration.

In patients submitted to SLIT, the visualization of the inflammatory activity is evident three minutes after the therapeutical extract's administration. In contrast to what was observed in SCIT patients, the inflammatory intensity, in the focalization, is relatively constant during the observation period, without an increase in later acquisitions. The SLIT also produced a very early systemic effect, namely with activity in the lateral-cervical region, where the presence of vascular-lymphatic structures have been reported. We admit that there is a descending drainage effect from the site of the extract's administration.

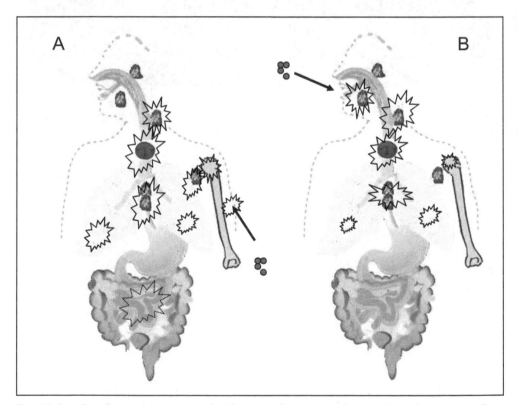

Fig. 16. Local and systemic events related to specific immunotherapy (A: subcutaneous; B: sublingual)

The visualization of the activity with intra-abdominal (intestinal) focalization was occasional, but exclusive to patients in SCIT. In patients undergoing SLIT, despite the swallowing of the extract, there was no focalization in this area three minutes after the extract's administration, Figure 16.

The anatomic regions reported to the central immune system (bone marrow and suprasternal area) evidenced a constant growth in UCCs during the experiment. The SIT triggers an early and continuous influx of leukocytes, from the circulation into the central immune organs, with potential implications in the immunomodulatory mechanism.

Regarding the response's magnitude in the bone marrow and functional thymic tissue, there were no apparent differences regarding the type of extract and the administration type during the first six hours after the administration of the therapeutical extract.

The persistence of the therapeutical extract administered subcutaneously indicates an inflammatory activity and a continuous influx of inflammatory cells. In the sublingual administration, the influx and local activity are lower, without any evidence of an increase in the inflammatory activity throughout the experiment. Therefore, patients under SLIT treatment will require administrations more frequent and with shorter breaks between administration in order to obtain a persistent therapeutic effect.

Our results reinforce the need for new and elective pharmacologic investigation strategies, focusing on the mainstay function of the central immune organs in the treatment of systemic inflammatory disease such as allergy. In fact, in face of the current knowledge of the immunological effects induced by SIT, namely the effect on T-regs with a long-lasting biological effect, this would only be possible if a central immune cellular modulation had occurred.

6. Acknowledgment

We would like to thank Dr Margarida Abrantes (IBILI, Medicine Faculty of Coimbra University. Portugal), Dr Daniel Machado (Immunoallergology Department, Coimbra University Hospital. Coimbra. Portugal), and Prof J Pedroso Lima (Nuclear Medicine Department, Coimbra University Hospital. Portugal) for all the performance and commitment to this project. The authors thank Dr Joana Branco and Dr André Faustino for the precious English writing assistance.

7. References

Agea, E.; et al. (2005). Human CD1-restricted T cell recognition of lipids from pollens. *The Journal Experimental Medicine,*.Vol.202, No.2, (July 2005), pp. 295-308, ISSN 0022-1007

Akdis, C.A. & Akdis, M. (2011) Mechanisms of allergen-specific immunotherapy. *The Journal of Allergy and Clinical Immunology,*.Vol.127, No.1, (January 2011), pp. 18-27, ISSN 0091-6749

Akdis, C.; et al. (2001). Mechanisms of IL10 induced T cell inactivation in allergic inflammation and normal response to allergens. *International Archives of Allergy and Immunology*, Vol.124, No.1-3, (January-March 2001), pp. 124: 180-182, ISSN 1018-2438

Allam, J.P.; et al. (2006). Comparative analysis of nasal and oral mucosa dendritic cells. *European journal of allergy and clinical immunology (Allergy)*, Vol.61, No.2, (February 2006), pp. 166-172, ISSN 0105-4538

Allam, J.P.; et al. (2003). Characterization of dendritic cells from human oral mucosa: a new Langerhans_ cell type with high constitutive FcepsilonRI expression. *The Journal of Allergy and Clinical Immunology*, Vol. 112, No.1, (July 2003), pp. 141-148, ISSN 0091-6749

Alvarez-Cuesta E.; et al, (2006). Standards for pratical allergen- specific immunotherapy. *Allergy*, 2006; Vol. 61, Suppl.82, (October 2006), pp. 1-20, ISSN 0105-4538

Alazraki, N.; et al. (2002). Procedure guideline for lymphoscintigraphy and the use of intraoperative gamma probe for sentinel lymph node localization in melanoma of intermediate thickness. *Journal Nuclear Medicine*, Vol. 43, No.43, (October 2002), pp. 1414-1418, ISSN 0161-5505

Ariano, R., et al. (1999). Long-term treatment with allergoid immunotherapy with Parietaria. Clinical and immunologic effects in a randomized, controlled trial. *European journal of allergy and clinical immunology (Allergy)*, Vol.54, No.4, (April 1999), pp. 313-319, ISSN 0105-4538

Arellano, M.V.; et al. (2006). Thymic Function-Related Markers Within the Thymus and Peripheral Blood: Are They Comparable? *Journal of Clinical Immunolology*, Vol.26, No.1, (January 2006), pp. 96-100, ISSN 0271-9142

Bagnasco, M.; et al. (2005). Pharmacokinetics of Der p 2 allergen and derived monomeric allergoid in allergic volunteers. *International Archives of Allergy and Immunology*, Vol.138, No.3, (November 2005), pp. 197–202, ISSN 1018-2438

Bagnasco, M.; et al. (1997). Absortion and distribution kinetics of the major Parietaria judaica (Par j 1) administered by noninjectable routes in healthy human beings. *The Journal of Allergy and Clinical Immunology*, Vol.100, No.1, (July 1997), pp. 122-129, ISSN 0091-6749

Bagnasco, M.; et al. (2001). Pharmacokinetics of an allergen and a monomeric allergoid for oromucosal immunotherapy in allergic volunteers. *Clinical and Experimental Allergy*, Vol.31, No.1, (January 2001), pp. 54-60, ISSN 0954-7894

Bienestock, J. & McDermott, M.R.. (2005). Bronchus- and nasal-associated lymphoid tissues. Immunological Reviews. Vol.206, (August 2005), pp. 22-31, ISSN 0105-2896

Bousquet, J.. (2006). Sublingual immunotherapy: validated! *Allergy*, Vol.61, Suppl.81, (July 2006), pp. 5-31, ISSN 0105-4538

Bousquet, J. & Fiocchi, A. (2006). Prevention of recurrent respiratory tract infections in children using a ribosomal immunotherapeutic agent: a clinical review. *Paediatric Drugs*, Vol.8, No.4, pp. 235-243, ISSN 1174-5878

Bousquet, J.; et al. (1998). Allergen immunotherapy: therapeutic vaccines for allergic diseases. A WHO position paper. *The Journal of Allergy and Clinical Immunology*, Vol.102, No.4, (October 1998), pp. 558-562, ISSN 0091-6749

Canónica, G.W. & Passalacqua, G. (2003). Noninjection routes for immunotherapy. *Journal of Allergy and Clinical Immunology*, Vol.111, No.3, (March 2003), pp. 437-448, ISSN 0091-6749

Casanovas, M.; et al. (2005). Comparative Study of Tolerance between Unmodified and High Doses of Chemically Modified Allergen Vaccines of *Dermatophagoides pteronyssinus*. *International Archives of Allergy and Immunology*, Vol.137, No.3, (July 2005), pp. 211–218, ISSN 1018-2438

Casanovas, M.; et al. (2007). Safety of immunotherapy with therapeutic vaccines containing depigmented and polymerized allergen extracts. *Clinical and Experimental Allergy*, Vol. 37, No.3, (March 2007), pp. 434-440, ISSN 0954-7894

Clot, J. (1997). Pharmacology of ribosomal immunotherapy. *Drugs*, Vol. 54, Suppl.1, pp. 33-36, ISSN 0012-6667

Cyr, M.M. & Denburg, J.A.. (2001). Systemic aspects of allergic disease: the role of the bone marrow. *Current Opinion in Immunology*, Vol.13), No.6, (December 2001), pp. 727-732, ISSN 0952-7915

Denburg, J.A.; et al.. (1998). Hemopoietic mechanisms in allergic airway inflammation. *International Archives of Allergy and Immunology*, Vol.117, No.3, (November 1998), pp. 155-159, ISSN 1018-2438

Denburg, J.A.; et al.. (2000). Systemic aspects of allergic disease: Bone marrow responses. *The Journal of Allergy and Clinical Immunology*, Vol.106, Suppl.5.2, (November 2000), pp. S242-6, ISSN 0091-6749

Denburg, J.A. & van Eeden, S.F.. (2006). Bone marrow progenitors in inflammation and repair: new vistas in respiratory biology and pathophysiology. *The European Respiratory Journal*, Vol. 27, No.3, (March 2006), pp. 441-445, ISSN 0903-1936

Francis, J.N.; et al.. (2003). Induction of IL-101CD41CD251 T cells by grass pollen immunotherapy. *The Journal of Allergy and Clinical Immunology*, Vol.111, No.6, (June 2003), pp 1255-1261, ISSN 0091-6749

Frew, A.J.. (2010). Allergen immunotherapy. *The Journal of Allergy and Clinical Immunology*, Vol.125, No.2 (Suppl 2), (February 2010), pp. S306-133, ISSN 0091-6749

Geijtenbeek, T.B. et al.. (2002). Engering A, Van KY. DC-SIGN, a C-type lectin on dendritic cells that unveils many aspects of dendritic cell biology. *Journal of Leukocyte Biology*, Vol. 71, No.6, (June 2002), pp. 921–931, ISSN 0741-5400

Hakim, F.T.; et al.. (2005). Age-dependent incidence, time course, and consequences of thymic renewal in adults.*The Journal of Clinical Investigation*, Vol.115, No.4, (April 2005), pp. 930-939, ISSN 0021-9738

Harris, J.M.; et al.. (2005). Multiparameter evaluation of human thymic function: interpretations and caveats. *Clinical Immunology*, Vol. 115, No.2, (May 2005), pp. 138-146, ISSN 1521-6616

Haselden, B.M.; et al.. (1999). Immunoglobulin E-independent major histocompatibility complex-restricted T cell peptide epitope-induced late asthmatic reactions. *The Journal of Experimental Medicine*, Vol.189, No.12, (June 1999), pp. 1885-1894, ISSN 0022-1007

Ibarrola, I.; et al.. (2004). Biological characterization of glutaraldehyde-modified Parietaria judaica pollen extracts. *Clinical Experimental Allergy*, Vol. 34, No.2, (February 2004), pp. 303–309, ISSN 0954-7894

Kelly, M.; et al.. (2007). Modulating leukocyte recruitment in inflammation. *The Journal of Allergy and Clinical Immunology*, Vol.120, No.1, (July 2007), pp. 3-10, ISSN 0091-6749

Kumar V.. (2005) Radiolabeled white blood cells and direct targeting of micro-organisms for infection imaging. *The Quarterly Journal of Nuclear Medicine and Molecular Imaging*, Vol.49, No.4. (December 2005), pp. 325-338, ISSN 1824-4785

Lambrecht, B.N. & Hammad, H.. (2002) Myeloid dendritic cells make it to the top. *Clinical Experimental Allergy*, Vol.32, No.6, (June 2002), pp. 805-810, ISSN 0954-7894

Larché, M.; et al.. (2006). Immunological mechanisms of allergen-specific immunotherapy. Nature Reviews Immunology, Vol. 6, No.10, (October 2006), pp. 761-71, ISSN 1474-1733

Lukacs, N.. (2000). Migration of helper T-lymphocyte subsets into inflamed tissues. *The Journal of Allergy and Clinical Immunology*, Vol.106, No.5(Part 2), (November 2000), pp. S264-269, ISSN 0091-6749

Mistrello, G.; et al.. (1994). Modified Par j I allergen from P judaica pollen and its rate of absorption in rats. Immunology Letter,s Vol. 40, No.1, (April 1994), pp 31-36, ISSN 0165-2478

Moingeon, P.; et al.. (2006). Immune mechanisms of allergen-specific sublingual immunotherapy. *Allergy*, Vol. 61, No.2, (February 2006), pp. 151-165, ISSN 0105-4538

Novak, N.; et al.. (2004). The role of antigen presenting cells at distinct anatomic sites: they accelarate and they slow down allergies. *Allergy*, Vol. 59, No.1, (January 2004), pp. 5-14, ISSN 0105-4538

Passalacqua, G.; et al.. (2005). Pharmacokinetics of radiolabelled Par j 1 administered intranasally to allergic and healthy subjects. *Clinical and Experimental Allergy*, Vol. 35, No.7, (July 2005), pp. 880–883, ISSN 0954-7894

Pereira C. Dinâmica da inflamação alérgica e da imunoterapia específica. Contribuição para o seu estudo in vivo. PhD Thesis. Medicine Faculty from the University of Coimbra. 2009 (pp:1-516); University of Coimbra, Portugal.

Pereira, C.; et al.. (2004). Kinetics and dynamic evaluation of specific immunotherapy. *European annals of allergy and clinical immunology*, Vol.36, No.10, (December 2004), pp. 375-386. ISSN 1764-1489

Peters, A.M.; et al.. (1986). Clinical experience with 99m Tc-hexamethyl propylene-amine oxime for labelling leucocytes and imaging inflammation. *Lancet*, Vol. 25, No.2(8513), (October 1986), pp. 946-949, ISSN 0140-6736

Sehmi, R.; et al.. (1996). Increased levels of CD34+ hemopoietic progenitor cells in atopic subjects. *American Journal of Respiratory Cell Molecular Biology*, Vol.15, No.5, (November 1996), pp. 645-654, ISSN 1044-1549

Senti, G.; et al.. (2008). Intralymphatic allergen administration renders specific immunotherapy faster and safer: a randomized controlled trial. *Proceedings of the National Academy of Sciences of the United States of America*, Vol.105, No.46, (November 2008), pp. 17908-17912, ISSN 0027-8424

Schmit-Weber, C.B. & Blaser, K.. (2002). T-cell tolerance in allergic response. *Allergy*, Vol. 57, No.9, (September 2002), pp. 762-768, ISSN 0105-4538

Schmit-Weber, C.B. & Blaser, K.. (2005). New insights into the mechanisms of allergen-specific immunotherapy. *Current Opinion in Allergy Clinical Immunology*, Vol. 5, No.6, (December 2005), pp. 525-530, ISSN 1528-4050

Spiller, H.A.; et al.. (1993), A five year evaluation of acute exposures to phenol disinfectant (26%). *Journal of toxicology. Clinical toxicology*, Vol.31, No.2, pp. 307-313, ISSN 0731-3810

Till, S.J.; et al.. (2004). Mechanisms of immunotherapy. *The Journal of Allergy and Clinical Immunology*, Vol.113, No.6, (June 2004), pp. 1025-1034, ISSN 0091-6749

Togias, A.. (2004). Systemic effects of local allergic disease *The Journal of Allergy and Clinical Immunology*, Vol.113, No.1(Suppl 1), (January 2004), pp. S8-14, ISSN 0091-6749

Upham, J.W.; et al. (2002). Rapid response of circulating myeloid dendritic cells to inhaled allergen in asthmatic subjects. *Clinical Experimental Allergy*, Vol. 32, No.6, (June 2002), pp. 818-823, ISSN 0954-7894

von Bubnoff, D.; et al.. (2002). Antigen-presenting cells and tolerance induction. *Allergy*, Vol. 57, No.1, (January 2002), pp. 2-8, ISSN 0105-4538

van Helvoort, J.M.; et al.. (2004). Preferential expression of IgG2b in nose draining cervical lymph nodes and its putative role in mucosal tolerance induction. *Allergy*, Vol. 59, No.11, (November 2004), pp. 1211–1218, ISSN 0105-4538

Wheeler, A.W. & Woroniecki, S.R..(2004). Allergy vaccines- new approaches to an old concept. *Expert opinion on biological therapy*, Vol. 4, No.9, (September 2004), pp. 1473–11481, ISSN 1471-2598

Woodfolk, J.A.. (2007). T-cell responses to allergens. *The Journal of Allergy and Clinical Immunology*, Vol.119, No.2, (February 2007), pp. 280-294, ISSN 0091-6749

8

Preventive Phytotherapy of Anaphylaxis and Allergic Reactions

Elaine A. Cruz[1], Michelle F. Muzitano[1],
Sonia S. Costa[2] and Bartira Rossi-Bergmann[3]
[1]*Faculdade de Farmacia, Macae Campus,*
[2]*Nucleo de Pesquisa de Produtos Naturais,*
[3]*Instituto de Biofísica Carlos Chagas Filho,*
Universidade Federal do Rio de Janeiro,
Brazil

1. Introduction

Anaphylactic shock is an extreme and life-threatening allergic reaction that requires immediate action to prevent death from airway and blood pressure collapse. The acute management comprises the use of epinephrine (adrenaline), the first-line medication of choice, and H1-antihistaminic drugs in doses that will depend on the severity of symptoms, in order to preserve the airway function and maintain the blood pressure and oxygenation at acceptable levels (Kemp & Lockey, 2002). On the other hand, long-term management comprises identification of precipitants (e.g.: Medications, foods, latex, insect venom) and their avoidance, and also immunotherapy.

One of the main mediators that are released and associated the many anaphylactic symptoms is histamine. H1-antihistamines are commonly used to relieve anaphylactic cutaneous symptoms such as itching, flushing, and urticaria, but play little role in the relief of bronchospasm or gastrointestinal symptoms, and fail to relieve upper airway edema or hypotension. Moreover, in usual doses, antihistamines alone do not prevent the explosive release of histamine and other mediators of inflammation from mast cells and basophils that culminate in the anaphylactic shock.

Since bronchospasm, hypotension and edema are not reversed immediately with antihistamines, a rapid administration of epinephrine is required to revert these symptoms. It has potent life-saving β-1 adrenergic vasoconstrictor effects on the small arterioles and precapillary sphincters leading to decreased mucosal edema, thereby preventing and relieving upper airway obstruction, and also to increased blood pressure, thereby preventing and relieving shock. (Kemp et al, 2008). Its strong effect on β-1 adrenergic receptors activation lead to increased rate and force of cardiac contractions, while activation of β-2 adrenergic receptors leads to increased bronchodilation and decreased release of histamine, tryptase, and other mediators of inflammation from mast cells and basophils (T.C. Westfall & D.P. Westfall, 2006). The adverse effects of epinephrine therapy involve pallor, headache (β -1 adrenergic receptors), palpitations (β-1 adrenergic receptors), tremor, vasodilation, increased release of mediators (β-2 adrenergic receptors) and anxiety (central CNS stimulation) that altogether may impose severe risk to patients with cardiac, central nervous system or thyroid diseases. On the other hand, glucocorticoids, that down-regulate β-2 while up-regulating β-1 adrenergic receptors and are mainstays in the treatment of asthma, have been shown not to reverse anaphylaxis symptoms (Simons, 2006). Therefore, in view of the hyper-acute nature of anaphylactic shock that limits adequate therapy, prevention is still the most adequate measure. Current prevention of anaphylaxis is based on allergen desensitization through specific immunotherapy of patients with high-risk of type I hypersensitivity reactions that involve immunoglobulin E (IgE)–mediated release of histamine and other mediators. The immunotherapy comprises the administration of increased doses of low-concentrated specific allergen solution that induce peripheral tolerance associated with differentiation of IL-10 and TGF-β - producing $CD4^+CD25^+$ regulatory T cells (Francis et al , 2003; Jutel et al, 2003). The efficacy of immunotherapy is also associated with an increase of antigen-specific IgG antibodies that block IgE effects on mast cells and basophils (Akdis & Blaser, 2000).

Table 1 summarizes the current measures available to treat and prevent anaphylactic shock:

DRUG	PHASE OF MANAGEMENT	EFFECTS
EPINEFRINE	Acute	Vasoconstriction, increased peripheral vascular resistance, increased blood pressure and relief of hypotension and shock; decreased mucosal edema and relief of upper airway obstruction and angioedema (effects through β-1 adrenergic receptors). Bronchodilation, decreased release of mediators (effects through β-2 adrenergic receptors).
H1-ANTIHISTAMINES	Acute	Relief of itching, flushing, urticaria, bronchospasm and gastrointestinal symptoms.
β2-ADRENERGIC AGONIST	Acute	Reversion of bronchospasm by relaxing of airway smooth muscle and reduction of asphyxia.
GLUCOCORTICOIDS	Acute	Inhibition of cytokine and arachidonic acid derivates production.
IMMUNOTHERAPY	Long-term	Induction of antigen-specific tolerance and increase of blockers antigen-specific IgG antibodies production.

Table 1. Summary of management of anaphylactic shock

2. Plants as sources of anti-allergic substances

Over the years, ethnobotanical studies allowed the association of plants with a diversity of biological activities and the discovery of new pharmaceutical drugs (Farnsworth et al., 1994). In the period 1981 to 2006, 52% of the small molecules discovered and in the development process were natural products or had their origins in natural products (Newman et al., 2007).

There have been many reports on the anti-allergic effects of some plants and natural compounds (Table 2).

SPECIES	EXTRACT	EXPERIMENTAL MODEL	EFFECT	REFERENCE
Ailanthus altissima	Swingle	Rat	Inhibits production of histamine, TNF, IL-6, and IL-8, and nuclear NF-κB/Rel A	Kang et al., 2010
Albizzia lebbeck	Bark aqueous extract	Guinea pig	Inhibits ileum contraction and bronchospasm	Barua et al.,1997
Baliospermu m montanum	Leaf chloroform and ethanol extracts	Rat	Inhibits mast cell degranulation	Venkatesh et al., 2010
Calotropis gigantea	Methanol extract	Rat	Inhibits paw edema	Ghaisas et al., 2011
Camellia japonica	Leaf extract. (quercetin and eugenol)	Rat	Inhibits Src-family kinase and degranulation in mast cells, and passive cutaneous anaphylaxis.	Lee et al., 2008
Crinum glaucum	Aqueous extract	Guinea pig	Inhibits ileum contractions	Okpo and Adeyemi, 2002
Euphorbia hirta	Ethanol extract	Rat and mouse	Inhibits paw edema, passive cutaneous and systemic anaphylaxis, TNF-α and IL-6.	Youssouf et al.,2007
Garcinia brasiliensis	7-epiclusianone	Guinea pig	Inhibits allergen-evoked intestinal spasm	Neves et al., 2007
Impatiens balsamina	Petal ethanol extract (flavonols and naphthoquinon es)	Mouse	Prevents blood pressure fall and fatal anaphylactic shock	Ishiguro et al.,1997; Fukumoto et al.,1996
Impatiens textori	Flower ethanol extract (apigenin, and luteolin)	Mouse	Inhibits scratching behavior and blood pressure decrease.	Ueda et al., 2005
Kalanchoe pinnata	Aqueous extract (quercitrin)	Mouse	Inhibits bronchospasm, fatal anaphylactic shock, IgE, eosinophilia, IL-5, IL-10, IL-13 and TNF-α, and histamine release.	Cruz et al, 2011, Cruz et al., 2008
Macrocystis pyrifera seaweed	Alginic acid	Rat	Inhibits histamine release, IL-1β and TNF-α, but not IL-6 or IL-8 production.	Jeong et al., 2006

SPECIES	EXTRACT	EXPERIMENTAL MODEL	EFFECT	REFERENCE
Matricaria recutita	Methanol extract	Rat	Reduces compound 48/80 induced anaphylaxis and histamine release	Chandrashekhar et al., 2011
Oryza sativa	Methanol extract	Rat	Reduces histamine release	Kim et al., 1999
Picrorhiza kurroa	Root and rhizome glycoside fraction	Guinea pig, mouse and rat.	Inhibits passive cutaneous anaphylaxis, ileum contraction but not bronchospasm induced by histamine.	Baruah et al., 1998
Porcirus trifoliata	Aqueous extract	Rat	Inhibits histamine release	Lee et al., 1996
Prunus mahaleb	Ethanol extract (oleic and linoleic acids)	Guinea pigs	Ovalbumin-induced bronchospasm	Shams et al., 2007
Rhus javanica	Gall aqueous extract	Rat and mouse	Decrease histamine release, TNF-α and IL-6 secretion.	Kim et al., 2005

Table 2. Anti-anaphylactic natural products

Chamomile (*Matricaria recutita*, Asteraceae) is one of the medicinal plants whose methanol extract containing flavonoids, tannins, terpenoids and coumarines has reported properties against compound 48/80 induced anaphylaxis in rats (Chandrashekhar et al., 2011). Not only plants but also seaweeds containing alginic acid (Jeong et al., 2006) and honeybees-produced propolis have been marketed for their anticipated anti-allergic effects (revised by Sforcin, 2007). Propolis consists of approximately 300 plant-derived compounds including flavonoids, phenolic acids, cinnamic acid derivatives, terpenoids, cellulose and amino acids. It has demonstrated protection against OVA-sensitized airway inflammatory reaction associated with inihibition of mast cell degranulation, and chrysin and kaempferol present in the ethanol extract appears to be the main anti-allergic compounds (Nakamura et al., 2010). Since 2005, there have been a number of double-blind, placebo-controlled clinical studies in China investigating the efficacy and safety of Chinese herbal products. The major findings of four promising herbal remedies, comprising at least three plant species, were revised by Li and Brown (2009).

Most of the plant products that fight inflammation belong to the chemical groups of alkaloids, coumarins, polyphenols, terpenoids and flavonoids. In particular, flavonoids such as quercetin, luteolin, fisetin and apigenin have been described with potent immunomodulatory properties. Studies on structure-activity relationship of 45 flavonoids showed that oberall they were more potent in inhibiting the production of IL-4 which is largely associated with allergic reactions (Revised by Kawai et al. 2007). Comalada et al. (2006) studied the structure–activity relationship for several flavonoids using primary bone marrow-derived mouse macrophages. They observed that some flavonoids inhibit TNF-α production as well as *i*NOS expression and nitric oxide (NO) production in LPS-activated macrophages, an effect that has been associated with the inhibition of the NF-κB pathway.

Suppression of of NF-κB nuclear factor activation by *Ailanthus altissima* swingle has also been associated with the reduced production of TNF-α, IL-6, and IL-8 pro-inflammatory cytokines and reduced histamine release during induced anaphylaxis (Kang et al., 2010). Flavonoids are known to have potent antiallergic activity (Kawai et al, 2007). For instance, luteolin and quercetin flavonoids (Figure 1) are potent inducers of the anti-inflammatory cytokine IL-10. Structure–activity relationship showed that four hydroxylations at positions 5, 7, 30 and 40, together with the double bond at C2–C3 and the position of the B ring at 2, seem to be necessary for the highest anti-inflammatory effect.

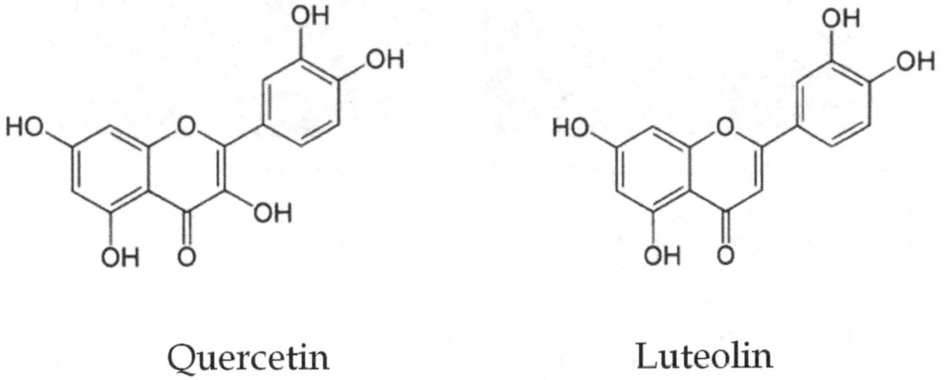

Quercetin   Luteolin

Fig. 1. Chemical structures of quercetin and luteolin flavonoids.

Due to the problematic curative therapeutics, preventive therapy may be an alternative life-saving therapy in highly allergic individuals prone to anaphylactic shock. It depends primarily on optimal management of risk factors, avoidance of allergen and other anaphylactic sensitizers (food, insect stings, plants and drugs), and immunomodulation. Since induced immunotolerance therapy involving the administration of increasing doses of a specific allergen has had limited success, and currently available immunosuppressive drugs are not safe enough to be continuously administered as a prophylactic measure, new anti-anaphylactic substances are highly needed in the market. In view of the enormous diversity of chemicals produced, medicinal plants are particularly interesting for the discovery of new anti-allergic agents as the safety of continuous consumption (e.g. herbal infusions) is popularly testified. This is the case of the plant *Kalanchoe pinnata*, whose potential use as source of anti-anaphylactic substances is described below in more detail.

3. The *Kalanchoe pinnata* example

Kalanchoe pinnata (Kp, syn *Bryophyllum pinnatum* Kentz., *Bryophyllum calycinum* Salisb., Crassulaceae) (Figure 2), is widely used in folk medicine in the form of infusions, juices and compresses to treat rheumatoid arthritis, gastric ulcer and in skin disorders (Lucas and Machado, 1946; Lorenzi and Abreu-Matos, 2008). It is native of Madagascar, Kp is now found in several countries such as India, China, and Brazil (Allorge-Boiteau, 1996).

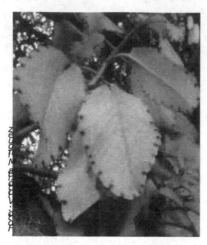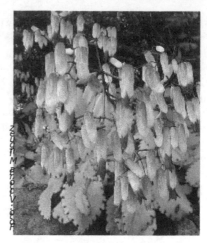

Fig. 2. *Kalanchoe pinnata* (Crassulaceae) : Leaves and Inflorescences

Antiparasitic (anti-leishmania), antibacterial, hepatoprotective and immunomodulatory activities have been described for Kp leaf extracts (Da Silva et al. 1995; Akinpelu, 2000; Muñoz et al. 2000; Yadav and Dixit, 2003; Rossi-Bergmann et al. 1994; Almeida et al., 2000). Exploratory toxicological studies in mice and humans have indicated absence of chronic and acute oral toxicity (Torres-Santos et al., 2003, Sousa et al., 2005). The clinical safety of Kp was also suggested during a study in 67 pregnant women (25 to 35 weeks of gestation) and their neonates (Plangger et al., 2006), corroborating its popular acceptance and pharmaceutical potential.

Kp contains substances belonging to different chemical classes, including: terpenes (Siddiqui et al. 1989; Gaind et al., 1972), bufadienolidos (Yamagishi et al., 1989; Supratman et al., 2001) and flavonoids (Gaind and Gupta, 1971; Ichikawa, 1986; Muzitano et al., 2006a, 2006b and 2009). Kp flavonoids are significantly more abundant when the leaves are collected during the summer (Muzitano et al., 2011). Quercitrin (quercetin 3-*O*-α-L-rhamnopyranoside), kaempferol 3-*O*-α-L-arabinopyranosyl (1→2)-α-L-rhamnopyranoside (kapinnatoside), quercetin 3-*O*-α-L-arabinopyranosyl (1→2)-α-L-rhamnopyranoside and 4′,5-dihydroxy-3′,8-dimethoxyflavone 7-*O*-β-D-glucopyranoside were isolated from a bioactive flavonoid fraction obtained from a Kp aqueous extract (Muzitano et al., 2006a, 2006b and 2009).

3.1 The anti-anaphylactic effect of the aqueous extract of *Kalanchoe pinnata*

The anti-anaphylactic activity of the aqueous extract of Kp leaves given orally to ovalbumin (OVA)-sensitized mice indicated the potent immunomodulatory action, preferentially inhibiting Th2-type immune responses known to be committed with enhanced susceptibility to cutaneous leishmaniasis and to allergies (Rossi-Bergmann et al, 1994; Da Silva et al 1999, Cruz et al 2008, Gomes et al 2009). Despite the early reports on the antihistaminic activity of Kp using the experimental models of isolated guinea pig ileum contraction and vasodilatation in rats (Nassis et al, 1992); its fatty acid associated suppressive activity on T cells (Rossi-Bergmann et al, 1994, Almeida *et al*, 2000).), and its Th2-suppressive and iNOS-suppressive association with oral protection against cutaneous and visceral leishmaniasis

(Da-Silva *et al*, 1995, Da-Silva *et al*, 1999, Gomes et al. 2009), only recently the therapeutic effect of Kp in allergy was more deeply explored.

The antianaphylactic activity o Kp was studied using a murine model of OVA-induced anaphylactic shock. The intraplantar injection of OVA (2.5 mg/kg) into pre-sensitised mice elicited a severe systemic anaphylactic response with death occurring within 15 min-30 min of allergen challenge. This extreme allergic reaction was effectively prevented with 400 mg/Kg of oral Kp during the 14-day sensitization process that maintained alive 100% for over 48 h of follow-up. Intraperitoneal injections with 200 mg/kg of Kp every other day during the same period of time was also effective, but to a lesser extent (80% of survival), similar to observed with 12.5 mg/Kg of i.p. cyclosporin A, an immunosuppressive drug also having anti-allergic effect. Interestingly, a single i.p. dose of 200 mg/Kg of Kp 3 h prior to OVA challenge was sufficient to protect 60% of the animals, suggesting that not only immunosuppression but also modulation of acute events related to shock was critical for protection.

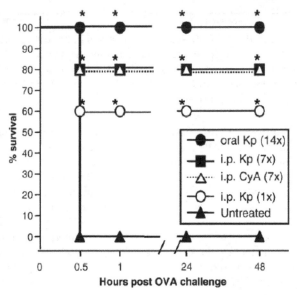

Fig. 3. Pre-treatment with Kp prevents fatal anaphylactic shock. BALB/c mice (n=5) were sensitized with OVA in adjuvant on days 1 and 7, and were challenged with 50 µg of OVA on day 14. During the sensitization period, they were treated as follows: i) by the oral route (daily doses of 400 mg/Kg of Kp for 14 days), ii) by the intraperitoneal route (7 doses of 200 mg/Kg of Kp or 12.5 mg/Kg of Cyclosporin in alternate days; or a single dose of 200 mg/Kg of Kp 3 h before OVA challenge). Controls were left untreated. Upon challenge on day 14, death events were monitored for up to 48 h and recorded as shown. The results are expressed as the percentage of surviving animals. *p<0.01 compared to untreated group.

As allergic parameters, the effect of Kp treatment on the number of circulating eosinophils and in allergen-specific IgE response was investigated. The OVA-induced enhanced eosinophilia was prevented by Kp, especially in animals receiving multiple oral or i.p. doses, although a single i.p. dose of Kp could be effective (Figure 4A). The raised production of OVA-specific IgE in sensitized mice was prevented by Kp therapy, particularly in animals on the oral regimen (Figure 4B).

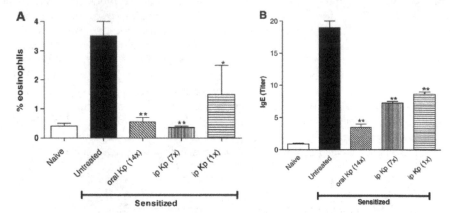

Fig. 4. Decreased eosinophilia and OVA-specific IgE levels in Kp-treated mice. Mice were sensitized and treated with Kp as for Fig. 1. A group of animals was bled 1 h before allergen challenge for the percentage of eosinophils in total leukocytes (top) and for individual assessment of the serum levels of anti-OVA IgE (bottom). Means±S.D (n=4). *$p \leq 0.05$ and **$p \leq 0.01$ in relation to untreated controls.

3.2 Quercitrin as an important anti-anaphylactic component of *Kalanchoe pinnata*

Like the aqueous extract, the isolated quercitrin flavonoid (Figure 5) was found to to be active in mice against cutaneous leishmaniasis caused by *Leishmania amazonensis* infection (Muzitano et al, 2006). Since cutaneous leishmaniasis, like allergy, is a disease driven by Th2-type immune responses, quercitrin was tested in the mouse model of OVA-induced anaphylactic shock. The animals were treated daily with oral quercitrin during the 14-day OVA-sensitization, with a dose 5% of that used with Kp (400 mg/Kg), compatible with its content in the aqueous extract. We observed that oral treatment with quercitrin conferred resistance to fatal anaphylactic shock in 75% of the animals, as compared with 0% of resistance in untreated sensitized animals (Figure 6), suggesting that quercitrin is an important anti-anaphylactic component of Kp.

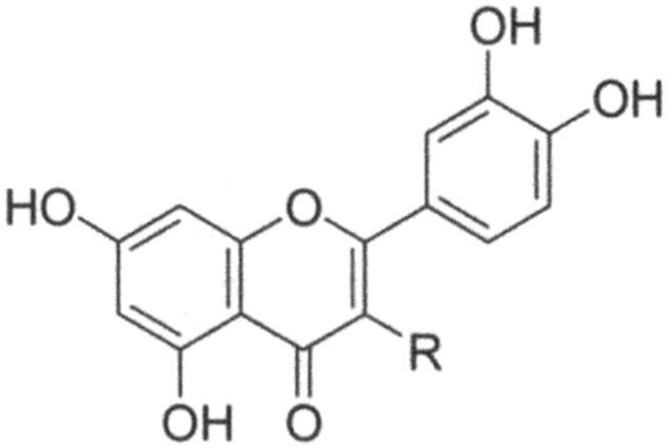

Quercitrin: R= O-α-ramnopyranose

Fig. 5. Chemical structure of quercitrin.

To better analyze the modulatory effect on Th2-type T cells, IL-5 and IL-10 cytokines were measured in the cell culture supernatants. Treatment of sensitized mice with oral or i.p. Kp reduced the capacity of their cells to respond to OVA with IL-5 and IL-10 production (Fig. 7). The production of TNF-α was also inhibited by Kp treatment, and like IL-10, this effect was more pronounced when the i.p. route was used, indicating that cytokines that contribute to allergy are down regulated during i.p, and to a lesser extent oral Kp treatments. The importance of the TNF-α was confirmed in mice deficient in TNFR1, and corroborated with other studies on *Ailanthus altissimain* and *Euphorbia hirta* (Table 2).

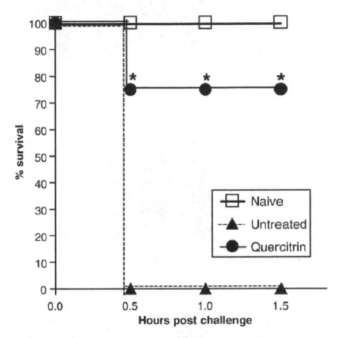

Fig. 6. Pre-treatment with quercitrin partially prevents death due to anaphylactic shock. BALB/c mice (n=8) were sensitized as for Fig. 1. During the sensitization period, they were daily treated with 20 mg/Kg of quercitrin by the oral route, during 14 days. Controls were left untreated. Naive were untreated non-immunized mice. Upon challenge on day 14, death events were monitored for up to 90 min and recorded as shown. The results are expressed as the percentage of surviving animals. *pb0.01 compared to untreated group.

The effect of Kp on histamine release by anti-DNP IgE-sensitized mast cells challenged with DNP was also investigated, and a significant inhibition of secreted histamine was found in cells that were pre-treated with Kp prior to DNP challenge (Fig. 8).
As mentioned above, cutaneous leishmaniasis and allergy are pathologies associated with expanded Th2-type immune responses, and they are benefited from the oral treatment with Kp. Although blockade of histamine release may ultimately contribute to the anti-anaphylactic effect of Kp, it is conceivable that downregulation of Th2-type immune responses is more critical for the resistance phenotype. The immunological effects of Kp are summarized in Figure 9.

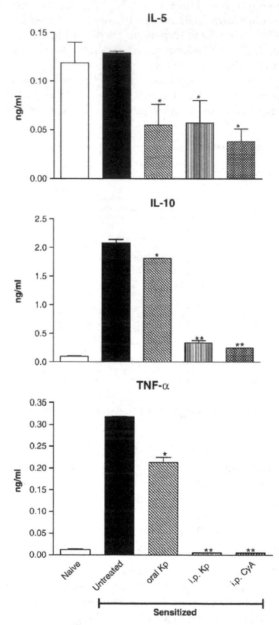

Fig. 7. Cytokine production in Kp-treated mice. Lymph nodes were obtained from mice that were sensitized and treated with Kp or Cyclosporin A (CyA) as indicated, and the cells restimulated in vitro with 1 mg/ml of OVA. After 48 h, the culture supernatants were collected for the determination of IL-5, IL-10 and TNF-α levels by ELISA.Means±S.D. (n=5). *p≤0.05 and **p≤0.01 in relation to untreated controls.

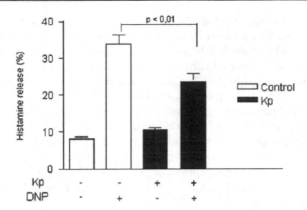

Fig. 8. Prevention of mast cell histamine release by Kp in vitro. Rat peritoneal mast cells were sensitized in vitro with anti-DNP IgE and then incubated with 500 µg/ml of Kp for 30 min prior to the 1-hour challenge with 50 µg/ml of DNP/BSA. Histamine was measured in the supernatants by a fluorimetric assay and expressed as the percentage of total histamine in cell lysates. Means±S.D (n=4).

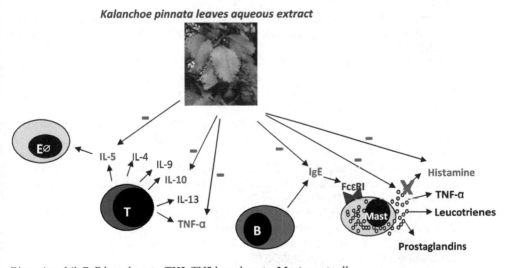

Eϕ: eosinophil, **B:** B lymphocyte, **TH2:** TH2 lymphocyte, **Mast:** mast cell.

Fig. 9. Anti-anaphylactic mechanisms of Kp. Anaphylactic shock is mediated by immunological mechanisms involving the production of Th2 cytokines (IL-4, IL-5, IL-9 and IL-13), the production of antigen-specific IgE antibodies, the recruitment and activation of eosinophils (through IL-5) and mast cells. The subsequent contact with antigen causes crosslinking of IgE molecules that are linked to the surface of mast cells via Fcε RI receptor and subsequent degranulation. After crosslinking, there is a systemic release of inflammatory mediators that responsible for the symptoms and the severity of anaphylaxis. Treatment with aqueous extract of Kp inhibits the production of IgE, the production of IL-10, IL-5 and TNF-α, degranulation of mast cells and histamine release.

The safety of Kp to humans is substantiated by the fact that it is widely consumed in the popular medicine, and that a human case of cutaneous leishmaniasis displayed unaltered serum toxicological parameters following oral treatment (Torres-Santos et al, 2003). For its effectiveness in mice and expected clinical safeness, quercitrin-containing Kp or quercitrin alone are potential candidates for clinical tests aiming at a prophylactic therapy for hypersensitive people under the risk of anaphylactic shock.

Anaphylaxis is a life-threatening allergic condition. Promising preventive measures include allergen nonspecific and allergen-specific immunotherapy. A range of plant species, including *Kalanchoe pinnata*, contain promising anti-allergic substances. Flavonoids extracted from *K. pinnata*, particularly quercitrin that down regulate Th2-type immune responses and also inflammatory reactions primarily induced by TNF-α, that together lead to overt release of histamine and other mediators by mast cells and basophils, culminating with anaphylactic shock.

4. References

Akdis, C.A. & Blaser, K. (2000). Mechanisms of allergen-specific immunotherapy. *Allergy*, 55, pp. (522-530).

Akinpelu, D.A. (2000). Antimicrobial activity of *Bryophyllum pinnatum* leaves. *Fitoterapia*, 71, pp. (193-194).

Allorge-Boiteau, L. (1996). Madagascar centre de spéciation et d'origine du genre *Kalanchoe* (Crassulaceae). In: *Biogéographie de Madagascar*. LOURENÇO, W.R. Editions de l'ORSTOM, Paris.

Almeida, A.P., Da Silva, A.G., Souza, M.L.M., Lima, L.M.T.R. Rossi-Bergmann, B., Gonçalves De Moraes, V.L. & Costa, S.S. (2000). Isolation and chemical analysis of a fatty acid fraction of *Kalanchoe pinnata* with a potent lymphocyte suppressive activity. *Planta Medica*, 66, pp. (134-137).

Barua, C.C., Gupta, P.P., Patnaik, G.K., Kulshrestha, D.K. & Dhawan, B.N. (1997). Studies on antianaphylactic activity of fractions of Albizzia lebbeck. *Current Science*, 72, 6, *pp.* (397-399).

Baruah, C.C., Gupta, P.P., Nath, A, Patnaik, L.G.K. &; Dhawan, B.N. (1998). Anti-allergic and anti-anaphylactic activity of picroliv - A standardised iridoid glycoside fraction of Picrorhiza kurroa. *Pharmacological Research*, 38, 6, pp. (487-492).

Chandrashekhara, V.M., Halagalia, K.S., Nidavania, R.B., Shalavadia, M.H., Ganapatyb, S., Biswasa, D. & Muchchandia, V.M. (2011). Anti-allergic activity of German chamomile (Matricaria recutita L.) in mast cell mediated allergy model. *Journal of Ethnopharmacology*, 137, 1, pp. (336-340).

Comalada, M., Ballester, I., Bailón, E., Sierra, S., Xaus, J., Gálvez, J., De Medina, F.S. & Zarzuelo, A. (2006). Inhibition of pro-inflammatory markers in primary bone marrow-derived mouse macrophages by naturally occurring flavonoids: Analysis of the structure-activity relationship. *Biochemical Pharmacology*, 72, pp. (1010-1021).

Costa, S.S., Muzitano, M.F., Camargo, L.M.M. & Coutinho, M.A.S. (2008). Therapeutic Potential of *Kalanchoe* Species: Flavonoids and other Secondary Metabolites. *Natural Product Communications*, 3, pp. (2151-2164).

Cruz, E.A., Da-Silva, S.A.G, Muzitano, M.F., E Silva, P.M.R., Costa, S.S. & Rossi-Bergmann, B. (2008). Immunomodulatory Immunomodulatory pretreatment with *Kalanchoe pinnata* extract and its quercitrin flavonoid effectively protects mice against fatal anaphylactic shock. *International Immunopharmacology*, 8, 12, pp. (1616-1621).

Cruz, E.A., Reuter, S., Martin, H., Dehzad, N., Muzitano, M.F., Costa, S.S., Rossi-Bergmann, B., Buhl, R., Stassen, M. & Taube, C. (2011). *Kalanchoe pinnata* inhibits mast cell activation and prevents allergic airway disease. *Phytomedicine*. (Jul 2011).

Da-Silva, S.A.G., Costa, S.S., Mendonça, S.C.F., Silva, E.M., Moraes, V.L.G. & Rossi-Bergmann B. (1995). Therapeutic effect of oral Kalanchoe pinnata leaf extract in murine leishmaniasis. *Acta Tropica*, 60, pp. (201–210).

Da-Silva, S.A.G., Costa, S.S. & Rossi-Bergmann, B. (1999). The anti-leishmanial effect of *Kalanchoe* is mediated by nitric oxide intermediates. *Parasitology*, 118, pp. (575-582).

Farnsworth, N.R. (1994). Ethnopharmacology and drug development. *Ciba Foundation Symptoms*, 185, pp. (42–51).

Francis, J.N., Till, S.J. & Durham, S.R. (2003). Induction of IL-10+CD4+CD25+ T cells by grass pollen immunotherapy. *J. Allergy Clin. Immunology*, 111, pp. (1255-1261).

Fukumoto, H., Yamaki, M., Isoi, K. & Ishiguro, K. (1996). Antianaphylactic effects of the principal compounds from the white petals of Impatiens balsamina L. *Phytotherapy Research*, 10, 3, pp. (202-206).

Gaind, K.N. & Gupta, R.L. (1972). Alkanes, alkanols, triterpenes and sterols of *Kalanchoe pinnata*. *Phytochemistry*, 11, pp. (1500-1502).

Gaind, K.N. & Gupta, R.L. Flavonoid glycosides from *Kalanchoe pinnata*. (1971). *Planta Medica*, 20, pp. (368-373).

Ghaisas, M.M., Kumar, D., Sarda, A.P. & Bhamre, S.S. (2011). Anti-anaphylactic and Mast Cell Stabilizing Effect of Calotropis gigantea Extract. *Latin American Journal of Pharmacy*, 30, 2, pp. (363-367).

Gomes, D.C.O., Muzitano, M.F., Costa, S.S. & Rossi-Bergmann, B. (2009). Effectiveness of the immunomodulatory extract of *Kalanchoe pinnata* against murine visceral leishmaniasis. *Parasitology*, 137, pp. (613-618).

Ichikawa, M., Ogura, M. & Iijima, T. Antiallergic flavone glycoside from *Kalanchoe pinnatum*. Patent 61, 118, 396 [86, 118, 319] (Cl. CO7H17/07), Apl 84/240, 282, 14 nov 1984; 4p-Chemical Abstracts, 105, 178423q, 1986.

Ishiguro, K. & Fukumoto, H. (1997). A practical and speedy screening method for murine anaphylaxis: On the antianaphylactic effect of Impatiens balsamina L. *Phytotherapy Research*, 11, 1, pp. (48-50).

Jeong, H.J., Lee, S.A., Moon, P.D., Na, H.J., Park, R.K., Um, J.Y., Kim, H.M. & Hong, S.H. (2006). Alginic acid has anti-anaphylactic effects and inhibits inflammatory cytokine expression via suppression of nuclear factor-kappa B activation. *Clinical and Experimental Allergy*, 36, 6, pp. (785-794).

Jutel, M., Akdis, M., Budak, F., Aebischer-Casaulta, C., Wrzyszcz, M., Blaser, K. & Akdis, C.A. (2003). IL-10 and TGF-beta cooperate in the regulatory T cell response to mucosal allergens in normal immunity and specific immunotherapy. *European Journal of Immunology*, 33, pp. (1205-1214).

Kang, T.H., Choi, I.Y., Kim, S.J., Moon, P.D., Seo, J.U., Kim, J.J., An, N.H., Kim, S.H., Kim, M.H., Um, J.Y., Hong, S.H., Kim, H.M. & Jeong, H.J. (2010). Ailanthus altissima swingle has anti-anaphylactic effect and inhibits inflammatory cytokine expression via suppression of nuclear factor-kappaB activation. *In Vitro Cellular & Developmental Biology-Animal*, 46, 1, pp. (72-81).

Kawai, M., Hirano, T., Higa, S., Arimitsu, J., Maruta, M., Kuwahara, Y., Ohkawara, T., Hagihara, K., Yamadori, T., Shima, Y., Ogata, A., Kawase, I. & Tanaka, T. (2007). Flavonoids and Related Compoundsas Anti-Allergic Substances. *Allergology International*, 56, pp. (113-123).

Kemp, S.F., Lockey, R.F. & Simons, F.E.R. (2008). Epinephrine: the drug of choice for anaphylaxis: a statement of the World Allergy Organization. *Allergy*, 63, pp. (1061–1070).

Kemp, S.F. & Lockey, R.F. (2002). Anaphylaxis: A review of causes and mechanisms. *Journal of Allergy and Clinical Immunology*, 110, pp. (341-348).

Kim, H.M., Yi, D.K. & Shin, H.Y. (1999). The evaluation of antianaphylactic effect of Oryza sativa L-in rats. *American Journal of Chinese Medicine*, 27, 1, pp. (63-72).

Kim, S.H., Park, H.H., Lee, S., Jun, C.D., Choi, B.J., Kim, S.Y., Kim, S.H., Kim, D.K., Park, J.S., Chae, B.S. & Shin, T.Y. (2005). The anti-anaphylactic effect of the gall of Rhus javanica is mediated through inhibition of histamine release and inflammatory cytokine secretion. *International Immunopharmacology*, 5, 13-14, pp. (1820-1829).

Lee, J.H., Kim, J.W., Ko, N.Y., Mun, S.H., Kim, D,K., Kim, J.D., Kim, H.S. Lee, K.R., Kim, Y.K., Radinger, M., Her, E. & Choi, W.S. (2008). Camellia japonica suppresses immunoglobulin E-mediated allergic response by the inhibition of Syk kinase activation in mast cells. *Clinical and Experimental Allergy*, 38, 5, pp. (794-804).

Lee, Y.M., Kim, D.K., Kim, S.H., Shin, T.Y. & Kim, H.M. (1996). Antianaphylactic activity of Poncirus trifoliata fruit extract. *Journal of Ethnopharmacology*, 54, 2-3, pp. (77-84).

Li, X.M. & Brown, L. (2009). Efficacy and mechanisms of action of traditional Chinese medicines for treating asthma and allergy. *Journal of Allergy and Clinical Immunology*, 123, pp. (297-306).

Li, X.M., Zhang, T.F., Sampson, H., Zou, Z.M., Beyer, K., Wen, M.C. & Schofield, B. (2004). The potential use of Chinese herbal medicines in treating allergic asthma. *Annals of Allergy, Asthma and Immunology*, 93, PP. (S35-S44).

Lorenzi, H. & Abreu-Matos, F.J. (2008). *Plantas Medicinais no Brasil – nativas e exóticas, (2a ed)*, Instituto Plantarum de Estudos da Flora Ltda, São Paulo, Brasil.

Lucas, V. & Machado, O. (1946). Contribuição ao estudo das plantas medicinais brasileiras - Saião. *Revista da Flora Medicinal*, 77, PP. (1-39).

Muñoz, V., Sauvain, M., Bourdy, G., Callapa, J., Rojas, I., Vargas, L. & Deharo, E. (2000). The search for natural bioactive compounds through a multidisciplinar approach in Bolivia: Part II. Antimalarial activity of some plants used by mosetane Indians. *Journal of Ethnopharmacology*, 69, pp. (139-155).

Muzitano, M.F., Cruz, E.A., Almeida, A.P., Da Silva, S.A., Kaiser, C.R., Guette, C., Rossi-Bergmann, B. & Costa, S.S. (2006a). Quercitrin: an antileishmanial flavonoid glycoside from *Kalanchoe pinnata*. *Planta Medica*, 72, pp. (81–83).

Muzitano, M.F., Tinoco, L.W., Guette, C., Kaiser, C.R., Rossi-Bergmann, B. & Costa, S.S. (2006b). Assessment of antileishmanial activity of new and unusual flavonoids from *Kalanchoe pinnata*. *Phytochemistry*, 67, pp. (2071-2077).

Muzitano, M.F., Bergonzi M.C., De Melo, G.O., Lage, C.L.S., Bilia A.R., Vincieri F.F., Rossi-Bergmann, B. & Costa, S.S. (2011). Influence of cultivation conditions, season of collection and extraction method on the content of antileishmanial flavonoids from *Kalanchoe pinnata*. *Journal of Ethnopharmacology*, 133, pp. (132-137).

Muzitano, M.F., Falcão, C.A.B., Cruz, E.A., Bergonzi M.C., Bilia A.R., Vincieri F.F., Rossi-Bergmann, B. & Costa, S.S. (2009). Oral Metabolism and Efficacy of Flavonoids in a Murine Model of Cutaneous Leishmaniasis. *Planta Medica*, 75, pp. (307-311).

Nakamura, R., Nakamura, R., Watanabe, K., Oka, K., Ohta, S., Mishima, S. & Teshima, R. (2010). Effects of propolis from different areas on mast cell degranulation and identification of the effective components in propolis. *International Immunopharmacology*, 10, pp. (1107–1112).

Nassis, C. Z., Haebisch, E.M. & Giesbrecht, A.M. (1992). Antihistamine activity of *Bryophyllum calycinum*. *Brazilian Journal of Biological Research*, 25, pp. (929-936).

Neves, J.S., Coelho, L.P., Cordeiro, R.S.B., Veloso, M.P., Silva, P.M.R.E, Dos Santos, M.H. & Martins, M.A. (2007). Antianaphylactic properties of 7-epiclusianone, a tetraprenylated benzophenone isolated from Garcinia brasiliensis. *Planta Medica*, 73, 7, pp. (644-649).

Newman, D.J. & Cragg, G.M. (2007). Natural products as sources of new drugs over the last 25 years. *Journal of Natural Products*, 70, pp. (461-477).

Okpo, S.O. & Adeyemi, O.O. (2002). The antianaphylactic effects of Crinum glaucum aqueous extract. *Journal of Ethnopharmacology*, 81, 2, pp. (187-190).

Plangger, N., Rist, L., Zimmermann, R. & Von Mandach, U. (2006). Intravenous tocolysis with *Bryophyllum pinnatum* is better tolerated than beta-agonist application. *European Journal of Obstetrics & Gynecology and Reproductive Biology*, 124, pp. (168–172).

Rossi-Bergmann, B., Costa, S.S., Borges, M.B.S., Da-Silva, S.A., Noleto, G.R., Souza, M.L.M & Moraes, V.L.G. (1994). Immunosuppressive effect of the aqueous extract of Kalanchoe pinnata in mice. *Phytotherapy Research*, 8, pp. (399–402).

Sforcin, J.M. (2007). Propolis and the immune system: a review. *Journal of Ethnopharmacology*, 113, pp. (1–14).

Shams, K.A. & Schmidt, R. (2007). Lipid fraction constituents and evaluation of anti-anaphylactic activity of Prunus mahaleb L. kernels. *African Journal of Traditional Complementary and Alternative Medicines*, 4, 3, pp. (289-293).

Siddiqui, S., Fazi, B.S. & Sultana, N. (1989). Triterpenoids and phenanthrenes from leaves of *Bryophullum pinnatum*. *Phytochemistry*, 28, pp. (2433-2438).

Sousa, P.J.C., Rocha, J.C.S., Pessoa, A.M., Alves, L.A.D. & Carvalho, J.C.T. (2005). Estudo preliminar da atividade antiinflamatória de *Bryophillum calycinum* Salisb. *Revista Brasileira de Farmacognosia*, 15, pp. (60-64).

Supratman, U., Fujita, T., Akiyama, K., Hayashi, H., Murakami, A., Sakai, H., Koshimizu, K. & Ohigashi, H. (2001). Anti-tumor promoting activity of bufadienolides from *Kalanchoe pinnata* and *K. daigremontiana* X tubiflora. *Bioscience Biotechnology and Biochemistry*, 65, 4, pp. (947-949).

Torres-Santos, E.C., Da-Silva, S.A.G, Santos, A.P.P.T., Almeida, A.P., Costa, S.S. &, Rossi-Bergmann, B. (2003). Toxicological analysis and effectiveness of oral Kalanchoe pinnata on a human case of leishmaniasis. *Phytotherapy Research* 17, pp. (801–803).

Ueda, Y., Oku, H., Iinuma, M. & Ishiguro, K. (2005). Antianaphylactic and antipruritic effects of the flowers of Impatiens textori MiQ. *Biological & Pharmaceutical Bulletin*, 28, 9, pp. (1786-1790).

Venkatesh, P., Mukherjee, P.K., Mukherjee, D., Bandyopadhyay, A., Fukui, H. & Mizuguchi, H. (2010). Potential of Baliospermum montanum against compound 48/80-induced systemic anaphylaxis. *Pharmaceutical Biology*, 48, 11, pp. (1213-1217).

Westfall, T.C. & Westfall, D.P. (2006). Adrenergic agonists and antagonists, In: *Goodman & gilman´s the basis of pharmacological therapeutics*. Brunton, L.L., Lazo, J.S., Parker, K.L., (11a ed.), pp. (237-295), McGraw-Hill, New York.

Yadav, N.P. & Dixit, V.K. (2003). Hepatoprotective activity of leaves of *Kalanchoe pinnata* Pers. *Journal of Ethnopharmacology*, 86, 2-3, pp. (197-202).

Yamagishi, T., Haruna, M., Yan, X.Z., Chang, J.J. & Lee, K.H. (1989). Antitumor agents, 110 1,2, Bryophilin B, a novel potent cytotoxic bufadienolide from *Bryophullum pinnatum*. *Journal of Natural Products*, 52, pp. (1071-1079).

Youssouf, M.S., Kaiser, P., Tahir, M., Singh, G.D., Singh, S., Shanna, V.K., Satti, N.K., Haque, S.E. & Johri, R.K. (2007). Anti-anaphylactic effect of Euphorbia hirta. *Fitoterapia*, 7-8, pp. (535-539).

9

Derived Products of Helminth in the Treatment of Inflammation, Allergic Reactions and Anaphylaxis

C.A. Araujo[1] and M.F. Macedo-Soares[2]
[1]Department of Immunology, St Jude Children's Research Hospital, Memphis, TN,
[2]Laboratory of Immunopathology, Butantan Institute, Sao Paulo, SP,
[1]USA
[2]Brazil

1. Introduction

Anaphylaxis is a life-threatening and systemic disorder that involves several organs and may lead to death. It is believed to be mostly triggered by release of mediators from activated mast cells, basophils and macrophages after allergen exposure. There are two major types of anaphylactic mechanisms: classical and alternative anaphylactic pathways. Classical anaphylactic pathway is triggered by cross-linking of IgE bound to FcεRI, high affinity IgE receptors, on mast cell and basophil surfaces to release pre-formed vasoactive amines (e.g. histamine), lipid mediators and neutral proteases from secretory granules upon allergen exposure. The alternative anaphylactic pathway is an IgE-independent mechanism and involves basophils and macrophages. Upon allergen exposure, IgG-immune complexes binds to FcγRIII, low affinity activating IgG receptor, and subsequent release PAF (platelet activating factor), but not histamine as major mediator. The understanding of immune mechanisms on triggering anaphylaxis is crucial for understanding how to manipulate the immune system to find better therapeutic interventions.

Helminth infection and their products have been demonstrated as potential therapeutic interventions in inflammatory disorders. Helminths use several imunomodulatory strategies to evade and/or modify the host immune response in order to survive in the host, including suppression or inactivation of host antigen-specific immune response. The modulation of the immune system has been considered beneficial for both host and parasites since it could avoid helminth eradication and protect the host from inflammatory responses which may damage host's tissues and organs. Several helminth immunomodulatory molecules and strategies have been identified and reported, such as eotaxin metalloproteinase, calreticulin, antioxidants and neutrophil inhibitory factor. They interfere with antigen processing and presentation, cell proliferation, cause T cell death, decrease IgE responses, reduce B cell activation and stimulate regulatory T cells. Therefore, these immunomodulatory factors can affect both the inductive and effector immune response, being suitable to modulate the inflammatory, allergic and anaphylactic responses.

Our studies have been focused in the immunossuppressive responses induced by roundworms *Ascaris suum* infection and a protein secreted by these worms named PAS-1 (protein from *Ascaris suum*). We have demonstrated that PAS-1 suppresses LPS-induced inflammation due to stimulating the secretion of IL-10 and TGF-β. Furthermore, PAS-1 was demonstrated suppressing B and T cell responses against OVA. Besides playing a down-modulatory effect in inflammatory responses induced by unrelated antigens, PAS-1 suppresses the acute and chronic lung allergic inflammation induced by APAS-3 (allergenic protein from *Ascaris suum*). In OVA/alum lung inflammation model, PAS-1 down-modulates the lung inflammatory response due CD4+CD25+FoxP3+ cells and CD8+γδTCR+ cells, which secretes IL-10/TGF-β and IFN-γ, respectively. In chronic lung inflammation model using OVA/alum or alum/APAS-3, besides inhibiting the inflammation into the lungs, PAS-1 also inhibits the airway remodeling by decreasing the activity of metaloproteinases and the production of angiogenic factors (IL-13 and VEGF). Taken together, these findings demonstrated that PAS-1 inhibits both acute and chronic lung inflammation in mouse models.

The understanding of immune modulatory mechanisms that control anaphylactic responses is critical to investigate therapeutic interventions for anaphylactic inflammatory disorders. The purpose of this chapter is to discuss the mechanisms triggered by allergic and anaphylactic reactions and potential therapeutic strategies using helminth products.

2. Immune responses triggered by anaphylactic reactions

2.1 Concept of anaphylaxis

Anaphylaxis is a systemic and immediate hypersensitivity with multi-organ system involvement that can progress potentially to a life-threatening reaction causing thousands deaths in the world. The term anaphylaxis was named by Dr Charles Robert Richet, a Nobel laureate in Physiology or Medicine in 1913. In 1902, Richet and his colleague Paul Portier reported that dogs immunized with non-lethal dose of sea anemone venom display fatal reactions to the second injection of the venom even in small doses. Shibasaburo Kitasato and Emil von Behring had previously demonstrated that animals immunized with bacterial toxins are able to produce anti-toxins (neutralizing antibodies). Since then, this phenomenon was named **anaphylaxis,** which term is derived from the Greek words "a-" (against) and "–phylaxis" (protection).

Anaphylaxis can occur following exposure to several allergen sources including food allergens, aeroallergens, venoms, drugs and vaccination. The most common symptoms include itching, erythema and urticaria after the exposure to allergens. The most severe cases of anaphylaxis involve cardiovascular and respiratory system with drop of cardiac pressure, bronchoconstriction, laryngeal edema and shock (Brown, 2004). The gastrointestinal system may be also involved featuring vomiting, abdominal pain and diarrhea. The central nervous system can be affected leading to a felling of impending doom and lack of consciousness related to hypotension and hypoxia. Once the anaphylactic reactions occur rapidly, an effective treatment (usually epinephrine injection) may avoid the occurrence of severe symptoms (Simons et al., 2003). Thus, it is crucial to understand the molecular mechanisms involved on anaphylactic reactions for strategically managing the risk and preventing recurrence.

2.2 Types of anaphylactic reactions

Anaphylaxis occurs due to release of vasoactive and inflammatory mediators from mast cells, basophils and macrophages upon allergen exposure. When antigens cross-link FcεRI-bound IgE or bind to IgGs, which are found as IgG-immune complexes attached to FcγRs, mainly FcγRIII, a signaling cascade is trigger to promote release of mediators which cause smooth muscle contraction and increase vascular permeability, leading to laryngeal edema (which may cause respiratory difficulty), hypotension, urticaria, abdominal muscular contraction, diarrhea (Ewan, 1998). It is reported that anaphylactic reactions in rodent models are induced by two different pathways: classical and alternative anaphylactic pathways (Figure 1).

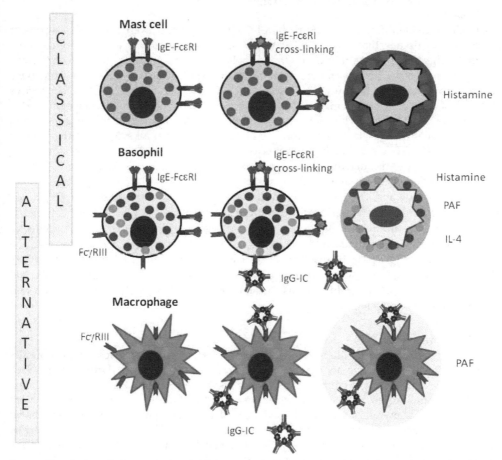

Fig. 1. Classical and alternative anaphylactic pathways. In the classical anaphylactic pathway, cross-linking among IgE-bound FcεRI and specific antigen leads to mast cell and basophil degranulation and secretion of histamine as major mediator. In the alternative anaphylactic pathway, IgG-immune complexes bind to FcγRIII on basophil and macrophage surfaces, triggering the secretion of PAF as major mediator. Basophils also secrete IL-4 that is crucial for IgE class-switching.

Classical anaphylactic pathway is triggered by cross-linking of antigen and antigen-specific IgE bound to FcεRI on mast cell and basophil surfaces, which stimulates these cells to degranulate and release histamine, serotonin, lipid mediators (such as leukotrienes) and cytokines (such as IL-4, TNFα, IL-1, VEGF) (Kumar & Sharma, 2010). Strait et al. (2003) have demonstrated that IgE-mediated anaphylaxis depends on IL-4/IL-4Rα, mast cells, FcεRI, IgE, histamine and H1 receptor but does not depend on macrophages, serotonin and leukotrienes. Alternative anaphylactic pathway is triggered by IgG-immune complexes bound to FcγRIII on basophils and macrophages, causing release of PAF (Mukai et al., 2009).

2.3 Cells involved in anaphylactic reactions
2.3.1 Mast cells
Mast cells were identified by Paul Ehrlich in 1879 (reviewed in Beaven, 2009) as cells present in connective tissues that reacts metachromatically with aniline dyes. He named them *Mastzellen* due the presence of granules that he believed to have a nutritional role on this cell type (the word *mast* denotes fattening in German). Mast cells are generated from bone marrow immature cells that migrate to skin and intestine and differentiate into connective tissue mast cells and mucosal mast cells, respectively (Arinobu et al., 2005; Galli et al., 2005). Stem cell factor (SCF or c-kit ligand) and c-kit play an important role in the growth and differentiation of mast cells, which express c-kit constitutively at all stages of differentiaton (Hu et al., 2007). They serve as important effector cells of the innate immune system along with other cell types (i.e. macrophages, dendritic cells, neutrophils, NK cells).

In anaphylactic reactions, mast cells are the effector cells in triggering the classical anaphylactic pathways. They express constitutively FcεRI, high affinity IgE receptor, which are usually bound to monomeric IgE upon antigen exposure. This receptor-IgE complex is cross-linked with multivalent antigens that consequently stimulate the release of effector mediators such as histamine, lipid mediators, and cytokines, which are pre-formed and stored in secretory granules of mast cells (Kumar & Sharma, 2010; Kemp & Lockey, 2002). These mediators act on many cellular types, including vascular endothelial cells and bronchial smooth muscle, inducing anaphylactic manifestations such as hypotension and dyspnea (Winbery & Lieberman, 2002).

2.3.2 Basophils
Similarly to mast cells, basophils were identified as cells that present metachromatic granules in the cytoplasm. Unlike human, mouse basophils are exceptionally rare (Urbina et al., 1981). They are the least common circulating cells that comprise less than 1% of total circulating granulocytes and are not normally present in tissues although are recruited to inflammatory sites. Basophils may contribute to IgE-mediated allergic inflammation and IgG1-mediated systemic anaphylaxis (Mukai et al., 2005; Tsujimura et al, 2008). They arise from bone marrow progenitors and complete their terminal differentiation in bone marrow (Arinobu et al., 2005).

Basophils constitutively express FcεRI, high affinity IgE receptor, and upon cross-linking of FcεRI-bound IgE with specific antigen, they release effector mediators such as histamine, leucotrienes, PAF and Th2 cytokines (IL-4, IL-5, IL-13) and TSLP (thymic stromal lymphopoietin) in response to protease allergens, causing immediate type hypersensitivity (Min, 2008). Mukai et al. (2009) have reported basophils as one of the major players in the IgG- but not IgE-mediated systemic anaphylaxis although basophils may function as initiator of allergic inflammation. Experiments from Tsujimura et al. (2008) demonstrated that mice passively transferred with anti-PenicillinV (PenV) monoclonal IgG1 antibody and challenged with PenV-conjugated BSA as allergen presented high drop of body temperature in both mast cell sufficient or deficient mice. They found that mainly basophils captured IgG1-immune complexes (they possessed highest amount of allergen per cell in comparison with other cell types), the binding was greatly inhibited by treatment with anti-FcγRIIb/FcγRIII antibody (against low affinity FcγRs), and they secrete high amount of PAF when stimulated by IgG1-immune complexes, indicating basophils as a good candidate to trigger IgG1-mediated anaphylatic reactions.

Besides their function as effector cells in IgG1-mediated anaphylaxis, basophils play a crucial role as early secretor of IL-4 that is essential to the development of anaphylactic reactions due to promoting class-switching to IgE. Sokol et al. (2008) have demonstrated that basophils are crucial for the initiation of Th2 cells in response to papain, a cystein protease, which activity is commonly found in most allergenic proteins. In addition, other findings reported that naïve CD4+ T cells stimulated with peptide-pulsed DCs could develop into Th2 cells when co-cultured with basophils from wild type mice but not IL-4-deficient mice (Oh et al, 2007), enforcing the role of basophils as early source of IL-4 in the immune responses.

2.3.3 Macrophages

Macrophages are long lived cells that function as a first line of defense in the body. These cells serve as early detector of invading pathogens through PAMPs, as antigen-presenting cells which initiate the immune responses, as effector cytotoxic cells to kill directly pathogens and also they play a role as regulatory and suppressor cells in parasitic infections and tumor-bearing hosts (Gordon, 2003). They arise from monocytes which are released in the blood stream and migrate to tissues to differentiate in macrophages or dendritic cells according to the stem cell factors milieu (Geissmann et al., 2010).

Macrophages have been involved in the development of IgG-dependent anaphylactic pathway (Oettgen et al., 1994; Miyajima et al., 1997; Strait et al., 2002). Passive immunization with allergen-specific monoclonal IgG1 antibody induce systemic anaphylaxis upon allergen exposure but this effect can be neutralized by treatment with anti-FcγRIIb/FcγRIII monoclonal antibodies (against low affinity FcγRs) and after depletion of macrophages with gadolinium (Strait et al, 2002), indicating the participation of macrophages in triggering IgG1-mediated anaphylactic reactions. Although platelets and neutrophils have been implicated in IgG-dependent anaphylaxis (Pinckard et al., 1977; Kimura et al., 1997), Strait et al. (2002) found in their studies that the techniques used for platelets and neutrophil depletion may inhibit IgE-independent anaphylaxis by producing immune complexes that desensitize macrophages, mimicking these cells as contributors of FcγRIII-dependent anaphylaxis.

Macrophages along with basophils also contribute to IgG-mediated anaphylaxis by releasing PAF upon antigen exposure. It has been demonstrated that the injection of anti-FcγRIIb/FcγRIII stimulates macrophages to release PAF by cross-linking FcγRIII on these cells and also inhibits IgG-dependent anaphylactic responses to antigen by blocking IgG-immune complex activation of macrophages through FcγRIII (Ujike et al., 1999; Strait et al., 2002).

2.4 Mediators involved in classical and alternative anaphylactic reactions
2.4.1 IgE and FcεRI

Ishizaka & Ishizaka (1976) discovered a new class of antibodies capable of transferring sensitivity to allergens. IgE antibodies are considered major players in allergic disorders such as anaphylaxis, asthma, atopic dermatitis, food allergy (Oettgen & Geha, 1999). It is considered the only antibody involved in classical anaphylactic reactions. It is also associated with protective immunity to parasitic infections (Capron et al., 1982). IgE consists of two identical heavy chains and two light chains with variable (V) and constant (C) regions and no hinge region which makes IgE to be less flexible. The ε-heavy chains contain one variable heavy chain and four constant region domains (Cε1-4) (Williams & Barclay, 1988) and are highly glycosylated (Arnold et al., 2007). IgE is the less abundant antibody class in serum with normal concentration of 50-200 ng/mL in nonallergic individuals (Gould et al., 2003). Even during helminth infections or allergic reactions, human serum IgE levels are lower than serum IgG levels; IgG peaks at around 30 μg/mL whereas IgG4 peaks at around 680 μg/mL (Bell, 1996). IgE has the shortest half-life of all immunoglobulins. Its half-life is about 3 days in serum (Iio et al., 1987), 16 hours on cells in suspension (Ishizaka & Ishizaka, 1971) and 2 weeks in tissues when is receptor-bound on cell surfaces (Geha et al., 1985). Its production requires class-switching from IgM, often via IgG to IgE by somatic recombination of germline genes in B cells", which depends on Th2 cytokines (IL-4/IL-13) and CD40 ligation (Poulsen & Hummelshoj, 2007).

It has been identified three IgE receptors in human (FcεRI($\alpha\beta\gamma2$ and $\alpha\gamma2$), galectin-3 and FcεRII) and four receptors in mice (FcεRI($\alpha\beta\gamma2$ and $\alpha\gamma2$), galectin-3, FcεRII and FcεRIV). Most of IgE bind to high affinity IgE receptor (FcεRI) that is present in mast cells, basophils (Gould et al., 2003) and antigen-presenting cells e.g. Langerhans cells (Bieber et al., 1992). FcεRI has a central role in mediating the allergic disorders (Kinet, 1999). Cross-linking of FcεRI associated to IgE with specific antigens induces the release of preformed mediators, newly formed lipid mediators and de novo synthesis of cytokines that potentially mediate anaphylactic reactions or prolonged allergic inflammation. FcεRI shares a common oligomeric structure, comprising a ligand binding immunoglobulin-like α-subunit associated to a β-subunit and two γ-subunits (Daeron, 1997). It binds stably monomeric IgE on mast cell surface (Kd ~ 10^{-10} M). The extracellular domain of α-subunit is glycosilated which seem to be crucial to appropriate maturation during FcεRI traffic through endoplasmic reticulum (Fiebiger et al., 2005) although is not required for monomeric IgE binding (Garman et al., 1999). The β- and γ-subunits bear ITAM (immunoreceptor tyrosine-based activation motif) that is phosphorylated in tyrosine residues by Lyn after cross-linking of FcεRI (Honda et al., 2000). The β-subunit possesses four transmembrane domains and the C-terminal domain has an ITAM motif. The γ-subunit belongs to T cell receptor (TCR) (gene family and is associated to Fc receptors including FcγRI, FcγRIIA, FcαRI (Takai, 2005). Other variant of FcεRI is constituted only by three chains (one α-subunit and two γ-subunits) that are expressed in monocytes, macrophages and neutrophils (Gould & Sutton, 2008). The low affinity IgE receptor (FcεRII) or CD23 is expressed in several cell types including B cells, activated T cells, monocytes, eosinophils, platelets, follicular dendritic cells, and thymic epithelial cells. CD23 facilitates the antigen presentation to T cells upon binding to IgE-antigen complex and also plays a role as negative regulator of IgE production (Gould & Sutton, 2008). Another IgE receptor is galectin-3 or ε-binding protein, which has been reported to be involved in neutrophil activation (Truong et al., 1993). In mice, it has been found a fourth type of IgE receptor, FcγRIV, which binds IgE-immune complexes on macrophage surface, inducing lung inflammation (Mancardi et al., 2008).

2.4.2 IgG and FcγRIII
IgG antibodies were identified by Tiselius and Kabat in 1939. They immunized rabbits with ovalbumin and fractionated the immune serum by electrophoresis into albumin, α-globulin,

β-globulin and γ-globluin fractions. The fact that this rabbit serum binds to ovalbumin γ-globulin fraction named the immune factor present in rabbit sera as immunoglobulin(Ig) or IgG (Tiselius & Kabat, 1939). Classically, there are four types of IgG subclasses in humans (IgG1-IgG4) and mice (IgG1, IgG2a, IgG2b, and IgG3). They are the most predominant antibody isotype (70-75% of total IgG) in the blood and extravascular compartments. Four different types of FcγRs have been identified in mice (FcγRI, FcγRIIb, FcγRIII, and FcγRIV). The human and primates FcγRs have several allelic variants that codify six types of FcγRs: FcγRI, FcγRIIa, FcγRIIc, FcγRIIb, FcγRIIIa, FcγIIIb.

Traditionally, these receptors belong to two different categories – they are classified in high or low affinity FcγRs according IgG affinity to them, and in activating or inhibitory FcγRs if the type of signaling pathway is triggered by ITAMs (immunoreceptor tyrosine-based activation motif) or ITIMs (immunoreceptor tyrosine-based inhibitory motif). Then, FcγRI is high affinity, activating FcγRs in both mice and humans; FcγRIII and FcγRIV (in mice) and FcγRIIa, FcγRIIc, FcγRIIIa, FcγRIIIb (in human) are categorized as low affinity, activating FcγRs; and FcγRIIb is the only low affinity, inhibitory FcγR in mice and humans. IgGs antibodies bind with different affinity and specificity to different FcγRs (Dijstelbloem et al., 2001). In general terms, monomeric IgG binds predominantly to high affinity FcγRs (FcγRI) and IgG-immune complexes binds to low affinity FcγR. These receptors are widely expressed in haematopoietic cells (except T cells), endothelial cells, osteoclasts, and mesangial cells. In mice, monocytes and macrophages express all activating and inhibitory FcγRs (FcγRI-IV), neutrophils express mainly FcγRIII, FcγRIV and FcγRIIb, dendritic cells express FcγRI, FcγRIII, FcγRIIb, NK cells only express FcγRIII and B cells only have FcγRIIb (Nimmerjhan & Ravetch, 2008).

IgG antibodies and FcγRIII have been implicated in triggering alternative anaphylaxis pathway. Mice lacking mast cells, IgE or FcεRI alpha chain still develop systemic anaphylactic responses upon antigen exposure (Jacoby et al., 1984; Oettgen et al., 1994; Dombrowicz et al., 1997) whereas FcRγ deficient mice that lack the expression of Fc(RI and activating Fcγ (receptors FcγRI, FcγRIII, FcγRIV) have no apparent signal of systemic anaphylaxis (Miyajima et al., 1997). Furthermore, it has been found that mice passively transferred with allergen-specific monoclonal IgG, particularly monoclonal IgG1, developed systemic anaphylaxis upon allergen exposure; when these mice were pre-treated with anti-FcγRIIb/FcγRIII, FcγRIV monoclonal antibodies, the systemic anaphylaxis was inhibited, indicating the role of FcγRIII in IgG-mediated anaphylaxis (Strait et al., 2002).

2.4.3 Histamine and H1 receptor

Histamine is an autacoid, also referred as 2-(1H-imidazol-4-yl)ethanamine, that modulates the cellular function in several tissues including dermis, small intestine, stomach, lungs and brain (Jones & Kearns, 2011). Its synthesis depends on histidine decarboxylase (HDC) that removes of carboxylic acid residue on the histidine side chain in the Golgi apparatus. It is stored basically in mast cells and basophils although it has been demonstrated that other cell types (e.g. neutrophils, lymphocytes, monocytes, dendritic cells, platelets, gastric cells and brain histaminergic cells) express HDC (MacGlashan, 2003). The release of histamine occurs in response to cross-link of antigen-specific IgE on mast cells and basophils surfaces upon antigen exposure during systemic anaphylaxis and the early phase of allergic responses. Large quantities of histamine (10^{-5} to 10^{-3} mol/L) are released within 30 minutes after allergen exposure (Simons, 2003). Histamine and other released mediators such as leukotrienes and prostaglandins produce the acute symptoms including pruritus of nasal mucosa, eyes, skin and increased vascular permeability, vasodilatation and edema resulting in nasal congestion, rhinorrea and conjuntival edema and erythema (Clough et al., 1998). Histamine can cause bronchoconstriction due to mucus accumulation by activated globet cells in the lung (Golightly & Greos, 2005) and may be involved in airway remodeling (Kunzmann et al, 2007). Histamine is responsible for mast cell activation by stimulating the secretion of cytokines and chemokines from T and B lymphocytes which up-regulates adhesion molecules in epithelial cells (Akdis & Blaser, 2003).

Histamine binds to four major receptors (H1, H2, H3 and H4) which belong to G-protein seven transmembrane receptor family. H1 receptor has been widely discussed in anaphylactic disorders. Histamine binds to H1R that activates inositol-1, 4, 5 pathway, mobilizing intracellular calcium which induces the vascular endothelium to release nitric oxide and stimulate guanyl cyclase to increase the production of cyclic GMP in vascular endothelial cells. This cascade promotes vasodilatation, erythema, vascular permeability and edema (Li et al, 2003). Activation of H1R produces direct effect in bronchial smooth muscle leading to bronchoconstriction. H1 and H2 receptors are overexpressed in patients with asthma in contrast to patients with rhinitis only (Botturi et al, 2010). The H2 receptor is expressed on gastric mucosa, vascular smooth muscle, brain, adipocytes and immune cells. Activation of H2 results in relaxation of smooth muscle in the airway and vasculature (Akdis & Simons, 2006). The stimulation of H3 receptor is been involved in pruritus (Sugimoto et al, 2004) and H4 receptor may play a role in inflammatory processes by inducing chemotaxis and calcium influx in bone marrow-derived and tracheal mast cells migration from connective tissue toward epithelium (Thurmond et al, 2004).

2.4.4 Platelet activation factor (PAF)

The term PAF was first used to describe the factors that aggregate and activate platelets (Benveniste et al., 1972). PAF is a potent proinflammatory phospholipid synthesized from the cleavage of glycerophospholipids by phospholipase A2 that binds to PAF receptor, a G-protein coupled seven-transmembrane receptor. It is active at concentration as low as 10^{-12}M (Stafforini et al, 2003). Since its discovery, pleiotropic effects of PAF have been demonstrated, including its role in bronchoconstriction, hypotension, vascular permeability, chemotaxis, degranulation of eosinophils and neutrophils (Hanahan, 1986). PAF is released from mast cells, basophils and macrophages upon antigen stimulation in human and experimental anaphylactic reactions (Vadas et al., 2008; Finkelman, 2007). Histamine, which can be secreted by mast cells and basophils, effectors cells in classical anaphylactic pathway, is a potent agonist for PAF synthesis by human endothelial cells (McIntyre et al., 1985). Circulating levels of PAF are controlled by the activity of PAF acetylhydrolase, enzyme that rapidly degrades PAF, making its half-life very short; it ranges from 3 to 13 minutes (Karasawa, 2006).

Vadas et al. (2008) have found that PAF levels positively correlate with the severity of anaphylaxis and may be pivotal for anaphylaxis outcome. Serum PAF levels is significantly elevated in allergic patients with severe anaphylaxis than those with milder manifestations of anaphylaxis. PAF has been identified as relevant vascular leak mediator in anaphylaxis (Camerer et al., 2009). The deletion of PAF receptor impairs anaphylactic responses in genetically manipulated mice (Ishii et al., 1998). In addition, recombinant PAF acetylhydrolase is protective and reduces mortality in experimental models of anaphylaxis (Fukuda et al., 2000; Gomes et al., 2006). Furthermore, PAF stimulate NO (nitric oxide) production by enhancing the activity of NOS (constitutive nitric oxide synthase), instead of iNOS (inducible nitric oxide synthase), which relaxes vascular smooth muscle, leading to hypotension and death (Cauwels et al., 2006).

2.4.5 IL-4 and IL-4Ralpha

IL-4 is a pleiotropic type I cytokine, recognized as signature cytokine of Th2 immune responses (Swain et al., 1990). It is produced by Th2 CD4+ T cells, basophils, mast cells, eosinophils and CD1-restricted NKT cells upon stimulation (Paul, 1997). IL-4 binds to IL-4 receptor, which is a heterodimer of IL-4 receptor α chain and common γ chain, resulting in phosphorylation of STAT6 (signal transducer and activator of transcription 6) (Nelms et al., 1999).

IL-4 exacerbates anaphylaxis through a direct effect on mast cell and basophils or through enhancing antibody production. Strait et al. (2003) have demonstrated that IL-4R signaling increase the responsiveness of mast cell- and macrophage-secreted mediators such as histamine, PAF, serotonin and leukotriene C4. IL-4 increases anaphylactic responses in a mouse model infected with *Thrichinella spiralis* by increasing histamine and PAF, but also enhances anaphylaxis at doses lower than those produced by helminth infections (Conrad et al., 1990). The contribution of IL-4/IL-4Rα in the anaphylaxis is also associated to their role in antibody production. IL-4 promotes class-switching to IgE antibodies (Finkelman et al., 1988) but it does not seem crucial to IgG1 production since high IgG1 levels is found in mice treated with anti-IL-4, and in IL-4 or STAT-6 deficient mice (Finkelman et al., 1989; Kuhn et al., 1991; Shimoda et al., 1996).

3. Helminth infections as predisposed factors to allergic and anaphylactic reactions

Helminths are known to cause widespread infections, mainly in tropical and subtropical areas in the developing world where the water suply and sanitation conditions are not adequate (De Silva et al., 2003). Although they did not cause high mortality, they tend to cause chronic infections in populations that live in endemic area, leading to iron-deficiency anemia and malnourishment and interfering with physical and mental growth in children (Stephenson et al., 2000).

The immune response against helminth infections is associated with high production of IgE levels and tissue infiltration of eosinophils, mast cells and Th2 cells which secrete IL-4, -5 and -13 (Fallon & Mangan, 2007). Th2 immune responses are believed to mediate protective immunity against these parasites (Anthony et al., 2007). Certain parasites such as *Schistosome mansoni* produce a strong Th2 immune response that is correlated with the formation of Th2 granuloma around schistosoma eggs (Wilson et al., 2007).

Several studies have demonstrated that helminth infection may increase allergic inflammation. Individuals exposed to helminthes for a short time often have allergic-like manifestations (Cooper, 2009). Lynch and collaborators (Lynch et al., 1984, 1987, 1992, 1997) have shown that the intensity of helminth transmission determines the effect of helminth infection on allergic reactivity - in high income urban areas where the transmission is low, the allergic reactivity is high whereas in urban and rural areas where people are chronically infected by helminthes, the allergic reactivity is low. Geohelminth parasite with pulmonary larval stages, such as *Ascaris lumbricoides, Necator americanus, Ancylostoma duodenale* and *Strongyloides stercoralis,* are found to cause Loeffler's syndrome which is characterized by eosinophilic infiltrate into the lungs after parasitic infection (Loefller, 1959).

Corroborating with Lynch's studies, it has been reported high association between dust mites and parasitic diseases in tropical allergies (Caraballo & Acevedo, 2011). Mites are important source of allergens in tropical areas (Fernandez-Caldas et al., 1993, 2008). The warm temperatures and high humidity facilitate the proliferation of dust mites such as *Blomia tropicalis* and *Dermatophagoides pteronyssinus* (Puerta et al., 1993). Likewise, nematodes are highly prevalent in tropical areas. *Ascaris lumbricoides* is the most prevalent, affecting around 1.5 million people worldwide (McSharry et al., 1999) by oral contamination with embryonated eggs that differentiate in migratory larvae, compromising intestine, liver, and lungs (Bradley & Jackson, 2004). Cross-reactivity between mites and *Ascaris* could explain why there is a positive correlation between allergies caused by dust mites and nematode infections in tropical areas. Acevedo et al. (2009) found cross-reactivity of specific IgE and tropomyosin from *B. tropicalis*, *D. pteronyssinus* and *A. lumbricoides* in asthmatic patients. It is postulated that high prevalence of specific IgE to mites in a tropical environment may be influenced by cross-reactivity with *Ascaris* spp. allergens (Acevedo et al., 2011). Another study also suggested that nematode infections may induce reactivity to tropomyosin in atopic individuals. Santiago et al. (2011) have demonstrated that there is 72% of amino acid identity between tropomyosin from *D. pteronyssinus* (Der p10) and *Onchocerca volvulus* in sera from *O. volvulus*-infected and non-infected atopic individuals and the prevalence of Der p10-specific IgE and IgG was increased in *O. volvulus*-infected individuals. Besides *Ascaris* infection, HDM (house dust mite) sensitization is strongly associated to wheeze symptoms in individuals from urban areas than in rural areas that had *Trichuris* infection (Scrivener et al., 2001).

Cooper (2009) and Smits et al. (2010) have listed four factors that may determine the effect of helminthic infections in promoting allergic responses (Figure 2): 1) **Timing** - periodic helminth infections in adult age (acute infections) may induce allergic manifestations whereas long-lasting helminthic infections in early age (childhood) (chronic infections) may suppress allergic inflammation due to inducing an immunomodulatory environment. 2) **Intensity of infection** – light parasite burden may induce allergic manifestations and heavy parasite burdens may induce down-modulation of allergic symptoms. 3) **Host genetics** – atopic individuals may be more likely to develop allergic manifestations than non-atopic individuals. 4) **Parasite** – different helminthes have different effects on atopy and allergies, parasites with larvae stages in the lung and skin than in other organs/tissues may be more predisposed to allergic manifestations.

4. Helminths and their products as anti-inflammatory modulators for allergic and anaphylactic disorders

Despite inducing strong Th2 and being considered predisposing factor to allergic manifestations, helminth infections can induce suppression of allergic diseases. Smits et al. (2010) related that chronic helminth infections may protect against allergic diseases by stimulating regulatory B and T cells and modulating dendritic cell functions. The immunosuppressive effect of helminthes and their products in the immune response have been widely reported in the literature (Smits et al., 2010; Hewitson et al., 2009; Soares & Araujo, 2008; Harnett & Harnett, 2008; Maizels et al., 2004). Helminth molecules can degrade some host molecules such as eotaxin and antibodies, inhibit the formation of reactive oxygen and nitrogen intermediates, interfere with macrophage activaction, down-modulate the antigen presentation by dendritic cell and macrophages, and mimic cytokines such as IFN-γ, TGF-β and MIF.

ALLERGIC MANIFESTATIONS

Adult people
Light parasite burden
Atopic individuals
Parasite with life cycle stage in the lungs

HELMINTH PARADIGM

Children
Heavy parasite burden
Non-atopic individuals
Parasite with life cycle stage in
organs/tissues other than lungs

SUPPRESSION OF
ANAPHYLACTIC RESPONSES

Fig. 2. Helminth paradigm. Helminthes can stimulate allergic manifestations or suppress inflammatory/anaphylactic responses depending on time and intensity of the infection, host genetic background and parasite life cycle.

Helminth infections can impair immune response toward heterologous antigen (Stewart et al., 1999), allografts (Liwski et al., 2000), viral infections (Actor et al., 1993) and other helminth infections (Jenkins, 1975). Helminths employ several immunomodulatory strategies in order to evade and/or modify the host immune response and, consequently, perpetuate their survival in the host (Playfair, 1982), including inactivation and/or modulation of the host protective immune response. The immunomodulation has been considered beneficial both to the host and the parasites since it could avoid helminth erradication and protect the host from inflammatory responses that may damage the host's tissue (van Riet et al., 2007).

It has been identified several immunomodulatory molecules and strategies by which the helminths evade the host immune system, permitting that the parasites subvert the host protective responses. Some of these molecules include eotaxin metalloproteinase (Culley et al., 2000), calreticulin (Pritchard et al., 1999), antioxidants (Brophy et al., 1995) and neutrophil inhibitory factor (Moyle et al., 1994). They can interfere with antigen processing and presentation (Dainichi et al., 2001), cell proliferation (Allen & MacDonalds, 1998), cause T cell death (Semnani et al., 2003), decrease IgE responses (Langlet et al., 1984), reduce B cell activation (Deehan et al., 1997) and stimulate regulatory T cells (Belkaid et al., 2006). In this section, we will discuss about some helminth products and their immunomodulatory effect in the immune system (Figure 3).

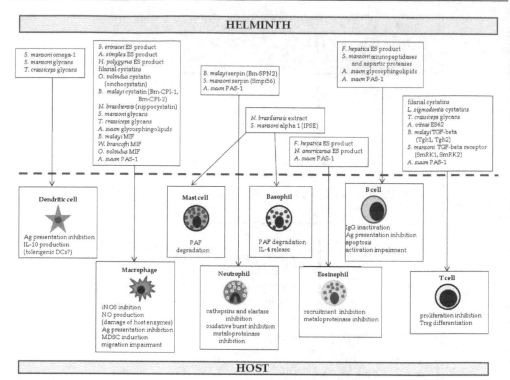

Fig. 3. Some immunosuppressive products secreted by helminthes that may be used as therapeutic strategies for anaphylactic disorders. Helminth can secrete molecules that possess down-modulatory effect on the host's immune system. The upper panel show some molecules secreted by helminthes and the lower panel show the cell targets of the helminth-secreted products. Abs, antibodies; Ag, antigen; ES, excretory/secretory products; MIF, macrophage-migration inhibition factor; MDSC, myeloid-derived suppressor cells; NO, nitric oxide; iNOS, inducible nitric oxide synthase; PAF, platelets-activating factor; PAS-1, protein from *Ascaris suum*; Treg, regulatory T cells.

4.1 Helminth products and their strategies to immunomodulate the host immune responses

4.1.1 Cleavage of host immune system molecules

It has been described several helminth defense mechanisms that can block host immune system by cleaving immune factors. The adult stage of *Nippostrongylus brasiliensis* releases in *in vitro* culture a product with acetylhydrolase activity that promotes cleavage of platelet-activating factor (PAF), promoting bronchoconstriction and increasing vascular permeability (Blackburn & Selkirk, 1992). Excretory/secretory (ES) products from hookworm *Necator americanus* cleave eotaxin (Culley et al., 2000), and in this way inhibit the recruitment of eosinophils, pivotal cells in development of the late phase of allergic responses.

Helminth serpins can also interfere in the immune response by cleaving immune factors. Serpins are an extensive family of serine proteinase inhibitors which regulate a wide variety of proteinase-dependent physiological functions, such as blood coagulation, fibrinolysis, activation of complement, and the inflammatory response (Potempa et al., 1994). A serpin produced by microfilarial stage of *Brugia malayi*, Bm-SPN-2, inhibits the enzymatic activity of serine proteinases, cathepsin G and elastase from human neutrophils (Zang et al., 1999). In addition, Smpi56, a serpin from *Schistosoma mansoni*, inhibits the neutrophil elastase (Ghendler et al., 1994), protecting the parasite from activated neutrophils during inflammation.

Besides promoting the cleavage of PAF, eotaxin and inactivation of neutrophil enzymes, helminth products also can cleave host antibody. Antibody cleavage is critical for the parasite evasion because it inhibits ADCC (antibody-dependent cell cytotoxity) and promotes IgG degradation, which blocks FcγR-mediated cytokine release. For instance, ES products from *Fasciola hepatica* cleave all human IgG subclasses at the hinge region (Berasain et al., 2000). In addition, *S. mansoni* schitosomula produces a trypsine-like proteinase or aminopeptidase that cleave Fab fragment when Fc receptor of the worm binds IgG (Auriault et al., 1981). Recombinant schistosome aspartic proteases from *S. japonicum* cleave specifically human IgG, suggesting that these proteases may play a role in the degradation of host serum proteins ingested as part of the schistosome bloodmeal (Verity et al., 2001).

4.1.2 Modulation of nitric oxide production

Nitric oxide (NO) is a potent microbicidal agent that plays a role in host defense against parasites. This effect has been demonstrated toward several helminthes. It has been found that ES products from parasites such as *Spirometra erinacei* (Fukumoto et al., 1997), *Anisakis simplex* (Cuellar et al., 1998), *Heligmosomoides polygyrus* (Rzepecka et al., 2006) suppress the expression of iNOS in LPS-activated macrophages in a dose dependent manner. However, filarial nematode cystatins (Hartmann et al., 2002) up-regulate NO production from IFN-γ-activacted macrophages. In spite of the susceptibility of parasites to NO, its stimulation in the host by helminth products is critical to promote nitration and oxidation of host´s molecules and damage several biological processes. Moreover, in filariasis murine model NO production was associated with suppression of T cell proliferation (O'Connor et al., 2000), suggesting that the secretion of NO is linked to microfilariae killing and T cell response inhibition.

4.1.3 Interference with antigen presentation and T cell responses

Helminth cystatins are thought to be the most important molecules that interfere with antigen presentation. Cystatins constitute a family of cysteine protease inhibitors that are widely distributed and play essential roles in a spectrum of physiological processes (Barrett, 1986). Nematode cystatins could lead to severe changes in antigen processing and inhibit efficient generation of peptide-MHC class II molecule, decreasing the antigen presentation by APC. These molecules target cysteine proteases such as cathepsins, which play a role in two catalytic processes (Hartmann & Lucius, 2003). First, cysteine proteases degrade proteins within the endosomal-lysosomal compartment of APC. Second, cysteine proteases are involved in the cleavage of the MHC class II-associated invariant chain, which leads to the formation of MHC molecules associated to CLIP (class II-associated invariant chain peptide). Then, synthesized CLIP molecules allow the binding of peptides to MHC class II molecules to promote antigen presentation. The invariant chain cleavage is promoted by cathepsins S in B cells and dendritic cells (Riese et al., 1996), cathepsins L in thymus epithelial cells (Nakagawa et al., 1998) and cathepsin F in macrophages (Shi et al., 2000).

Nematode cystatins are homologous to mamalian cystatin C, which are highly expressed by immature dendritic cells and are down-regulated during dendritic cells maturation process to permit the transport of MHC II molecules to cell surface. Parasite cystatins maintain dendritic cells in immature state, preventing the antigen presentation by these cells and also down-regulate *in vitro* cellular proliferation (Pierre & Mellman, 1998). The first described parasite cystatin was onchocystatin, derived from *Onchocerca volvulus* (Lustigman et al., 1992), that down-regulates the HLA-DR expression by human monocytes after 72 hours of co-culture (Hartman et al., 1997). *Brugia malayi* nematodes secrete two homologues cystatins (Schonemeyer et al., 2001; Manoury et al., 2001): Bm-CPI-1, which is selectively expressed by L2 and L3 stage into the mosquito vector and Bm-CPI-2, which is constitutively expressed during the parasite life and interferes with two classes of proteases in the MHC class II antigen presentation: cathepsins B, L and S and asparagine endopeptidase. Also, Bm-CPI-2 blocks the presentation of peptide derived from tetanus toxoid by human B cells. Nippocystatin, a cysteine protease inhibitor found in ES products from *N. brasiliensis*, modulate the antigen processing and interfere with antigen presentation due to inhibiting multiple cysteine protease activities found in endosomes/lysosomes of B cells (Dainichi et al., 2001). In addition, *Litomosoides sigmodontis* cystatins upregulate the production of tumor necrosis factor alpha (TNF-α) and decrease antigen-specific proliferation of spleen cells in mice (Pfaff et al., 2002). Besides inhibiting proteases from MHC classe II pathway, cystatins can also down-modulate T cell proliferation and up-regulate IL-10 production (Hartmann et al., 1997; Schonemeyer et al., 2001). ES62, a phosphorylcholine-bearing filarial product, secreted by *Acanthocheilonema viteae*, desensitizes LPS-stimulated mouse peritoneal macrophages to produce IFN-γ (Goodridge et al., 2001). ES-62 also reduces lymphocyte proliferation and stimulates anti-inflammatory properties (Harnett & Harnett, 2001). Phosphorylcholine(PC)-containing glycosphingolipids from *Ascaris suum* are immunomodulatory molecules due to the fact that they inhibit BCR-mediated B cell proliferation by causing apoptosis, inhibit LPS-induced activation of B cells by decreasing Erk phosphorylation, modulate IL-12p40 production in LPS/IFN-γ-induced peritoneal macrophages (Deehan et al., 2002) indicating the PC moiety is important to induce the immunomodulatory effect. In addition, lysophosphatidylserine from *S. mansoni* can specifically target the immune system via TLR-2, interacts to dendritic cells and induce IL-10-producing regulatory T cells involved in immunosuppression (van der Kleij et al., 2002).

4.1.4 Stimulation of myeloid-derived suppressor cells

Several carbohydrate components derived from helminthes also modulate the immune response by stimulating myeloid-derived suppressor cells (MDSC) (Reyes & Terazas, 2007) These cells are a heterogeneous population of cells that express CD11b and Gr-1 and consists of early myeloid progenitors and immature myeloid cells (macrophages, granulocytes and dendritic cells) at different stages of differentitation (Gabrilovich & Nagaraj, 2009). The basic concept about suppressor cells is based on the findings of Gordon's group who observed a direct in vitro effect of IL-4 on the expression of mannose receptor in macrophages (reviewed in Gordon, 2003). This observations lead to macrophages being categorized in classically-activated (CA) macrophages which are NO- and IFN-γ-dependent (Kusmartsev et al., 2000) and alternatively-activated (AA) macrophages which are IL-4- or IL-13-dependent (Kreider et al., 2007; Goerdt et al., 1999). In this regard, Mantovani et al. (2004) proposed that macrophages can be polarized in inflammatory (M1) or anti-inflammatory (M2) conditions. Besides, M2 macrophages can be classified into subpopulations M2a (which are AA macrophages) and M2b (which are IL-10-secreting cells upon immune complex activation), and M3c (which are IL-10-induced deactivated macrophages). All these type of macrophages (and other suppressor cells) can be found in several different of immunological situations, including tumors, autoimmunity, intracellular pathogen infections, helminthic infections.

Two glycans derived from *Schistosoma* eggs, lacto-N-fucopentaose III and lacto-N-neotetraose, have been related to induce IL-10 production, suppressing T cell proliferation (Terrazas et al., 2001). Soluble egg antigens (SEA) from *S. mansoni*, which are rich in lacto-N-fucopentaose III, suppress the LPS-induced inflammation by inducing Th2 responses (Pearce & MacDonald, 2002), by enhancing production of IL-10 and impairing dendritic cell (DC) activation. This latter property is due to the fact that SEA inhibit MyD88-independent, but not dependent-, pathways which result in IL-10 production (Kane et al., 2004), suggesting that SEA regulate multiple signaling pathways downstream and may target the initiation signaling in DC. The suppression of DC activation could be through the ligation of mannose receptor or DC-SIGN (DC-specific intercellular adhesion molecule-grabbing non-integrin) that results in inhibition of DC to secrete IL-12 in response to TLR ligands (Nigou et al., 2001). DC-SIGN ligation leads to IL-10 production, which has been implicated in suppression of DC function (Geijtenbeek et al., 2001). It has been found that lacto-N-fucopentaose III presents an anti-inflammatory effect due to inducing Th2 response and functioning as an adjuvant (Okano et al., 2001). High levels of IL-4, IL-5, IL-10, but not IFN-γ, are secreted by nasal lymphocytes from mouse immunized with human serum albumin conjugated to lacto-N-fucopentaose III. Lacto-N-fucopentaose III is also able to expand peritoneal macrophages that bear Gr1+ marker and act as suppressor cells, inhibiting CD4+ T cell proliferation via NO- and IFN-γ-dependent mechanisms (Atochina et al., 2001).

Carbohydrate components from *Taenia crassiceps* also favor Th2 responses, stimulating IgG1 and polyclonal IgE responses, IL-4, IL-5, IL-10 production to a bystander antigen and are critical to induce gene expression in AA macrophages (Gomes-Garcia et al., 2006), indicating that these components enhance Th2 responses as an adjuvant and trigger anti-inflammatory responses by stimulating AA macrophages. Glycans from *Taenia crassiceps* in their conformational structure recruit F4/80+ Gr1+ peritoneal exudate cells and suppresses proliferation of CD90+ cells (T cells) via cell-to-cell contact, not via IFN-γ and NO (Gomes-Garcia et al., 2005). Moreover, *T. crassiceps* glycans did not activate F4/80+ Gr1+ cells (M2a macrophages) through TLR-4 as has been proposed to synthetic and natural glycoconjugates (Terrazas et al., 2001; Atochina et al., 2001). In addition, the treatment of intact glycans with sodium periodate, which removes glycosilation, decrease M2a macrophages indicating that intact glycans are essential to recruit F4/80+ Gr1+ cells.

4.1.5 Inititation of Th2 immune responses

S. mansoni eggs secrete two proteins that have been implicated in Th2 differentiation: alpha-1 and omega-1. Alpha-1 is a dimer that cross-link IgE-FcεRI complex on basophils, in an antigen-dependent manner, hence being named IL-4 inducing principle of schistosoma eggs (IPSE). It induces the degranulation of mouse and human basophils and releases of IL-4 release (Schramm et al., 2003, 2007), initiating Th2 differentiation. Omega-1 is a ribonuclease also secreted by schistosoma eggs which is necessary to egg transit into the host tissues (Fitzsimmons et al., 2005). It is believed to be involved in Th2 responses by conditioning human monocyte-derived dendritic cells to drive Th2 polarization (Everts et al., 2009; Steinfelder et al., 2009).

4.1.6 Mimicry of cytokines and other mediators

Helminthes can produce homologous proteins to immune system mediators/receptors, such as TGF-β, IFN-γ, TNF-αR and histamine that play a role in regulating anti-parasite responses. Parasite-encoded TGF-β molecules have been characterized in filarial nematodes *Brugia malayi* and *B. pahrangi*. They are two TGF-β homologues that show to be differentially regulated during the filarial life cycle: tgh-1 in *Brugia malayi* and *B. pahangi* (Gomez-Escobar et al., 1997), and tgh-2 in *B. malayi* (Gomes-Escobar et al., 2000). Tgh-1 molecule is required for filarial development within the human host (Gomes-Escobar et al., 1998) and Tgh-2 is predominantly expressed in adult stages and binds to the human TGF-β receptor (Hirata et al., 2005), mimicking human TGF-β and stimulating regulatory responses in the host. In addition to *Brugia* species, TGF-β immunorective molecules have been detected at the surface of cervical bodies, in tegument and subtegumental cells of other parasite stages of *Schistosoma japonicum*, during the whole life cycle (eggs, cercariae, schistosomula and adult worms), although being distinctly regulated at each developmental stage (Davies et al., 1998).

Besides TGF-β homologues, TGF-β receptor homologues have also been described in *Brugia* and *Schistosoma* species. SmTβR1 or SmRK1, a homologue of type I TGF-β receptor and a type of TGF-β family of receptor serine/threonine kinase, have been shown in *Schistosoma mansoni* surface following its entry into the mammalian host (Forrester et al., 2004). In addition to expressing SmRK1, *S. mansoni* expresses another type I TGF-β receptor, SmRK2, from schistosomula and adult stages and it is located predominantly to the tegumental surface of parasite (Grencis & Entwistle, 1997). Type I TGF-β receptor (Bp-trk-1) has been also isolated from the filarial parasitic nematode *Brugia pahangi* in the three main stages of its life cycle: microfilariae, infective larvae and adults; although the ligand remains unknown, it may likely act as a receptor for host TGF-β rather than for parasite ligands (Gomes-Escobar et al., 2000).

Helminths also produce homologues that mimic IFN-γ. *Trichuris muris*-derived molecules share cross reactive epitopes with the host IFN-γ. Moreover, these molecules can be shown to bind to IFN-γ receptor and induce change in lymphoid cells similar to those induced by murine IFN-γ (Calandra & Bucala, 1997). Thus, it possible that the host immune system produces IL-4 to expulse the worms, the IFN-γ homologue production may perpetuate the parasite survival into the host.

Other types of molecules that mimic the host cytokines are macrophage-migration inhibition factors (MIFs), which are produced by several nematodes. Mammalian MIFs are small proteins produced by non-haematopoietic cells that act as pro-inflammatory cytokines and induce TNF production by macrophages in acute settings, such as septic shock (Pastrana et al, 1998). The first MIF homologue to be characterized from a nematode was BM-MIF-1 identified in the filarial parasite *Brugia malayi*, but *Wuchereria bancrofti* and *O. volvulus* also encode MIF family proteins (Reyes & Terrazas, 2007). It may play multiple roles in host-parasite interaction due being located in several tissue types and being found in both cell-associated and secreted forms. Possibly, helminthes may secrete MIF molecules down-modulate the inflammatory response, mainly by stimulating myeloid-derived suppressor cells that has been found to play down-regulatory functions in helminth infections, such as T cell proliferation inhibition and IL-10 and TGF-β release.

5. PAS-1, an anti-inflammatory protein from *Ascaris suum*

Our research group has been investigating the effect of *Ascaris suum* infection and secreted products in the inflammatory response. We have been demonstrated that components from *Ascaris suum* body extract modulate the antibody response and the cell-mediated response in mice. Soares et al. (1987) have demonstrated that, besides inhibiting the IgE production, *A. suum* extract suppresses the IgG1 and IgG2a antibody production. Ferreira et al. (1995) have shown that DBA/2 mice immunized subcutaneouly with OVA + *A. suum* extract and challenged with OVA in the footpad present suppression of immediate (3 hour after challenge) and late (24 hours after challenge) type IV hypersensitivity reaction. The isolation of protein fractions from *A. suum* extract by Sephacryl S-300 gel filtration chromatography yields three peaks (PI, PII, and PIII). PI is constituted by high weight components that suppress anti-OVA IgE antibody production in mice immunized with OVA + PI (Soares et al., 1992; Faquim-Mauro & Macedo, 1998). Thus, the suppressive effect observed in *A. suum* extract is due to high molecular weight components. PI protein fraction was used to obtain the monoclonal antibody MAIP-1, which recognizes one of the suppressive components in the *A. suum* extract; it is a 200-kDa-protein named PAS-1 (protein from *Ascaris suum*) (Oshiro et al., 2004).

PAS-1 suppresses the LPS-induced leukocyte migration and pro-inflammatory (IL-1β, IL-6 and TNF-α) cytokines production in air pouches exudates and macrophage culture supernatant; moreover, it stimulates the production of IL-10 and TGF-β (Oshiro et al., 2005), indicating that the modulatory effect of PAS-1 in LPS-induced inflammation is likely due to these two cytokine. Furthermore, PAS-1 was demonstrated modulating the humoral and cellular immune response against OVA. It inhibits the production of IgM, IgG1, IgG2a, IgE and anaphylactic IgG1 toward T-dependent but not T-independent, antigens and anti-OVA type IV hypersensitivity reaction in mouse footpad injected with carrageenan (Oshiro et al., 2006), suggesting that PAS-1 suppresses B and T cell responses.

PAS-1 also down-modulates antibody production, Th2 cytokine secretion, cellular recruitment and airway hyperresponsiveness induced by APAS-3, allergenic protein from *A. suum* (Itami et al., 2005). We have demonstrated that regulatory T CD4+CD25+ cells and T CD8+ cells secrete IL-10/TGF-β and IFN-γ, respectively and they are involved in the mechanisms by which PAS-1 down-modulate the acute lung allergic inflammation in mice since OVA-induced inflammation is reverted when PAS-1-primed regulatory T CD4+CD25+ cells or T CD8+ cells are adoptively transferred to OVA-immunized mice (Araujo et al., 2008; De Araujo et al., 2010). Besides playing an immunosuppressive role in the acute lung inflammation, we recently found that PAS-1 decreases the airway remodeling and angiogenesis in a mouse chronic lung inflammation model induced by OVA or APAS-3 by inhibiting metaloproteinases (MMP-2, MMP-9, ADAM-33) and angiogenic factors (VEGF and IL-13) (Araujo et al., manuscript in preparation).

6. Conclusion

In conclusion, anaphylaxis is a life-threatening and systemic disorder that involves two different pathways: classical anaphylactic pathway which is IgE-dependent mechanism triggered by IgE-FcεRI signaling on mast cell and basophils to secrete histamine, and alternative anaphylactic pathway which is IgG-dependent triggered by IgG-immune complex bound to FcγRIII on basophils and macrophages to secrete PAF. The understanding of molecular and cellular mechanisms involved in the anaphylactic disorders is crucial to investigate terapeuthic strategies for preventing anaphylaxis risk and recurrence.

Helminths secrete several immmunomodulatory factors that can modulate inflammatory response. Some helminth products can cleave host molecules, such as chemokines, antibodies, and enzymes; modulate the NO production; interfere with antigen presentation and T cell responses by down-modulating DC functions; mimic cytokines such as IFN-γ and TGF-β and MIF. Other potent immunodulatory molecule from helminth is PAS-1, a protein from *A. suum*, that down-modulate acute inflammatory responses and chronic lung allergic inflammation, decreasing IgG1 and IgE production, eosinophil infiltrate, and Th2 cytokines and interfering with metaloproteinase activity and production of angiogenic factors. Thus, due to their capacity to induce immunomodulation, these helminth products may be useful for therapeutic interventions in inflammatory, allergic and anaphylactic disorders.

7. References

Acevedo, N.; Sanchez, J.; Erler, A.; Mercado, D.; Briza, P; Kennedy, M; Fernandez, A; Gutierrez, M; Chua, KY; Cheong, N; Jimenez, S; Puerta, L & Caraballo, L. (2009). IgE cross-reactivity between Ascaris and domestic mites: the role of tropomyosin and the nematode polyprotein ABA-1. *Allergy*, Vol.64, No. 11, (November 2009), pp. 1635-1643, ISSN0105-4538

Acevedo, N.; Erler, A.; Briza, P.; Puccio, F.; Ferreira, F. & Caraballo, L. (2011). Allergenicity of Ascaris lumbricoides tropomyosin and IgE sensitization among asthmatic patients in a tropical environment. *International Archives of Allergy and Immunology*, Vol.154, No.3, (September 2011), pp.195-206, ISSN1018-2438

Actor, J.K.; Shirai, M.; Kullberg, M.C.; Buller, R.M.; Sher, A. & Berzofsky, J.A. (1993). Helminth infections results in decreased virus-specific CD8+ cytotoxic T cell and Th1 cytokine responses as well as delayed virus clearance. *Proceedings of the National Academy of Sciences USA*, Vol.90, No.3, (February 1993), pp.948-952, ISSN0027-8424

Akdis, C.A. & Blaser, K. (2003). Histamine in the immune regulation of allergic inflammation. *Journal of Allergy and Clinical Immunology*, Vol.112, No.1, (July 2003), pp.15-22, ISSN0091-6749

Akdis, C.A. & Simons, F.E. (2006). Histamine receptors are hot in immunopharmacology. *European Journal of Pharmacology*, Vol.533, No.1-3, (March 2006), pp.69-76, ISSN0014-2980

Allen, J.E. & MacDonalds, A.J. (1998). Profound suppression of cellular proliferation mediated by the secretions of nematodes. *Parasite Immunology*, Vol.20, No.5, (May 1998), pp.241-247, ISSN0141-9838

Anthony, R.M.; Rutitzky, L.I.; Urban, J.F. Jr; Stadecker, M.J. & Gause, W.C. (2007). Protective immune mechanisms in helminth infection. *Nature Reviews Immunology*, Vol.7, No.12, (December 2007), pp.975-987, ISBN1474-1733

Araujo, C.A.; Perini, A.; Martins, M.A.; Macedo, M.S. & Macedo-Soares, M.F. (2008). PAS-1, a protein from Ascaris suum, modulates allergic inflammation via IL-10 and IFN-gamma, but not IL-12. *Cytokine*, Vol.44, No.3, (December 2008), pp.8308-8314, ISSN1043-4666

Arinobu, Y.; Iwasaki, H.; Gurish, M.F.; Mizuno, S.; Shigematsu, H.; Ozawa, H.; Tenen, D.G.; Austen, K.F. & Akashi, K. (2005) Developmental checkpoints of the basophils/mast cell lineages in adult murine hematopoiesis. *Proccedings of the National Academy of Science USA*, Vol.102, No.50, (December 2005), pp.18105-18110, ISSN0027-8424

Arnold, J.N.; Wormald, M.R.; Sim, R.B.; Rudd, P.M. & Dwek R.A. (2007). The impact of glycosilation on the biological function and structure of human immunoglobulins. *Annual Reviews of Immunology*, Vol.25, (2007), pp.21-50, ISSN0732-0582

Atochina, O.; Daly-Engel, T.; Piskorska, D.; McGuire, E. & Harn, D.A Jr. (2001). A schistosome-expressed immunomodulatory glycoconjugate expands peritoneal Gr1(+) macrophages that suppress naïve CD4(+) T cell proliferation via an IFN-gamma and nitric oxide mechanism. *Journal of Immunology*, Vol.167, No.8, (October 2001), pp.4293-4302, ISSN0022-1467

Auriault, C.; Ouaissi, M.A.; Torpier, G.; Eisen, H.; Capron, A. (1981). Proteolytic cleavage of IgG bound to the Fc receptor of Schistosoma mansoni schistosomula. *Parasite Immunology*,Vol.3, No.1, (Spring 1981), pp.33-44, ISSN0141-9838

Barrett, A.J. (1986). The cystatins: a civerse superfamily of cysteinase peptidadase inhibitors. *Biomedica Biochimica Acta*,Vol.45, No.11-12, (1986), pp.1363-1374, ISSN0232-766X

Beaven, M.A. (2009). Our perception of the mast cell from Paul Ehrlich to now. *European Journal of Immunology*, Vol.39, No.1, (January 2009), pp.11-25, ISSN0014-2980

Belkaid, Y.; Sun, C.M. & Bouladoux, N. (2006). Parasites and immunoregulatory T cells. *Current Opinion in Immunology*, Vol.18, No.4, (August 2006), pp.406-412, ISSN0952-7915

Bell, R.G. (1996). IgE, allergies and helminth parasites: a new perspective on an old conundrum. *Immunology and Cell Biology*, Vol.74, No.4, (August 1996), pp.337-345, ISSN0818-9641

Benveniste, J.; Henson, P.M & Cochrane, C.G. (1972). Leukocyte dependent histamine release from rabbit platelets. The role of IgE, basophils, and a platelet-activating factor. *Journal of Experimental Medicine*, Vol.136, No.6, (December 1972), pp.1356-1377, ISSN0022-1007

Berasain, P.; Carmona, F.; Frangione, B.; Dalton, J.P. & Goni, F. (2000). Fasciola hepatica: parasite-secreted proteinases degrade all human IgG subclasses: determination of the specific cleavage sites and identification of the immunoglobulin fragments produced. *Experimental Parasitology*, Vol.94, No.2, (February 2000), pp.99-110, ISSN0014-4894

Bieber, T.; De La Salle, H.; Wollenberg, A.; Hakimi, J.; Chizzonite, R.; Ring, J.; Hanau, D. & De la Salle, C. (1992). Human epidermal Langerhans cells express the high affinity receptor for immunoglobulin E (Fc epsilon RI). *Journal of Experimental Medicine*, Vol.175, No.5, (May 1992), pp.1285-1290, ISSN0022-1007

Blackburn, C.C. & Selkirk, M.E. (1992). Inactivation of platelet-activation factor by a putative acetylhydrolase from the gastrointestinal nematode parasite Nippostrongylus brasiliensis. *Immunology*, Vol,75, No.1, (January 1992), pp.41-46, ISSN0019-2805

Botturi, K.; Lacoeuille, Y.; Vervloet, D.;& Magnan A. (2010). Histamine induces Th2 activation through the histamine receptor 1 in house dust mite rhinitic but asmathic patients. *Clinical and Experimental Allergy*, Vol.40, No.5, (May 2010), pp.755-762, ISSN0954-7894

Bradley, J.E & Jackson, J.A. (2004). Immunity immunoregulation and the ecology of trichuris and ascariasis. *Parasite Immunology*, Vol.26, No.11-12, (November-December 2004), pp.429-441, ISSN0141-9838

Brophy, P.M.; Patterson, L.H.; Brown, A. & Pritchard, D.I. (1995). Glutathione S-transferase (GST) expression in the human hookworm Necator americanus: potential roles for excretory-secretory forms of GST. *Acta Tropica*, Vol.59, No.3, (June 1995), pp.259-263, ISSN0001-706X

Brown, S.G. (2004). Clinical features and severity grading of anaphylaxis. *Journal of Allergy and Clinical Immunology*, Vol.114, No.2, (August 2004), pp.371-376, ISSN0091-6749

Calandra, T. & Bucala, R. (1997) Macrophage migration inhibitory factor (MIF): a glucocorticoid counter-regulator within the immune system. *Critical Reviews in Immunology*, Vol.17, No.1, (1997), pp.77-88, ISSN1040-8401

Camerer, E.; Regard, J.B.; Cornelissen, I.; Srinivasan, Y.; Duong, D.N.; Palmer, D.; Pham, T.H.; Wong, J.S.; Pappu, R. & Coughlin, S.R. (2009). Sphingosine-1 phosphate in the plasma compartment regulates basal and inflammation-induced vascular lead in mice. *Journal of Clinical Investigation*, Vol.119, No.7, (July 2009), pp.1871-1879, ISSN0021-9738

Caraballo, A. & Acevedo, N. (2011). Allergy in the tropics: the impact of cross-reactivity between mites and Ascaris. *Frontiers in Bioscience*, Vol. E3, (January 2011), pp.51-64, ISSN1093-9946

Capron, A.; Dessaint, J.P.; Haque, A. & Capron, M. (1982). Antibody-dependent cell-mediated cytotoxicity against parasites. *Progress in Allergy*, Vol. 31, (1982), pp.234-267, ISSN0079-6034

Cauwels, A.; Janssen, B.; Buys, E.; Sips, P. & Brouckaert, P. (2006). Anaphylactic shock depends on PI3K and eNOS-derived NO. *Journal of Clinical Investigation*, Vol.116, No.8, (August 2006), pp.2244-2251, ISSN0021-9738

Clough, G.F.; Bennett, A.R. & Church, M.K. (1998). Effects of H1 antagonist on the cutaneous vascular response to histamine and bradykinin: a study using scanning laser Doppler imaging. *British Journal of Dermatology*, Vol.138, No.5, (May 1998), pp.806-814, ISSN0007-0963

Conrad, D.H.; Ben-Sasson, S.Z.; Le Gros, G.; Finkelman, F.D. & Paul, W.E. (1990). Infection with Nippostrongylus brasiliensis or injection of anti-IgD antibodies markedly enhances Fc-receptor-mediated interleukin 4 production by non-B, non-T cells. *Journal of Experimental Medicine*, Vol.171, No.5, (May 1990), pp.1497-1508, ISSN0022-1007

Cooper, P.J. (2009). Interactions between helminth parasites and allergy. *Current Opinion in Allergy and Clinical Immunology*, Vol.9, No.1, (February. 2009), pp.29-37, ISSN1528-4050

Cuellar, C.; Pertequer, M.J. & de Las Heras, B. (1998). Effect of Anisakis simplex on nitric oxide production in J774 macrophages. *Scandinavian Journal of Infectious Diseases*, Vol.30, No.6, (1998), pp.603-606, ISSN0300-9475

Culley, F.J.; Brown, A.; Conroy, D.M.; Sabroe, I.; Pritchard, D.I. & Williams, T.J. (2000). *Journal of Immunology*, Vol.165, No.11, (December 2000), pp.6447-6453, ISSN0022-1767

Daeron M. (1997). Fc receptor biology. *Annual Reviews of Immunology*, Vol.15, (1997), pp.203-234, ISSN0732-0582

Dainichi, T.; Maekawa, Y.; Ishii, K.; Zhang, T.; Nashed, B.F.; Sakai, T.; Takashima, M. & Himeno, K. (2001). Nippocystatin, a cystein protease inhibitor from Nippostrongylus brasiliensis, inhibits antigen processing and modulates antigen-specific immune responses. *Infecion and Immunity*, Vol.69, No.12, (December 2001), pp.730-7386, ISSN0019-9567

Davies, S.J.; Shoemaker, C.B. & Pearce, E.J. (1998). A divergent member of the transforming factor beta receptor family from Schistosoma mansoni is expressed on the parasite surface membrane. *Journal of Biological Chemistry*, Vol.273, No.18, (May 1998), pp.11234-11240, ISSN1178-6264

De Araujo, C.A.; Perini, A.; Martins, M.A.; Macedo, M.S. & Macedo-Soares, M.F. (2010). PAS-1, an Ascaris suum protein, modulates allergic airway inflammation via CD8+γδTCR+ and CD4+CD25+FoxP3+ T cells. *Scandinavian Journal of Immunology*, Vol.72, No.6, (December 2010), pp.491-503, ISSN0300-9475

Deehan, M.R.; Harnett, M.M. & Harnett, W. (1997). A filarial nematode secreted product differentially modulates expression and activation of protein kinase C isoforms in B lymphocytes. *Journal of Immunology*, Vol.159, No.12, (December 1997), pp.6105-6111, ISSN0022-1767

Deehan, M.R.; Goodridge, H.S.; Blair, D.; Lochnit, G.; Dennis, R.D.; Geyer, R.; Harnett, M.M. & Harnett, W. (2002). Immunomodulatory properties of Ascaris suum glycosphingolipids – phosphorylcholine and non-phosphorylcholine- dependent effects. *Parasite Immunology*, Vol.24, No.9-10, (September-October 2002), pp.463-469, ISSN0141-2980

De Silva, N.R.; Brooker, S.; Hotez, P.J.; Montresor, A.; Engels, D. & Savioli, L. (2003). Soil-transmitted helminth infections: updating the global picture. Trends of Parasitology, *Vol.19, No.12, (December* 2003), pp.547-551, ISSN1471--4906

Dijstelbloem, H.M.; van de Winkel, J.G. & Kallenberg, C.G. (2001). Inflammation in autoimmunity: receptors for IgG revisited. *Trends in Immunology*, Vol..22, No.9, (September 2001), pp.510-516, ISSN1471-4906

Dombrowicz, D.; Flamand, V.; Miyajima, I.; Ravetch, J.V.; Galli, S.J. & Kinet, J.P. (1997) Absence of Fc epsilon RI alpha chain results in upregulation of Fc gamma RIII-dependent mast cell degranulation and anaphylaxis. Evidence of competition between Fc epsilon RI and Fc gamma RIII for limiting amounts of FcR beta and gamma chains. *Journal of Clinical Investigation*, (March 1997), Vol.99, No.5, pp.915-922, ISSN0021-9738

Everts, B.; Perona-Wright, G.; Smits, H.H.; Hokke, C.H.; van der Ham, A.J.; Fitzsimmons, C.M.; Doenhoff, M.J.; van der Bosch, J.; Mohrs, K.; Haas, H.; Mohrs, M.; Yazdanbakhsh, M. & Schramm, G. (2009). Omega-1, a glycoprotein secreted by Schistosoma mansoni eggs, drives Th2 responses. *Journal of Experimental Medicine*, Vol.206, No.8, (August 2009), pp.1673-1680, ISSN0022-1007

Ewan, P.W. (1998). ABC of Allergies-Anaphylaxis. *BMJ*, Vol.316, No.7142, (May 1998), pp.1442-1445, ISSN0958-8146

Fallon, P.G. & Mangan, N.E. (2007). Suppression of Th2 type allergic reactions by helminth infections. *Nature Reviews Immunology*, Vol.7, (March 2007), pp. 220-230, ISSN1474-1733

Faquim-Mauro, E.L. & Macedo, M.S. (1998). The immunosuppressive activity of Ascaris suum is due to high molecular weight components. *Clinical and Experimental Immunology*, Vol.114, No.2, (November 1998), pp.245-251, ISSN0009-9104

Fernandez-Caldas, E.; Puerta, L.; Mercado, D.; Lockey, R.F. & Caraballo, L.R. (1993). Mite fauna, Der p1, Der f1 and Blomia tropicalis allergen levels in a tropical environment. *Clinical and Experimental Allergy*, Vol.23, No.4, (April 1993), pp.292-297, ISSN0954-7894

Fernandez-Caldas, E.; Puerta, L.; Caraballo, L. & Lockey, R.F. (2008). Mite allergens. *Clinical Allergy and Immunology*, Vol.21, (2008), pp.161-182, ISSN1075-7910

Ferreira, A.P.; Faquim-Mauro, E.S.; Abrahamsohn, I.A. & Macedo, M.S. (1995). Immunization with Ascaris suum extract impairs T cell functions in mice. *Cellular Immunology*, Vol.162, No.2, (May 1995), pp.202-210, ISSN0008-8749

Fiebiger, E.; Tortorella, D.; Jouvin, M.H.; Kinet, J.P. & Ploegh, H.L. (2005). Cotranslational endoplasmic reticulum assembly of FcεRI controls the formation of functional IgE-binding receptors. *Journal of Experimental Medicine*, Vol.201, No.2, (January 2005), pp.267-277, ISSN0022-1007

Finkelman, F.D.; Katona, I.M.; Urban, J.F. Jr; Holmes, J.; Ohara, J.; Tung, A.S.; Sample, J.V. & Paul, W.E. (1988). IL-4 is required to generate and sustain in vivo IgE responses. *Journal of Immunology*, Vol.141, No.7, (October 1988), pp.2335-2341, ISSN0022-1767

Finkelman, F.D.; Holmes, J.; Urban, J.F. Jr; Paul, W.E. & Katona, I.M. (1989). T help requirements for the generation of an in vivo IgE response: a late acting form of T cell help other than IL-4 is required for IgE but not for IgG1 production. *Journal of Immunology*, Vol.142, No.2, (January 1989), pp.403-408, ISSN0022-1767

Finkelman, F.D. (2007). Anaphylaxis: lessons from mouse models. *Journal of Allergy and Clinical Immunology*, Vol.120, No.3, (September 2007), pp.506-515, ISSN0091-6749

Fitzsimmons, C.M.; Schramm, G.; Jones, F.M.; Chalmers, I.W.; Hoffman, K.F.; Grevelding, C.G.; Wuhrer, M.; Hokke, C.H.; Haas, H.; Doenhoff, M.J. & Dunne, D.W. (2005). *Molecular and Biochemical Parasitology*, Vol.144, No.1, (November 2005), pp.123-127, ISSN0166-6851

Forrester, S.G.; Warfel, P.W. & Pearce, E.J. (2004). Tegumental expression of a novel type II receptor serine/threonine kinase (SmRK2) in Schistosoma mansoni. *Molecular and Biochemical Parasitology*, Vol.136, No.2, (August 2004), pp.149-156, ISSN0166-6851

Fukuda, Y.; Kawashima, H.; Saito, K.; Inomata, N.; Matsui, M. & Nakanishi, T. (2000). Effect of human plasma-type platelet-activating factor acetylhydrolase in two anaphylactic shock models. *European Journal of Pharmacology*, Vol.390, No.1-2, (February 2000), pp.203-207, ISSN0021-8219

Fukumoto, S.; Hirai, K.; Tanikata, T.; Ohmori, Y.; Stuehr, D.J. & Hamilton, T.A. (1997). Excretory/secretory products from plerocercoids of Spirometra erinacei reduce iNOS and chemokine mRNA levls in peritoneal macrophages stimulated with cytokines and/or LPS. *Parasite Immunology*, Vol.19, No.7, (July 1997), pp.325-332, ISSN0141-2980

Gabrilovich, D.I. & Nagaraj, S. (2009). Myeloid-derived suppressor cells as regulators of the immune system. *Nature Reviews Immunology*, Vol.9, No.3, (March 2009), pp.162-174, ISSN1474-1733

Galli, S.J.; Kalesnikoff, J.; Grimbaldeston, M.A.; Piliponsky, A.M.; Williams, C.M. & Tsai, M. (2005). Mast cells as "tunable" effector and immunoregulatory cells: recent advances. *Annual Reviews of Immunology*, Vol.23, (2005), pp.749-786, ISSN0732-0582

Garman, S.C.; Kinet, J.P. & Jardetzky, T.S. (1999). The crystal structure of the human high affinity IgE receptor (FcεRI α). *Annual Reviews of Immunology*, Vol.17, (1999), pp.973-976, ISSN0732-0582

Geijtenbeek, T.B.; Kroosshoop, D.J.; Bleijs, D.A.; van Vliet, S.J.; Koppel, E.A.; van Duijnhoven, G.C.; Alon, R.; Figdor, C.G .& van Kooyk, Y. (2001). DC-SIGN-ICAM-2 interaction mediates dendritic cell trafficking. *Journal of Experimental Medicine*, Vol.193, No.6, (March 2001), pp.671-678, ISSN0022-1007

Geha, R.S.; Helm, B. & Gould, H. (1985). Inhibition of the Prausnitz-Kustner reaction by an immunoglobulin epsilon-chain fragment synthesized in E. coli. *Nature*, Vol. 315, No.6020, (June 1985), pp.577-578, ISSN0028-0836

Geissmann, F.; Manz, M.G.; Jung, S.; Sieweke, M.H.; Merad, M. & Ley, K. (2010). Development of monocytes, macrophages and dendritic cells. *Science*, Vol.327, No.5966, (February 2010), pp.656-661, ISSN0272-4634

Ghendler, Y.; Arnon, R. & Fishelson, Z. (1994). Schistosoma mansoni: isolation and characterization of Smpi56, a novel serine protease inhibitor. *Experimental Parasitology*, Vol.78, No.2, (March 1994), pp.121-131, ISSN0014-4894

Goerdt, S.; Politz, O.; Schledzewski K.; Birk, R.; Gratchev, A.; Guillot, P.; Hakiy, N.; Klembe C.D.; Dippel, E.; Kodelja, V. & Orfanos, C.E. (1999). Alternative versus classical activation of macrophages. *Pathobiology*, Vol.67, No.5-6, (1999), pp.222-226, ISSN1015-2008

Golightly, L.K. & Greos, L.S. (2005). Second generation antihistamines: actions and efficacy in the management of allergic disorders. *Drugs*, Vol.65, No.3, (2005), pp.341-384, ISSN0012-6667

Gomes, R.N.; Bozza, F.A.; Amancio, R.T.; Japiassu, A.M.; Vianna, R.C.; Larangeira, A.P.; Gouveia, J.M.; Bastos, M.S.; Zimmerman, G.A.; Stafforini, D.M.; Prescott, S.M.; Bozza, P.T. & Castro-Faria-Neto, H.C. (2006). Exogenous platelet-activating factor acetylhydrolase reduces mortality in mice with systemic inflammatory response syndrome and sepsis. *Shock*, Vol.26, No.1, (July 2006), pp.41-49, ISSN1073-2322

Gomez-Escobar, N.; van der Biggelaar, A. & Maizels, R. (1997). A member of the TGF-beta receptor gene family in the parasitic nematode Brugia parangi. *Gene*, Vol.199, No.1-2, (October 1997), pp.101-109, ISSN0378-1119

Gomez-Escobar, N.; Lewis, E. & Maizels, R.M. (1998). A novel member of the transforming growth factor-beta (TGF-beta) superfamily from the filarial nematodes Brugia malayi and B. parangi. *Experimental Parasitology*, Vol.88, No.3, (March 1998), pp.200-209, ISSN0014-4894

Gomez-Escobar, N.; Gregory, W.F. & Maizels, R.M. (2000). Identification of tgh-2, a filarial nematode homolog of Caenorhabditis elegans daf-7 and human transforming growth factor beta, expressed in microfilarial and adult stages of Brugia malayi. *Infection and Immunity*, Vol.68, No.11, (November 2000), pp.6402-6410, ISSN0019-9567

Gomez-Garcia, L.; Lopez-Marin L.M.; Saavedra, R.; Rodriguez-Sosa, M. & Terrazas, L.I. (2005). Intact glycans from cestode antigens are involved in innate activation of myeloid suppressor cells. *Parasite Immunology*, Vol.27, No.10-11, (October-November 2005), pp.395-405, ISSN0141-2980

Gomez-Garcia, L.; Rivera-Montoya, I.; Rodriguez-Sosa, M. & Terrazas, L.I. (2006). Carbohydrate components of Taenia crassiceps metacestodes display Th2-adjuvant and anti-inflammatory properties when co-injected with bystander antigen. *Parasitology Research*, Vol.99, No.4, (September 2006), pp.440-448, ISSN0932-0113

Goodridge, H.S.; Wilson, E.H.; Harnett, W.; Campbell, C.C.; Harnett, M.M. & Liew, F.Y. (2001). Modulation of macrophage cytokine production by ES-62, a secreted product of the filarial nematode Acanthocheilonema viteae. *Journal of Immunology*, Vol.167, No.2, (July 2001), pp.94-945, ISSN0022-1767

Gordon S. (2003). Alternative activation of macrophages. *Nature Reviews Immunology*, Vol.3, No.1, (January 2003), pp.23-35, ISSN1474-1733

Gould, H.J.; Sutton, B.J.; Beavil, A.J.; Beavil, R.L.; McCloskey, N.; Coker, H.A.; Fear, D. & Smuthwaite, L. (2003). The biology of IgE and the basis of allergic diseases. *Annual Reviews of Immunology*, Vol.21, (2003), pp.579-628, ISSN0732-0582

Gould, H.J. & Sutton, B.J. (2008). IgE in allergy and asthma today. *Nature Reviews Immunology*, Vol. 8, No.3, (March 2008), pp.205-217, ISSN1474-1733

Grencis, R.K. & Entwistle, G.M. (1997). Production of an interferon-gamma homologue by an intestinal nematode: functionally significant or interesting artifact? *Parasitology*, Vol.115, No. Suppl, (1997), pp.S101-106, ISSN0031-1820

Hanahan, D.J. (1986). Platelet activating factor: a biologically active phosphoglyceride. *Annual Reviews of Biochemistry*, Vol.55, (1986), pp.483-509, ISSN0066-4154

Harnett, W. & Harnett, M.M. (2001). Modulation of the host immune system by phosphorylcholine-containing glycoproteins secreted by parasitic filarial nematodes. *Biochimica et Biophysica Acta*, Vol.1539, No.1-2, (May 2001), pp.7-15, ISSN0006-3002

Harnett W & Harnett MM. (2008). Parasitic nematode modulation of allergic disease. *Current Allergy and Asthma Reports*, Vol.8, No.5, (September 2008), pp.392-397, ISSN1529-7322

Hartmann, S.; Kyewski, B.; Sonnenburg, B. & Lucius, R. (1997). A filarial cysteine protease inhibitor down-regulates T cell proliferation and enhances interleukin-10 production. *European Journal of Immunology*, Vol.27, No.9, (September 1997), pp.2253-2260, ISSN0014-2980

Hartmann, S.; Schonemeyer, A.; Sonnenburg, B.; Vray, B. & Lucius, R. (2002). Cystatins of filarial nematodes up-regulate the nitric oxide production of interferon-gamma activated murine macrophages. *Parasite Immunology*, Vol.24, No.5, (May 2002), pp.253-262, ISSN0141-9838

Hartmann, S. & Lucius, R. (2003). Modulation of hsot immune responses by nematode cystains. *International Journal of Parasitology*, Vol.30, No.11, (September 2003), pp.1291-1303, ISSN0020-7519

Hewitson, J.P.; Grainer, J.R. & Maizels, R.M. (2009). Helminth immunoregulation: the role of parasite secreted proteins in modulating host immunity. *Molecular and Biochemical Parasitology*, Vol.167, No.1, (September 2009), pp.1-11, ISSN0166-6851

Hirata, M.; Hirata, K.; Hara, T.; Kawabuchi, M. & Fukuma, T. (2005). Expression of TGF-beta-like molecules in the life cycle of Schistosoma japonicum. *Parasitology Research*, Vol.95, No.6, (April 2005), pp.367-373, ISSN0932-0113

Honda, Z.; Suzuki, T.; Kono, H.; Okada, M.; Yamamoto, T.; Ra, C.; Morita, Y. & Yamamoto, K. (2000). Sequential requirements of the N-terminal palmytoylation site and SH2 domain of Src family kinases in the initiation and progression of FcεRI signaling. *Molecular and Cellular Biology*, Vol.20, No.5, (March 2000), pp.1759-1771, ISSN0270-7306

Hu, Z.Q.; Zhao, W.H. & Shimamura, T. (2007). Regulation of mast cell development by inflammatory factors. *Current Medicinal Chemistry*, Vol.14, No. 28, (2007), pp.3044-3050, ISSN0929-8673

Iio, A.; Waldmann, T.A. & Strober, W. (1987). Metabolic study of human IgE: evidence for an extravascular catabolic pathway. *Journal of Immunology*, Vol.120, No.5, (May 1987), pp.1696-1701, ISSN0022-1767

Ishii, S.; Kuwaki, T.; Nagase, T.; Maki, K.; Tashiro, F.; Sunaga, S.; Cao, W.H.; Kume, K.; Fukuchi, Y., Ikuta, K.; Miyazaki, J.; Kumada, M. & Shimizu, T. (1998). *Journal of Experimental Medicine*, Vol.187, No.11, (June 1998), pp.1779-1788, ISSN0022-1007

Ishizaka, K. & Iszhizaka, T. (1971). Mechanism of reaginic hypersensitivity: a review. *Clinical Allergy*, Vol. 1, No.1, (March 1971), pp.9-25, ISSN0009-9090

Ishizaka, K. & Ishizaka, T. (1976). Identification of gamma-E-antibodies as a carrier of reaginic activity. *Journal of Immunology*, Vol.99, No.6, (1976), pp.1187-1198, ISSN0022-1767

Itami, D.M.; Oshiro, T.M.; Araújo, C.A.; Perini, A.; Martins, M.A.; Macedo, M.S. & Macedo-Soares, M.F. (2005). Modulation of murine experimental asthma by Ascaris suum components. *Clinical and Experimental Allergy*, Vol.35, No.7, (July 2005), pp.873-879, ISSN0954-7894

Jacoby, W.; Cammarata, P.V.; Findlay, S. & Pincus, S.H. (1984). Anaphylaxis in mast cell-deficient mice. *Journal of Investigative Dermatology*, Vol.83,No.4, (October 1984), pp.302-304, ISSN0022-202X

Jenkins, D.C. (1975). The influence of Nematospiroides dubius on subsequent Nippostrongylus brasiliensis infections in mice. *Parasitology*, Vol.71, No.2, (October 1975), pp.349-355, ISSN0031-1820

Jones BL & Kearns GL. (2011). Histamine: new thoughts about a familiar mediator. *Clinical Pharmacology and Therapeutics*, Vol.89, No.2, (February 2011), pp.189-197, ISSN0009-9325

Kane, C.M.; Cervi, L; Sun, J; McKee, A.S.; Masek, K.S.; Shapira, S.; Hunter, C.A. & Pearce, E.J. (2004). Helminth antigens modulate TLR-initiated dendritic cell activation. *Journal of Immunology*, Vol.173, No.12, (December 2004), pp.7454-7461, ISSN0022-1767

Karasawa, K. (2006). Clinical aspects of plasma platelets-activating factor- acetylhydrolase. *Biochimica et Biophysica Acta*, Vol.1761, No.11, (November 2006), pp.1359-1372, ISSN0006-3002

Kemp, S.F. & Lockey, R.F. (2002). Anaphylaxis: a review of causes and mechanisms. *Journal of Allergy and Clinical Immunology*, Vol. 110, No. 3, (September 2002), pp.341-348, ISSN0091-6749

Kumar, V. & Sharma, A. (2010). Mast cells; emerging sentinel innate immune cells with diverse role in immunity. *Molecular Immunology*, Vol.48, No.1-3, (November-December 2010), pp.14-25, ISSN0161-5890

Kimura, S; Nagata, M.; Takeuchi, M.; Takano, K. & Harada, M. (1997). Anti-granulocyte antibody suppression of active and passive anaphylactic shock in WBB6F1-W/Wv mice. *Cellular and Molecular Life Sciences*, Vol.53, No.8, (August 1997), pp.663-669, ISSN1420-682X

Kinet, J.P. (1999). The high –affinity IgE receptor (FcεRI): from physiology to pathology. *Annual Reviews of Immunology*, Vol.17, (1999), pp.931-972, ISSN0732-0582

Kreider, T.; Anthony, R.M.; Urban Jr, J.F.& Gause, W.C. (2007). Alternativelly activated macrophages in helminth infections. *Current Opinion in Immunology*, Vol.19, No.4, (August 2007), pp.448-453, ISSN0952-7915

Kuhn, R.; Rajewsky, K. & Muller, W. (1991). Generation and analysis of interleukin-4 deficient mice. *Science*, Vol.254, No.5032, (November 1991), pp.707-710, ISSN0272-4634

Kunzmann, S.; Schmidt-Weber, C.; Zingg, J.M.; Azzi, A.; Kramer, B.W.; Blaser, K.; Akdis, C.A. & Speer, C.P. (2007). Connective tissue growth factor expression is regulated by histamine in lung fibroblast: potential role of histamine in airway remodeling. *Journal of Allergy and Clinical Immunology*, Vol.119, No.6, (June 2007), pp.15-22, ISSN0091-6749

Kusmartsev, S.A.; Li, Y.& Chen, S.H. (2000). Gr-1+ myeloid cells derived from tumor-bearing mice inhibit prmary T cell activation induced through CD3/CD28 costimulation. *Journal of Immunology*, Vol.165, No.2, (July 2000), pp.779-785, ISSN0022-1767

Langlet, C.; Mazingue, C.; Dessaint, J.P. & Capron, A. (1984). Inhibition of primary and secondary IgE response by a schistosome-derived inhibitory factor. *International Archives of Allergy and Applied Immunology*, Vol.73, No.3, (1984), pp.225-230, ISSN0020-5915

Li, H.; Burkhardt, C.; Heinrich, U.R.; Brausch, I.; Xia, N. & Forstermann, U. (2003). Histamine upregulates gene expression of endothelial nitric oxide synthase in human vascular endothelial cells. *Circulation*, Vol.107, No.18, (May 2003), pp.2348-2354, ISSN0009-7322

Liwski, R.; Zhou, J.; McAlister, V.& Lee, T.D. (2000). Prolongation of allograft survival by Nippostrongylus brasiliensis is associated with decreased allospecific cytotoxic T lymphocyte activity and development of T cytotoxic cell type 2. *Transplantation*, Vol.69, No.9, (May 2000), pp.1912-1922,ISSN0041-1337

Loffler, W. (1956). Transient lung infiltrations with blood eosinophilia. *International Archives of Allergy and Applied Immunology*, Vol.8, No.1-2,(1956), pp.54-59, ISSN0020-5915

Loke, P.; MacDonald, A.S. & Allen, J.E. (2000). Antigen-presenting cells recruited by Brugia malayi induce Th2 differentiation of naïve CD4(+) T cells. *European Journal of Immunology*, Vol.30, No.4, (April 2000), pp.1127-1135, ISSN0014-2980

Lustigman, S.; Brotman, B.; Huima, T.; Prince, A.M. & McKerrow, J.H. (1992). Molecular cloning and characterization of onchocystatin, a cysteine proteinase inhibitor of Onchoceerca volvulus. *Journal of. Biological Chemistry*, Vol.267, No.24, (August 1992), pp.17339-17146, ISSN1178-6264

Lynch, N.R.; Medouze, L.P.F.; DiPrisco-Fuenmayor, M.C.; Verde, O.; Lopez, R.I. & Malave, C. (1984). Incidence of atopic disease in a tropical environment: partial independence from intestinal helminthiasis. *Journal of Allergy and Clinical Immunology*, Vol.73, No.2, (February 1984), pp.229-233, ISSN0091-6749

Lynch, N.R.; Lopez, R.I.; Di Prisco-Fuenmayor, M.C.; Hagel, I.; Medouze, L.; Viana, G.; Ortega, C. & Prato, G. (1987). Allergic reactivity and socio-economic level in a tropical environment. *Clinical Allergy*, Vol.17, No.3, (May 1987), pp.199-207, ISSN0009-9090

Lynch, N.R.; Hagel, I.; Perez, M.; DiPrisco, M.; Alvarez, N. & Rojas, E. (1992). Bronchoconstriction in helminthic infection. *International Archives of Allergy and Immunology*, Vol. 98, No.1, (1992), pp.77-79, ISSN1018-2438

Lynch, N.R.; Palenque, M.; Hagel, I. & DiPrisco, M.C. (1997). Clinical improvement of asthma after antihelminthic treatment in a tropical situation. *American Journal of Respiratory and Critical Care*, Vol.156, No.1, (July 1997), pp.50-54, ISSN1073-449X

MacGlashan, D. Jr. (2003). Histamine: a mediator of inflammation. *Journal of Allergy and Clinical Immunology*, Vol.112, No.4, (October 2003), pp.S53-S59, ISSN0091-6749

Maizels, R.M.; Balic, A.; Gomez-Escobar, N.; Nair, M.; Taylor, M.D. & Allen, J.E. (2004). Helminth parasites: masters of regulation. *Immunological Reviews*, Vol.201, (October 2004), pp. 89-116, ISSN0105-2896

Mancardi, D.A.; Iannascoli, B.; Hoos, S.; England, P.; Daeron, M. & Bruhns, P. (2008). FcgammaRIV is a mouse IgE receptor that resembles macrophage FcepsilonRI in human and promotes IgE-induced lung inflammation. *Journal of Clinical Investigation*, Vol.118, No.11, (November 2008), pp.3738-3750, ISSN0021-9738

Manoury, B.; Gregory, W.F.; Maizels, R.M. & Watts, C. (2001). Bm-CPI-2, a cystatin homolog secreted by the filarial parasite Brugia malayi, inhibits classII MHC-restricted antigen processing. *Current Biology*, Vol11, No.6, (March 2001), pp.447-451, ISSN0960-9822

Mantovani, A.; Sica, A.; Sozzani, S.; Allavena, P.; Vechii, A. & Locati, M. (2004). The chemokine system in diverse forms of macrophage activation and polarization. *Trends in Immunology*, Vol.25, No.12, (December 2004), ISSN1471-4906

McIntyre, T.M.; Zimmerman, G.A.; Satoh, K. & Prescott, S.M. (1985). Cultured endothelial cells synthesize both platelet-activating factor and prostacyclin in response to histamine, bradykinin, and adenosine triphosphate. *Journal of Clinical Investigation*, Vol.76, No.1, (July 1985), pp.271-280, ISSN0021-9738

McSharry, C.; Xia, Y.; Holland, C.V. & Kennedy, M.W. (1999). Natural immunity to Ascaris lumbricoides with immunoglobulin E antibody to ABA-1 allergen and inflammation indicators in children. *Infection and Immunity*, Vol.67, No.2, (February 1999), pp.484-489, ISSN0019-9567

Min, B. (2008). Basophils: what they "can do" versus what they "actually do". *Nature Immunology*, Vol.9, No.12, (December 2008), pp.1333-1339, ISSN1529-2908

Miyajima, I.; Dombrowicz, D.; Martin, T.R.; Ravetch, J.V.; Kinet, J.P. & Galli, S.J. (1997). Systemic anaphylaxis in the mouse can be mediated largely through IgG1 and FcgammaRIII. Assessment of cardiopulmonary changes, mast cell degranulation, and death associated with active or IgE- or IgG1-dependent passive anaphylaxis. *Journal of Clinical Investigation*, Vol. 99, No.5, (March 1997), pp.901-914, ISSN0021-9738

Moyle, M.; Foster, D.L.; McGrath, D.E, Brown, S.M.; Laroche, Y.; De Meutter, J.; Stanssens, P.; Bogowitz, C.A.; Fried, V.A. & Ely, J.A. (1994). A hookworm glycoprotein that inhibits neutrophil functions is a ligandof the integrin CD11b/CD18. *Journal of Biological Chemistry*,Vol.269, No.13, (April 1994), pp.10008-10015, ISSN1178-6264

Mukai, K.; Matsuoka, K.; Taya, C.; Suzuki, H.; Yokozeki, H.; Nishioka, K.; Hirokawa, K.; Etori, M.; Yamashita, M.; Kubota, T.; Minegishi, Y.; Yonekawa, H.; Karasuyama, H. (2005). Basophils play a critical role in the development of IgE-mediated chronic allergic inflammation independently of T cells and mast cells. *Immunity*, Vol. 23, No. 2, (August 2005), pp.191-202, ISSN1074-7613

Mukai, K.; Obta, K.; Tsujimura, Y. & Karasuyama, H. (2009). New insights into the roles for basophils in acute and chronic allergy. *Allergology International*, Vol.58, No.1, (March 2009), pp.11-19, ISSN1323-8930

Nakagawa, T.; Roth, W.; Wong, P.; Nelson, A.; Farr, A.; Deussing, J.; Villadangos, J.A.; Ploegh, H.; Peters, C. & Rudensky, A.Y. (1998). Cathepsin L: critical role in Ii degradation and CD4 T cell selection in the thymus. *Science*, Vol.280,No.5362, (April 1998), pp.450-453, ISSN0272-4634

Nelms, K.; Keegan, A.D.; Zamorao, J.; Ryan, J.J. & Paul, W.E. (1999). The IL-4 receptor: signaling mechanisms and biologic functions. *Annuals Reviews of Immunology*, Vol.17, (1999), pp.701-738, ISSN0732-0582

Nigou, J.; Zelle-Rieser, C.; Gilleron, M.; Thurnher, M. & Puzo, G. (2001). Mannosylated lipoarabinomannans inhibit IL-12 production by human dendritic cells: evidence for a negative signal delivered through the mannose receptor. *Journal of Immunology*, Vol.166, No.12, (June 2001), pp.7477-7485, ISSN0022-1767

Nimmerjahn, F. & Ravetch, J.V. (2008). Fcγ receptors as regulators of immune responses. *Nature Reviews of Immunology*, Vol.8, No.1, (January. 2008), pp.34-47, ISSN1474-1733

O'Connor, R.A.; Jenson, J.S. & Devaney, E. (2000). No contributes to proliferative suppression in a murine model of filariasis. *Infection and Immunity*, Vol.68, No.11, (November 2000), pp.6101-6107, ISSN0019-9567

Oettgen, H.C.; Martin, T.R.; Wynshaw-Boris, A.; Deng, C.; Drazen, J.M. & Leder, P. (1994). Active anaphylaxis in IgE-deficient mice. *Nature*, Vol.370, No.6488, (August 1994), pp.367-370, ISSN0028-0836

Oettgen, H.C. & Geha, R.S. (1999). IgE in asthma and atopy: cellular and molecular connections. Journal of Clinical Investigation, Vol.104, No.7, (October 1999), pp.829-835, ISSN0021-9738

Oh, K.; Shen, T.; Le Gros, G. & Min, B. (2007). Induction of Th2 type immunity in a mouse system reveals a novel immunoregulatory role of basophils. *Blood*, Vol. 109, No.7, (April 2007), pp.2921-2927, ISSN0006-4971

Okano, M.; Satoskar, A.R.; Nishizaki, K. & Harn, D.A Jr. (2001). Lacto-N-fucopentaose III found on Schistosome mansoni egg antigens functions as adjuvant for proteins by inducing Th2-type response. *Journal of Immunology*, Vol.167, No.1, (July 2001), pp.442-450, ISSN0022-1767

Oshiro, T.M.; Rafael, A.; Enobe, C.S.; Fernandes, I. & Macedo-Soares, M.F.(2004). Comparison of different monoclonal antibodies against immunosuppressive proteins of Ascaris suum. *Brazilian Journal of Medical and Biological Research*, Vol.37, No.2, (February 2004), pp.223-226, ISSN0100-879X

Oshiro, T.M.; Macedo, M.S. & Macedo-Soares, M.F. (2005). Anti-inflammatory activity of PAS-1, a protein component of Ascaris suum. *Inflammation Research*, Vol.54, No.1, (January 2005), pp.17-21, ISSN1023-3830

Oshiro, T.M.; Enobe, C.S.; Araújo, C.A.; Macedo, M.S. & Macedo-Soares, M.F. (2006). PAS-1, a protein affinity purified from Ascaris suum worms, maintain the ability to modulate the immune response to a bystander antigen. *Immunology and Cell Biology*, Vol.84, No.2, (April 2006), pp.138-144, ISSN0818-9641

Paul, W.E. (1997). Interleukin 4: signaling mechanisms and control of T cell differentiation. *Ciba Foundation Symposium*, Vol.204, (1997), pp.208-216, ISSN0300-5208

Pastrana, D.V.; Raghavan, N.; FitzGerald, P.; Eisinger, S.W.; Metz, C.; Bucala, R.; Schleimer, R.P.; Bickel, C & Scott, A.L. (1998). Filarial nematode parasites secrete a homologue of the human cytokine macrophage migration inhibitory factor. *Infection and Immunity*, Vol.66, No.12, (December 1998), pp.5955-5963, ISSN0019-9567

Pearce, E.J. & MacDonald A.S. (2002). The immunobiology of schistosomiasis. *Nature Reviews Immunology*, Vol.2, No.7, (July 2002), pp.499-511, ISSN1474-1733

Pfaff, A.W.; Schulz-Key, H.; Soboslay, P.T.; Taylor, D.W.; MacLennan, K. & Hoffmann, H.W. (2002). Litomosoides sigmodontis cystain acts as an immunomodulator during experimental filariasis. *International Journal of Parasitology*, Vol.32, No.2, (February 2002), pp.171-178, ISSN0020-7519

Playfair, J.H.L. (1982). Immunity to malaria. *British Medical Bulletin*, Vol.38, No.2, (May 1982), pp.153-159, ISSN0007-1420

Pierre, P. & Mellman, I. (1998). Developmental regulation of invariant chain proteolysis controls MHC classII trafficking in mouse dendritic cells. *Cell*,Vol.93, No.7, (June 1998), pp.1135-1145, ISSN0092-8674

Pinckard, R.N.; Halonen, M.; Plamer, J.D.; Butler, C.; Shaw, J.O. & Henson, P.M. (1977). Intravascular aggregation and pulmonary sequestration of platelets during IgE-induced systemic anaphylaxis in the rabbit: abrogation of lethal anaphylactic shock by platelet depletion. *Journal of Immunology*, Vol. 119, No.6, (December 1977), pp. 2185-2193, ISSN0022-1767

Potempa, J.; Korzus, E. & Travis J. (1994).The serpin superfamily of proteinase inhibitors: structure, function and regulation. *Journal of Biological Chemistry*, Vol.269, No.23, (June 1994), pp.15957-15960, ISSN1178-6264

Poulsen, L.K. & Hummelshoj, L. (2007). Triggers of IgE switching and allergy development. *Annals of Medicine*, Vol.39, No.6, (July 2007), pp.440-456, ISSN0785-3890

Pritchard, D.I.; Brown, A.; Kasper, G.; McElroy, P.; Loukas, A.; Hewitt, C.; Berry, C.; Füllkrug, R. & Beck, E. A hookworm allergen which strongly resembles calreticulin. *Parasite Immunology*, Vol.21, No.9, (September 1999), pp.439-450, ISSN0141-9838

Puerta, L.; Fernandez-Caldas, E.; Lockey, R.F. & Caraballo, L.R. (1993). Mite allergy in the tropics: sensitization to six domestic mite species in Cartagena, Colombia. *Journal of Investigational Allergology and Clinical Immunology*, Vol. 3, No.4, (July-August 1993), pp.198-204, ISSN1018-9068

Reyes, J.L. & Terrazas, L.I. (2007). The divergent roles of alternatively acitvated macrophages in helminthic infections. *Parasite Immunology*, Vol.29, No.12, (December 2007), pp.609-619, ISSN0141-9838

Riese, R.J.; Wolf, P.R.; Bromme, D.; Natkin, L.R.; Villadangos, J.A.; Ploegh, H.L. & Chapman, H.A. (1996). Essential role for cathepsin S in MHC classII-associated invariant chain processing and peptide loading. *Immunity*, Vol.4, No.4, (April 1996), pp.357-366, ISSN1074-7613

Rzepecka, J.; Lucius, R.; Dolegalska, M.; Beck, S.; Rausch, S. & Hartmann, S. (2006). Screening for immunomodulatory proteins of the intestinal parasitic nematode Heligmosomoides polygyrus. *Parasite Immunology*, Vol.28, No.9, (September 2006), pp.463-472, ISSN0141-9838

Santiago, H.C.; Bennuru, S.; Boyd, A.; Eberhard, M. & Nutman, T.B. (2011). Structural and immunological cross-reactivity among filarial and mite tropomyosin: implications for the hygiene hypothesis. *Journal of Allergy and Clinical Immunology*, Vol. 127, No. 2, (February 2011), pp.479-486, ISSN0091-6749

Schramm, G.; Mohrs, K.; Wodrich, M.; Doenhoff, M.J.; Pearce, E.J., Haas, H. & Mohrs, M. (2007). IPSE/alpha-1, a glycoprotein from *Schistosoma mansoni* eggs, induces IgE-dependent, antigen-independent IL-4 production by murine basophils in vivo. *Journal of Immunology*, Vol.178, No.10, (May 2007), pp.6023-6027, ISSN0022-1767

Schramm, G.; Falcone, F.H.; Gronow, A.; Haisch, K.; Mamat, U.; Doenhoff, M.J.; Oliveira, G.; Galle, J.; Dahinden, C.A. & Haas, H. (2003). Molecular characterization of an interleukin-4-inducing factor from Schistosoma mansoni eggs. *Journal of Biological Chemistry*, Vol.278, No.20, (May 2003), pp.18384-18392, ISSN1178-6264

Schönemeyer, A.; Lucius, R.; Sonnenburg, B.; Brattig, N.; Sabat, R.; Schilling, K.; Bradley, J. & Hartmann S. (2001). Modulation of human T cell responses and macrophage functions by onchocystatin, a secreted protein of the filarial nematode Onchocerca volvulus. *Journal of Immunology*, Vol.167, No.6, (September 2001), pp.3207-3215, ISSN0022-1767

Scrivener, S.; Yemaneberhan, H.; Zebenigus, M.; Tilahun, D.; Girma, S.; Ali, S.; McElroy, P.; Custovic, A.; Woodcock, A.; Pritchard, D.; Venn, A. & Britton, J. (2001). Independent effects of intestinal parasite infection and domestic allergen exposure on risk of wheeze in Ethiopia: a nested case-control study. *Lancet*, Vol.358, No.9292, (November 2001), pp.1493-1499, ISSN0099-5355

Semnani, R.T.; Liu, A.Y.; Sabzevari, H.; Kubofcik, J.; Ahou, J.; Gilden, J.K. & Nutman, T.B. Brugia malayi microfilariae induce cell death in human dendtric cells, inhibit their ability to make IL-12 and IL-10, and reduce their capacity to activate CD4+ cells. *Journal of Immunology*, Vol.171, No.4, (August 2003), pp.1950-1960, ISSN0022-1767

Shi, G.P.; Bryant, R.A.; Riese, R.; Verhelst, S.; Driessen, C.; Li, Z.; Bromme, D.; Ploegh, H.L. & Chapman, H.A. Role for cathepsin F in invariant processing and major histocompatibility complex classII peptide loading by macrophages. *Journal of Experimental Medicine*, Vol.19, No.7, (April 2000), pp.1177-1186, ISSN0022-1007

Shimoda, K.; van Deursen, J.; Sangster, M.Y.; Sarawar, S.R.; Carson, R.T.; Tripp, R.A.; Chu, C.; Quelle, F.W.; Nosaka, T.; Vignali, D.A.; Doherty, P.C.; Grosveld, G.; Paul, W.E. & Ihle, J.N. (1996). Lack of IL-4 induced Th2 response and IgE class switching in mice with disrupted Stat6 gene. *Nature*, Vol.380, No.6575, (April 1996), pp.630-633, ISSN0028-0836

Simons, F.E.; Frew, A.J.; Ansotegui, I.J.; Bochner, B.S.; Golden, D.B.; Finkelman, F.D.; Leung, D.Y.; Lotvall, J.; Marone, G.; Metcalfe, D.D.; Muller, U.; Rosenwasser, L.J.; Sampson, H.A.; Schwartz, L.B.; van Hage, M. & Walls, A.F. (2007). Risk assessement in anaphylaxis: current and future approaches. *Journal of Allergy and Clinical Immunology*, Vol. 120, No. 1, (July. 2007), pp.S2-24, ISSN0091-6749

Simons, F. (2003). H1-antihistamines: more relevant than ever in the treatment of allergic disorders. *Journal of Allergy and Clinical Immunology*, Vol.112, No.4(Suppl), (October 2003), pp.S42-52, ISSN 0091-6749

Smits, H.H.; Everts, B.; Hartgers, F.C. & Yazdanbakhsh, M. (2010). Chronic helminth infections protect against allergic diseases by active regulatory processes. *Current Allergy and Asthma Reports*, Vol.10, No.1, (January 2010), pp.3-12, ISSN1529-7322

Soares, M.F.M.; Macedo, M.S. & Mota, I. Suppressive effect of an Ascaris suum extract on IgE and IgG antibody responses in mice. *Brazilian Journal of Medical and Biological Research*, Vol., No.2, (1987), pp.203-211, ISSN0100-879X

Soares, M.F.M.; Mota, I. & Macedo, M.S. Isolation of Ascaris suum components which suppress IgE antibody responses. *International Archives of Allergy and Immunology*, Vol.97, No.1, (1992), pp.37-43, ISSN1871-5281

Soares MFM & Araujo CA. Helminth products as a potential therapeutic strategy for inflammatory diseases. *Inflammation and Allergy Drug Targets*, Vol.7, No.2, (June 2008), pp.113-118, ISSN1871-5281

Sokol, C.L.; Barton, G.M.; Farr, A.G. & Medzhitov, R. (2008). A mechanism for the initiation of allergen-induced T helper type 2 responses. *Nature Immunology*, Vol.9, No.3, (Mar 2008), pp.310-8, ISSN1529-2908

Stafforini, D.M.; McIntyre, T.M.; Zimmermann, G.A. & Prescott, S.M. (2003). Platelet-activating factor, a pleiotrophic mediator of physiological and pathological processes. *Critical Reviews in Clinical Laboratory Sciences*, Vol.40, No.6, (2003), pp.643-672, ISSN1040-8363

Steinfelder, S.; Andersen, J.F.; Cannons, J.L.; Feng, C.G.; Joshi, M.; Dwyer, D.; Caspar, P.; Schwartzberg, P.L.; Sher, A. & Jankovic, D. (2009) The major component in schistosome eggs responsible for conditioning dendritic cells for Th2 polarization is a T2 ribonuclease (omega-1). *Journal of Experimental Medicine*, Vol.206, No.8, (August 2009), pp.1681-1690, ISSN0022-1007

Stephenson, L.S.; Latham, M.C. & Ottesen, E.A. (2000). Global malnutrition. Parasitology, *Vol.121, (2000)*, pp.S5-22, ISSN0031-1820

Stewart, G.R.; Boussinesq, M.; Coulson, T.; Elson, L.; Nutman, T. & Bradley, J.E. (1999). Onchocerciasis modulates the immune response to mycobacterial antigens. *Clinical and Experimental Immunology*,Vol.117, No.3, (September 1999), pp.571-523, ISSN0009-9104

Strait, R.T.; Morris, S.C.; Yang, M.; Qu, X.W. & Finkelman, F.D. (2002). Pathways of anaphylaxis in the mouse. *Journal of Allergy and Clinical Immunology*, Vol.109, No.4, (April 2002), pp.658-668, ISSN0091-6749

Strait, R.T.; Morris, S.C.; Smiley, K.; Urban, J.F. Jr & Finkelman, F.D. (2003). IL-4 exarcebates anaphylaxis. *Journal of Immunology*, Vol.170, No.7, (April 2003), pp.3835-3842, ISSN0022-1767

Sugimoto, Y.; Iba, Y.; Nakamura, Y.; Kayasuga, R. & Kamei, C. (2004). Pruritus-associated response mediated by cutaneous histamine H3 receptors. *Clinical and Experimental Allergy*, Vol.34, No.3, (March 2004), pp.456-459, ISSN0954-7894

Swain, S.L.; Weinberg, A.D.; English, M. & Huston, G. (1990). IL-4 directs the development of Th2 like helper effectors. *Journal of Immunology*, Vol.145, No.11, (December 1990), pp.3796-3806, ISSN0022-1767

Takai, T. (2005). Fc receptors and their role in immune regulation and autoimmunity. *Journal of Clinical Immunology*, Vol. 25, No.1, (January 2005), pp.1-18, ISSN0271-9142

Terrazas, L.I.; Walsh, K.L.; Piskorska, D.; McGuire, E.& Harn, D.A Jr. (2001). The schistosome oligosaccharide lacto-N-neotetraose expands Gr1(+) cells that secrete anti-inflammatory cytokinse and inhibit proliferation of naive CD4(+) cells: a potential mechanism for immune polarization in helminth infections. *Journal of Immunology*, Vol.167, No.9, (September 2001), pp.5412-5416, ISSN0022-1767

Tiselius A & Kabat EA. (1939). An eletrophoretic study of immune sera and purified antibody preparations. *Journal of Experimental Medicine*, Vol.69, No.1, (January 1939), pp.119-131, ISSN0022-1007

Thurmond, R.L.; Desai, P.J.; Dunford, P.J.; Fung-Leung, W.P.; Hofstra, C.L., Jiang, W.; Nguyen, S.; Riley, J.P.; Sun, S.; Williams, K.N.; Edwards, J.P. and Karlsson, L. (2004). A potent and selective histamine H4 receptor antagonist with anti-inflammatory properties. *Journal of Pharmacology and Experimental Therapeutics*, Vol.309, No.1, (April 2004), pp.401-413, ISSN0022-3565

Truong, M.J.; Gruart, V.; Kusnierz, J.P.; Papin, J.P.; Loiseau, S.; Capron, A. & Capron M. (1993). Human neutrophils express immunoglobulin E (IgE)-binding proteins (Mac-2/epsilon BP) of the S-type lectin family: role in IgE-dependent activation. *Journal of Experimental Medicine*, Vol.177, No.1, (January 1993), pp.243-248, ISSN0022-1007

Tsujimura, Y.; Obata, K.; Mukai, K.; Shindou, H.; Yoshida, M.; Nishikado, H.; Kawano, Y.; Minegishi, Y.; Shimizu, T. & Karasuyama, H. (2008). Basophils play a pivotal role in immunoglobulin-G-mediated but not immunoglobulin-E-mediated systemic anaphylaxis. *Immunity*, Vol.28, No.4, (April 2008), pp.581-589, ISSN1074-7613

Ujike, A.; Ishikawa, Y.; Ono, M.; Yuasa, T.; Yoshino, T.; Fukumoto, M.; Ravetch, J.V. & Takai, T. (1999). Modulation of immunoglobulin(Ig)E-mediated systemic anaphylaxis by low-affinity Fc receptor for IgG. *Journal of Experimental Medicine*, Vol.189, No.10, (May 1999), pp.1573-1519, ISSN0022-1007

Urbina, C.; Ortiz, C. & Hurtado, I. (1981). A new look at basophil in mice. *International Archives of Allergy and Applied Immunology*, Vol. 66, No.2, (1981), pp.158-160, ISSN0020-4793

Vadas, P.; Gold, M.; Perelman, B.; Liss, G.M.; Lack, G.; Blyth, T.; Simons, F.E.; Simons, K.J.; Cass, D. & Yeung, J. (2008). Platelet-activating factor, PAF acetylhydrolase, and severe anaphylaxis. *New England Journal of Medicine*, Vol.358, No.1, (January 2008), pp.28-35, ISSN0028-4793

van der Kleij, D.; Latz, E.; Brouwers, J.F.; Kruize, Y.C.; Schmitz, M.; Kurt-Jones, E.A.; Espervik, T.; de Jong, E.C.; Kapsenberg, M.L.; Golenbock, D.T.; Tielens, A.G. & Yazdanbakhsh, M. (2002). A novel host-parasite lipid cross-talk. Schistosomal lyso-phosphatideylserine activates toll-like receptor 2 and affects immune polarization. *Journal of Biological Chemistry*, Vol.277, No.50, (December 2002), pp.48122-48129, ISSN1178-6264

van Riet, E.; Hartgers, F.C. & Yazdanbakhsh, M. (2007). Chronic helminth infections induce immunomodulation: consequences and mechanisms. *Immunobiology*, Vol.212, No.6, (April 2007), pp.475-490, ISSN0175-2985

Verity, C.K.; Loukas, A.; McManus, D.P. & Brindley, P.J. (2001). Schistosoma japonicum cathepsin D aspartic protease cleaves human IgG and other serum components. *Parasitology*, Vol.122, No.4, (April 2001), pp.415-421, ISSN0031-1820

Williams, A.F. & Barclay, A.N. (1998). The immunoglobulin superfamily – domains for cell surface recognition. *Annual Reviews of Immunology*, Vol.6, (1988), pp.381-405, ISSN0732-0582

Wilson, M.S.; Mentink-Kane, M.M.; Pesce, J.T.; Ramalingam, T.R.; Thompson, R. & Wynn, T.A. (2007). Immunopathology of schistosomiasis. *Immunology and Cell Biology*, Vol.85, No.2, (February-March. 2007), pp.148-154, ISBN0818-9641

Winbery, S.L. & Lieberman, P.L. (2002). Histamine and antihistamines in anaphylaxis. *Clinical Allergy and Immunology*, Vol. 17, (2002), pp. 287-317, ISSN1075-7910

Zang, X.; Yazdanbakhsh, M.; Jinag, H.; Kanost, M.R & Maizels, R.M. (1999). A novel serpin expressed by blood-borne microfilariae of the parasitic nematode Brugia malayi inhibits human neutrophil serine proteinase. *Blood*, Vol.94, No.4, (August 1999), pp.1418-1428, ISSN0006-4971

10

Parasite-Derived Proteins Inhibit Allergic Specific Th2 Response

Hak Sun Yu

Department of Parasitology, School of Medicine,
Pusan National University, Yangsan-si,
South Korea

1. Introduction

The prevalence of allergic disease and asthma has increased dramatically during the last 30-40 years. Atopic disorders comprise a range of allergic diseases including asthma, anaphylaxis, allergic rhinitis, and atopic dermatitis; these diseases have been seen a precipitous increase in the last four decades. Intriguingly, geographic regions with a high helminth infection burden tend to have a lower incidence of asthma (1). The effects of parasitic infections on the incidence of allergic disease has been receiving increased attention from researchers of late, with studies conducted in Ethiopia and Gabon demonstrating that parasitic infestation is associated with reduced atopic sensitization and dust mite skin test sensitivity (2-4). Children treated repeatedly for *Trichuris trichiura* and *Ascaris lumbricoides* exhibited increased dust-mite skin responses as compared with children that had not been treated for asymptomatic soil-associated helminthic infections (5). Several molecules from helminthes induce pronounced Th2 responses in a manner similar to that seen in cases of full-blown parasitic infection. Excretory-secretory (ES) glycoproteins isolated from the rodent nematode, *Nippostrongylus brasiliensis*, have been shown to evidence Th2-promoting activity on dendrite cells, however, the exact nature of the molecules involved in *N. brasiliensis* ES proteins remain to be clearly elucidated. This activity is heat-labile and protease-sensitive, thereby suggesting that the active component is proteinaceous in nature (6). Also, in schistosomiasis, the soluble extract of *Schistosoma mansoni* eggs (SEA) was shown to induce SEA-specific Th2 responses when injected into mice (7), and SEA was also demonstrated to condition human dendrite cells (DCs) to polarize Th response in a Th2 direction *in vitro* (8). When exposed to Th2 cytokines, these molecules can also activate host CD4+CD25+Foxp3+ T cells (regulatory T cells, T_{reg}) which subsequently release IL-10 and tumor growth factor β (TGF-β), which may be functionally involved in the suppression of the level of Th2 cytokines IL-4, IL-5, and IL-13. These parasites can establish a chronic infection, which highlights important issues (9), in that the presence of these metabolically active pathogens indicates that the immune system is being relentlessly challenged with foreign antigens; this continuous immune reactivity, if uncontrolled, could eventuate severe pathology. In addition, these pathogens may have developed evolutionary strategies by which they may evade the immune system for long-term survival in an immunocompetent host (10).

In order to ascertain, then, whether parasitic infections can reduce allergic reactions and whether their infective stage influences the immune system of the host, we have mimicked chronic infection conditions in our experiment via treatment with parasite-derived proteins for one month prior to allergen treatment. We attempted to determine whether or not these parasite-derived proteins suppressed allergy-specific Th2 reactions.

2. Immunization of parasite derived proteins inhibits allergic specific Th2 response

Long-lived parasites are highly accomplished practitioners of immune evasion and manipulation, utilizing strategies honed during their long co-evolutionary interaction with the mammalian immune system (10, 11). How is the host affected by these parasitic strategies? Although many hypotheses have been advanced, until the present time there has been little evidence to support these theories. Th2 host response as the result of parasitic infection was apparent, although this is the result of parasitic strategies to escape from the host immune system or the result of a human protective system associated with parasitic infection. Additionally, we could readily detect Th2 responses in allergic patients. Thus, until now, there has been considerable controversy regarding the relationship between parasites and allergic reactions; particularly, whether parasites can evoke some allergic-specific response or can reduce allergen-specific responses (12-14).

We have attempted to determine whether parasite-derived proteins can accelerate or reduce asthma symptoms in accordance with the treatment period (15). We have mimicked chronic infection conditions in our experiment via treatment with parasite (*Toxascaris leonina* adult worm)-derived proteins [ES protein (Tl-ES) and total proteins (Tl-TP)] for one month prior to the administration of allergen treatment. We mentioned this group as Immunized group; also Challenged with OVA group were mentioned which were administrated Tl-ES and Tl-TP at the same challenge days in airway allergic reaction procedure. As results, the immunized Tl-ES and Tl-TP groups evidenced a thinning of the bronchial epithelial and muscle layer, a disruption and shedding of the epithelial cells, a reduction in the number of goblet cells as compared to the OVA-challenged groups (Fig. 1). When the airway functions of these mice were monitored, we detected that the Penh values by methacholine treatment (from 2.5 mg/ml to 25 mg/ml) were significantly higher in the OVA-inhalation mice than those of Tl-TP and Tl-ES immunized group (Fig. 2A). The numbers of most inflammatory cells (macrophages, eosinophils, lymphocytes and neutrophils) in the BAL fluids were significantly increased in all of the OVA-challenged groups (Fig. 2B & 2C). The administration of Tl-ES and Tl-TP prior to asthma induction (immunized group) and the Tl-ES and Tl-TP with OVA challenge (challenged with OVA groups) evidenced inhibited recruitment of inflammatory cells into the airway (Fig. 2B & 2C). In particular, neutrophils and lymphocytes were significantly reduced by the parasite proteins at any administration time (p value < 0.05). The total number of eosinophils of the immunized and OVA-challenged group were slightly reduced; however, this reduction was not statistically significant (P value > 0.05).

Although some articles have previously asserted that nematodes can induce allergic reactions during their larval migration period (16, 17), many articles have reported that parasitic infections, particularly chronic parasitism, help to reduce host allergic reactions and to modulate host immune responses (14, 18, 19). We have determined that immunization with *T. leonina* adult worm ES and total proteins induces a down-regulation of asthma-associated cytokines, including IL-4 and IL-5, in the bronchial alveolar lavage (BAL) fluids (Fig. 3). However, these proteins did not significantly influence allergic airway inflammation response as the result of simultaneous OVA challenge, as compared to the immunization method. In particular, the Tl-ES treatment with OVA challenge group exhibited more severe lung inflammation than was observed in the immunized group. We believe that certain allergens or proteases might be included in the ES proteins, and parasitic proteases have also been identified as allergens (20-23). Sokol *et al.* previously suggested that a host-derived sensor of proteolytic activity might involve cleavage via parasite or allergic proteases. This sensor, once cleaved, activates the cells of the innate immune system to induce a Th2 response (13).

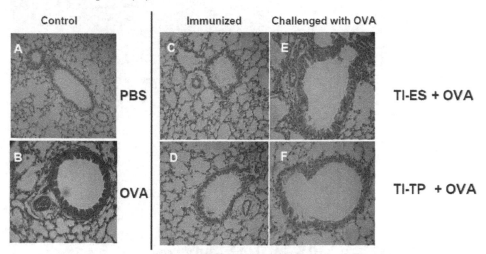

Fig. 1. **Histological findings of airway inflammation in ova-challenged control mice and the effect of immunization and challenge with OVA groups.** Female and 6 weeks of age mice were induced airway allergic reaction using intraperitoneally (I.P.) sensitizing with 75 ug of ovalbumin (OVA, Sigma, Grade V) and 2 mg of aluminium hydroxide gel, on days 0 and 7. One week after the final sensitization, the mice were intra nasal challenged with 50 ug of OVA on 4 consecutive days (days 13, 14, 19, and 20). We mentioned "Immunized group" that were injected by I.P. with 100 ul of 10 ug/ml *Toxascaris leonina* excretory-secretory (Tl-ES) and *T. leonina* total protein (Tl-TP), respectively, on 7 and 14 days before airway allergic reaction procedure. Also "Challenged with OVA" group were mentioned which were injected by I.P. with 100 ul of 10 ug/ml of Tl-ES and Tl-TP respectively at the same challenge days in airway allergic reaction procedure. The negative control group was challenged with PBS (I.N.) on the same challenge day in airway allergic reaction procedure. A; PBS-treated, B-F; OVA+ alum-treated (induced asthma), (C) immunized Tl-ES protein, (D) immunized Tl-TP, (E) Tl-ES protein treatment with OVA challenge, (F) Tl-TP protein with OVA challenge.

IL-4 has been demonstrated to regulate isotype class switching in B cells to IgE synthesis, and IL-5 stimulates eosinophil growth, activates these cells, and prolongs eosinophil survival. *T. leonina*-derived proteins could inhibit increases in the levels of IL-4 and IL-5 from OVA challenge. In particular, the level of IL-4 in the BAL fluid in the immunized group was almost half of that observed in the OVA-only challenge group. This result was consistent with the results regarding the IgE concentration in the blood (15). Although levels of the IL-5 cytokine of *T. leonina* ES and total protein-immunized mice were lower than those observed in asthma control mice, this effect was not remarkable. Also, the total number of eosinophils was not substantially reduced as the result of immunization. Eosinophils and IgE proved vitally important in allergy-induced Th2 response; additionally, the elevation of the numbers of these cells and IgE levels were identified as specific responses to parasite infection and this response was shown to be elicited only by treatment with parasite total proteins (24, 25).

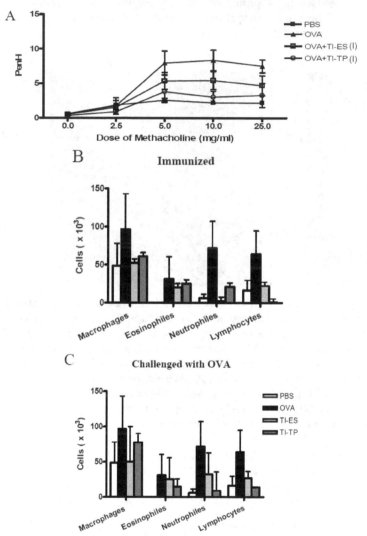

Fig. 2. **Airway hyperresponsiveness measurements and comparison of differential cell counts obtained via airway inflammation in ova-sensitized PBS mice and the effects in immunized and OVA-challenged groups**. Total protein of *T. leonina* immunization group [Tl-TP (I)] has lower penh value than those of OVA challenge group (A). The numbers of inflammatory cells were significantly lower in the parasite-derived protein-treated mice (B & C). The data were expressed as the means ± SD of individual mice.

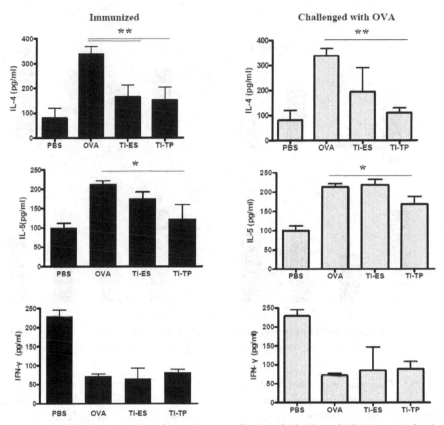

Fig. 3. **Th1 and Th2 cytokines levels in the BAL fluids of Tl-ES and Tl-TP treated mice.** The levels of all Th2 cytokines of the immunized group were contrasted with those of the OVA-challenged control mice. The data were expressed as the means $\pm$ SD of individual mice (* ; p value <0.05, **; p value <0.01).

How does helminth infection protect against allergy? Many hypotheses have been advanced thus far regarding this theme. One of these hypotheses is that non-specific IgE generated as the result of helminthic infection may inhibit allergen-specific IgE binding sites on mast cells or basophils. Although Jarrett suggested in 1980 that parasite-induced 'nonspecific' IgE does not protect against host allergic reactions (26). However, other scientists have suggested that nonspecific IgE can modulate host immune responses, as in the case of insulin-dependent diabetes, as well as Th2 response by allergens (25, 27-29). The other hypothesis states that helminth parasites stimulate the production of immunoregulatory mediators, which are likely to perform a function in the maintenance of the chronicity of infection, with no marked induction of pathology. In particular, elevated IL-10 levels have been associated previously with protection against allergic diseases in helminth-infected African children (4). Helminth infections can induce T_{reg} cells from hosts, and these cells secrete IL-10 and suppress the proliferation of other CD4+ T cells (30-32). We also found that parasite proteins could also induce the IL-10 cytokine, particularly in the Tl-TP immunized group (Fig. 4).

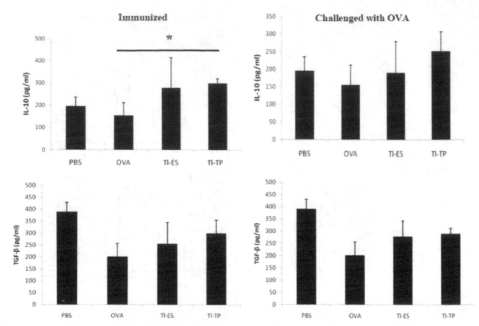

Fig. 4. T_reg cell related cytokines levels in the BAL fluids of Tl-ES and Tl-TP treated mice. The data were expressed as the means ± SD of individual mice (* ; p value <0.05, **; p value <0.01).

Finally, the data presented herein demonstrate that *T. leonina*-derived proteins may perform a crucial function in resistance against Th2 immune responses. We suggested that this inhibition may be related to the IL-10 cytokine, which was induced by parasite proteins. Further steps are currently being taken in an effort to gain a greater understanding of the molecular basis of immune evasion by nematodes. Thus, we are attempting to gain new insights into the immune regulation strategies of nematodes, and the growing number of new strategies employed by parasites to exert their marked down-regulatory effects.

3. Macrophage migration inhibitory factor homologues of parasite suppress Th2 response in allergic airway inflammation model via T_reg cell recruitment

A number of parasite-derived proteins, glycoconjugates, and small lipid moieties have been demonstrated to perform known or hypothesized functions in immune interference. Other researchers have already isolated several other immune downregulatory molecules from parasites, and these molecules have been identified as mammal cytokine homologues, protease inhibitors, abundant larval transcript antigens, glyco-networks, and venom allergen-like proteins (33-39). The cytokine network is a crucial component of host defense against pathogens. It is not, therefore, surprising to find that one of the immune evasion strategies utilized by infectious organisms is the generation of mammalian cytokine homologues, including TGF-β and the macrophage migration inhibitory factor (MIF) (40, 41).

MIF was described initially as one of the earliest cytokines to be derived from activated T-cells, and was believed to prevent the random migration of macrophages (42). MIF has also been demonstrated to be generated abundantly by monocytes/macrophages and to function in an autocrine/paracrine manner in the upregulation and sustenance of the activation of diverse cell types (43). The profile of the activities of MIF, both *in vivo* and *in vitro*, is reflective of a role for MIF in the pathogenesis of a variety of inflammatory diseases, including rheumatoid arthritis, inflammatory bowel disease, ankylosing spondylitis, and psoriasis (44). MIF performs a crucial function in airway inflammation and airway hyper-responsiveness in asthma (45).

Recently, several MIF homologues have been isolated from parasitic nematodes. Two types of MIF homologues have thus far been identified in nematodes (34). The type 1 MIF homologues bear a greater amino acid similarity with the mammalian MIFs than do the type 2 MIF homologues (46). The type 1 MIF homologues isolated from *Brugia malayi* (Bm-MIF1) induce eosinophil recruitment, and alternatively activated macrophage recruitment *in vivo* when injected into the peritoneal cavities of mice. Mutation of the conserved proline residue induces the abrogation of this activity (47). This ability of parasite MIF homologues was similar to those of mammalian MIF. However, recently Cho et al. reported that hookworm MIF (structurally type 2 MIF) functions differently from mammalian MIF (48, 49).

We have cloned another type 2 MIF homologue (As-MIF) from *Anisakis simplex* (whale worm) 3rd stage larva, which causes anisakidosis in humans (50). Recombinant As-MIF (rAs-MIF) proved highly effective with regard to the inhibition of goblet cell hyperplasia and inflammatory responses in the airways of OVA-induced asthma model mice (Fig. 5). Increasing concentrations of rAs-MIF induced an increase in the anti-inflammatory effects on asthma model mice. Additionally, the function of rAs-MIF was antagonized as compared to the function of host MIF (59).

How does As-MIF suppress allergy responses in mice? There have been many reports demonstrating that Th2-type effector responses may be regulated by T_{reg} cells (51-53). Additionally, nematode infections can induce and expand naturally occurring T_{reg} cells in both humans and mice (4, 54), thereby suggesting a role for these T_{reg} cells in the helminth-induced modulation of inflammatory diseases (55, 56). In particular, the clinical symptoms of allergic airway inflammation in the mouse model was clearly modulated by T_{reg} cell mediated immune suppression, which was itself activated by helminth infection or antigen treatment (57, 58). We could determine the increase in T_{reg} cells as the result of rAs-MIF treatment in OVA-alum asthma-induced mice (Fig. 6).

IL-10 and TGF-β were produced primarily by T_{reg} cells, and they are known to suppress immune response effects. The IL-10 and TGF-β levels measured in BALFs from rAs-MIF-treated asthma-induced mice were higher than those of the asthma-induced mice; the IL-10 and TGF-β levels occurred in accordance with their treated concentrations (59). The helminthic parasites stimulate the production of immunoregulatory mediators, which likely perform a function in the maintenance of the chronicity of infection, without any marked induction of pathology. In particular, elevated IL-10 levels have been associated with responses against allergic diseases in helminth-infected individuals (4). Also, Nagler-Anderson et al. showed that in mice sensitized with peanut plus cholera toxin, anti-IL-10 treatment abrogated the ability of helminths to protect against allergic symptoms and to downregulate allergen-specific IgE. IL-10, which is referred to as the cytokine synthesis inhibitory factor, is an anti-inflammatory cytokine, which is capable of inhibiting the synthesis of pro-inflammatory cytokines (60). The IL-10 requirement is critical to several important human diseases, including schistosomiasis, wherein marked increases in host morbidity and mortality are observed when IL-10 levels are low or absent (61). In cases of murine *S. mansoni* infection, IL-10 attenuates the hepatocyte damage induced by the eggs of the parasite. IL-10 is also essential for the maintenance of non-lethal chronic infections, in addition to the inhibition of inappropriate immune responses in experimental models (62). TGF-β1 is also a strong candidate for immune suppression by T_{reg} cells from helminth-infected mice, and has already been recognized to alleviate experimental airway allergy symptoms (63) and to instruct peripheral T cells to develop their regulatory capacities (64). Thus, the inhibition of asthma response by rAs-MIF may be associated with the principal T_{reg} cell–associated downregulatory cytokines, including TGF-β1 and IL-10.

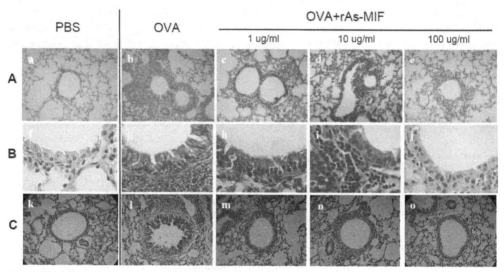

Fig. 5. **Histologic appearance of lungs after challenge with PBS, OVA, and rAs-MIF by concentration (H-E stain).** (A; x 100, B; x 600; C; PAS stain), C; **a**, **f**, and **k**; phosphate-buffered saline (PBS) treated, **b-e**, **g-j**, and **l-o**; OVA plus alum-treated (induced asthma), **c**, **h** and **m**; challenged with 1 μg/ml rAs-MIF, **d**, **i**, and **n**; challenged with 10 μg/ml rAs-MIF. **e**, **j**, and **o**; challenged with 100μg/ml rAs-MIF. In asthma-induced mice, a massive peri-bronchial infiltration with immune-related cells and hyperplasia of bronchial epithelial cells were observed. Upon challenge with 1μg/ml rAs-MIF treatment (**c**, **h** and **m**), asthma-induced mice evidenced thinner bronchial epithelial cells than were observed in the asthma-induced mice (**b**, **g**, and **l**). Mice challenged with treatment with 10 and 100μg/ml rAs-MIF evidenced thinner than normal bronchial epithelial cells and decreased numbers of immune-related cells. Goblet cells and immune-related cells in the airway walls of mice exposed to PBS, OVA and OVA challenge with 1, 10, and 100 μg/ml rAs-MIF. In asthma-induced mice (**g**), a massive peri-bronchial infiltration of inflammatory cells and hyperplasia of bronchial epithelial cells were detected. However, goblet cell hyperplasia was reduced in the bronchial epithelial cells of the rAs-MIF-treated mice (**h-j**).

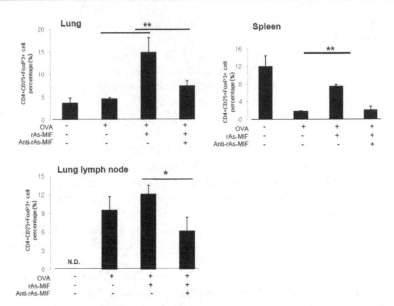

Fig. 6. T$_{reg}$ cell production could be induced by rAs-MIF treatment. T$_{reg}$ cell populations in the lungs and spleen were significantly increased by rAs-MIF treatment, but this effect was inhibited by rAnti-As-MIF. (*; $p < 0.05$, **; $p < 0.01$, n = 5 mice per group, 3 independent experiments).

4. Conclusion

We showed that parasite derived proteins may perform a crucial function in resistance against allergic airway inflammation via IL-10 cytokine induction and Treg cell recruitment. Parasites regulate or suppress their host immune response, maintaining their parasitism for a prolonged period, using unknown molecules. As-MIF might be one of the molecules that affect host immune regulation. The further characterization of parasite derived proteins might ultimately result in the design of novel therapeutic intervention strategies for the treatment of asthma.

5. References

[1] Zaccone, P., Z. Fehervari, J. M. Phillips, D. W. Dunne, and A. Cooke. 2006. Parasitic worms and inflammatory diseases. *Parasite immunology* 28:515-523.

[2] Scrivener, S., H. Yemaneberhan, M. Zebenigus, D. Tilahun, S. Girma, S. Ali, P. McElroy, A. Custovic, A. Woodcock, D. Pritchard, A. Venn, and J. Britton. 2001. Independent effects of intestinal parasite infection and domestic allergen exposure on risk of wheeze in Ethiopia: a nested case-control study. *Lancet* 358:1493-1499.

[3] Dagoye, D., Z. Bekele, K. Woldemichael, H. Nida, M. Yimam, A. Hall, A. J. Venn, J. R. Britton, R. Hubbard, and S. A. Lewis. 2003. Wheezing, allergy, and parasite

infection in children in urban and rural Ethiopia. *Am J Respir Crit Care Med* 167:1369-1373.

[4] van den Biggelaar, A. H., R. van Ree, L. C. Rodrigues, B. Lell, A. M. Deelder, P. G. Kremsner, and M. Yazdanbakhsh. 2000. Decreased atopy in children infected with Schistosoma haematobium: a role for parasite-induced interleukin-10. *Lancet* 356:1723-1727.

[5] van den Biggelaar, A. H., L. C. Rodrigues, R. van Ree, J. S. van der Zee, Y. C. Hoeksma-Kruize, J. H. Souverijn, M. A. Missinou, S. Borrmann, P. G. Kremsner, and M. Yazdanbakhsh. 2004. Long-term treatment of intestinal helminths increases mite skin-test reactivity in Gabonese schoolchildren. *J Infect Dis* 189:892-900.

[6] Balic, A., Y. Harcus, M. J. Holland, and R. M. Maizels. 2004. Selective maturation of dendritic cells by Nippostrongylus brasiliensis-secreted proteins drives Th2 immune responses. *Eur J Immunol* 34:3047-3059.

[7] MacDonald, A. S., A. D. Straw, B. Bauman, and E. J. Pearce. 2001. CD8- dendritic cell activation status plays an integral role in influencing Th2 response development. *J Immunol* 167:1982-1988.

[8] de Jong, E. C., P. L. Vieira, P. Kalinski, J. H. Schuitemaker, Y. Tanaka, E. A. Wierenga, M. Yazdanbakhsh, and M. L. Kapsenberg. 2002. Microbial compounds selectively induce Th1 cell-promoting or Th2 cell-promoting dendritic cells in vitro with diverse th cell-polarizing signals. *J Immunol* 168:1704-1709.

[9] Allen, J. E., and R. M. Maizels. 1996. Immunology of human helminth infection. *Int Arch Allergy Immunol* 109:3-10.

[10] Behnke, J. M., C. J. Barnard, and D. Wakelin. 1992. Understanding chronic nematode infections: evolutionary considerations, current hypotheses and the way forward. *Int J Parasitol* 22:861-907.

[11] Maizels, R. M., D. A. Bundy, M. E. Selkirk, D. F. Smith, and R. M. Anderson. 1993. Immunological modulation and evasion by helminth parasites in human populations. *Nature* 365:797-805.

[12] Demirturk, N., E. Kozan, T. Demirdal, F. Fidan, O. C. Aktepe, M. Unlu, and Z. Asci. 2007. Effect of parasitosis on allergic sensitization in rats sensitized with ovalbumin: interaction between parasitosis and allergic sensitization. *Adv Ther* 24:1305-1313.

[13] Sokol, C. L., G. M. Barton, A. G. Farr, and R. Medzhitov. 2007. A mechanism for the initiation of allergen-induced T helper type 2 responses. *Nat Immunol*.

[14] van Riet, E., F. C. Hartgers, and M. Yazdanbakhsh. 2007. Chronic helminth infections induce immunomodulation: consequences and mechanisms. *Immunobiology* 212:475-490.

[15] Lee, K. H., H. K. Park, H. J. Jeong, S. K. Park, S. J. Lee, S. H. Choi, M. K. Cho, M. S. Ock, Y. C. Hong, and H. S. Yu. 2008. Immunization of proteins from Toxascaris leonina adult worm inhibits allergic specific Th2 response. *Veterinary parasitology* 156:216-225.

[16] Kim, J. S., K. H. Kim, S. Cho, H. Y. Park, S. W. Cho, Y. T. Kim, K. H. Joo, and J. S. Lee. 2005. Immunochemical and biological analysis of allergenicity with excretory-

secretory products of anisakis simplex third stage larva. *Int Arch Allergy Immunol* 136:320-328.

[17] Baeza, M. L., A. Rodriguez, V. Matheu, M. Rubio, P. Tornero, M. de Barrio, T. Herrero, M. Santaolalla, and J. M. Zubeldia. 2004. Characterization of allergens secreted by Anisakis simplex parasite: clinical relevance in comparison with somatic allergens. *Clin Exp Allergy* 34:296-302.

[18] Flohr, C., L. N. Tuyen, S. Lewis, R. Quinnell, T. T. Minh, H. T. Liem, J. Campbell, D. Pritchard, T. T. Hien, J. Farrar, H. Williams, and J. Britton. 2006. Poor sanitation and helminth infection protect against skin sensitization in Vietnamese children: A cross-sectional study. *The Journal of allergy and clinical immunology* 118:1305-1311.

[19] Wang, C. C., T. J. Nolan, G. A. Schad, and D. Abraham. 2001. Infection of mice with the helminth Strongyloides stercoralis suppresses pulmonary allergic responses to ovalbumin. *Clin Exp Allergy* 31:495-503.

[20] Kobayashi, Y., S. Ishizaki, K. Shimakura, Y. Nagashima, and K. Shiomi. 2007. Molecular cloning and expression of two new allergens from Anisakis simplex. *Parasitology research* 100:1233-1241.

[21] Shaw, R. J., M. M. McNeill, D. R. Maass, W. R. Hein, T. K. Barber, M. Wheeler, C. A. Morris, and C. B. Shoemaker. 2003. Identification and characterisation of an aspartyl protease inhibitor homologue as a major allergen of Trichostrongylus colubriformis. *International journal for parasitology* 33:1233-1243.

[22] Furmonaviciene, R., H. F. Sewell, and F. Shakib. 2000. Comparative molecular modelling identifies a common putative IgE epitope on cysteine protease allergens of diverse sources. *Clin Exp Allergy* 30:1307-1313.

[23] Holt, D. C., K. Fischer, G. E. Allen, D. Wilson, P. Wilson, R. Slade, B. J. Currie, S. F. Walton, and D. J. Kemp. 2003. Mechanisms for a novel immune evasion strategy in the scabies mite sarcoptes scabiei: a multigene family of inactivated serine proteases. *The Journal of investigative dermatology* 121:1419-1424.

[24] Ishizaka, T., J. Urban, Jr., K. Takatsu, and K. Ishizaka. 1976. Immunoglobulin E synthesis in parasite infection. *The Journal of allergy and clinical immunology* 58:523-538.

[25] Ehigiator, H. N., A. W. Stadnyk, and T. D. Lee. 2000. Extract of Nippostrongylus brasiliensis stimulates polyclonal type-2 immunoglobulin response by inducing De novo class switch. *Infection and immunity* 68:4913-4922.

[26] Jarrett, E., S. Mackenzie, and H. Bennich. 1980. Parasite-induced 'nonspecific' IgE does not protect against allergic reactions. *Nature* 283:302-304.

[27] Imai, S., H. Tezuka, Y. Furuhashi, R. Muto, and K. Fujita. 2001. A factor of inducing IgE from a filarial parasite is an agonist of human CD40. *The Journal of biological chemistry* 276:46118-46124.

[28] Imai, S., H. Tezuka, and K. Fujita. 2001. A factor of inducing IgE from a filarial parasite prevents insulin-dependent diabetes mellitus in nonobese diabetic mice. *Biochemical and biophysical research communications* 286:1051-1058.

[29] Lynch, N. R., M. Palenque, I. Hagel, and M. C. DiPrisco. 1997. Clinical improvement of asthma after anthelminthic treatment in a tropical situation. *American journal of respiratory and critical care medicine* 156:50-54.

[30] Nagler-Anderson, C. 2006. Helminth-induced immunoregulation of an allergic response to food. *Chemical immunology and allergy* 90:1-13.

[31] Maloy, K. J., L. Salaun, R. Cahill, G. Dougan, N. J. Saunders, and F. Powrie. 2003. CD4+CD25+ T(R) cells suppress innate immune pathology through cytokine-dependent mechanisms. *The Journal of experimental medicine* 197:111-119.

[32] Mottet, C., H. H. Uhlig, and F. Powrie. 2003. Cutting edge: cure of colitis by CD4+CD25+ regulatory T cells. *J Immunol* 170:3939-3943.

[33] Gomez-Escobar, N., E. Lewis, and R. M. Maizels. 1998. A novel member of the transforming growth factor-beta (TGF-beta) superfamily from the filarial nematodes Brugia malayi and B. pahangi. *Experimental parasitology* 88:200-209.

[34] Gregory, W. F., M. L. Blaxter, and R. M. Maizels. 1997. Differentially expressed, abundant trans-spliced cDNAs from larval Brugia malayi. *Molecular and biochemical parasitology* 87:85-95.

[35] Yenbutr, P., and A. L. Scott. 1995. Molecular cloning of a serine proteinase inhibitor from Brugia malayi. *Infection and immunity* 63:1745-1753.

[36] Joseph, G. T., T. Huima, and S. Lustigman. 1998. Characterization of an Onchocerca volvulus L3-specific larval antigen, Ov-ALT-1. *Molecular and biochemical parasitology* 96:177-183.

[37] Thomas, P. G., M. R. Carter, O. Atochina, A. A. Da'Dara, D. Piskorska, E. McGuire, and D. A. Harn. 2003. Maturation of dendritic cell 2 phenotype by a helminth glycan uses a Toll-like receptor 4-dependent mechanism. *J Immunol* 171:5837-5841.

[38] Murray, J., W. F. Gregory, N. Gomez-Escobar, A. K. Atmadja, and R. M. Maizels. 2001. Expression and immune recognition of Brugia malayi VAL-1, a homologue of vespid venom allergens and Ancylostoma secreted proteins. *Molecular and biochemical parasitology* 118:89-96.

[39] Beall, M. J., S. McGonigle, and E. J. Pearce. 2000. Functional conservation of Schistosoma mansoni Smads in TGF-beta signaling. *Molecular and biochemical parasitology* 111:131-142.

[40] Gomez-Escobar, N., A. van den Biggelaar, and R. Maizels. 1997. A member of the TGF-beta receptor gene family in the parasitic nematode Brugia pahangi. *Gene* 199:101-109.

[41] Maizels, R. M., N. Gomez-Escobar, W. F. Gregory, J. Murray, and X. Zang. 2001. Immune evasion genes from filarial nematodes. *International journal for parasitology* 31:889-898.

[42] Bloom, B. R., and B. Bennett. 1966. Mechanism of a reaction in vitro associated with delayed-type hypersensitivity. *Science (New York, N.Y* 153:80-82.

[43] Baugh, J. A., and R. Bucala. 2002. Macrophage migration inhibitory factor. *Crit Care Med* 30:S27-S35.

[44] Morand, E. F. 2005. New therapeutic target in inflammatory disease: macrophage migration inhibitory factor. *Internal medicine journal* 35:419-426.

[45] Kobayashi, M., Y. Nasuhara, A. Kamachi, Y. Tanino, T. Betsuyaku, E. Yamaguchi, J. Nishihira, and M. Nishimura. 2006. Role of macrophage migration inhibitory factor in ovalbumin-induced airway inflammation in rats. *Eur Respir J* 27:726-734.

[46] Pastrana, D. V., N. Raghavan, P. FitzGerald, S. W. Eisinger, C. Metz, R. Bucala, R. P. Schleimer, C. Bickel, and A. L. Scott. 1998. Filarial nematode parasites secrete a homologue of the human cytokine macrophage migration inhibitory factor. *Infection and immunity* 66:5955-5963.

[47] Falcone, F. H., P. Loke, X. Zang, A. S. MacDonald, R. M. Maizels, and J. E. Allen. 2001. A Brugia malayi homolog of macrophage migration inhibitory factor reveals an important link between macrophages and eosinophil recruitment during nematode infection. *J Immunol* 167:5348-5354.

[48] Cho, Y., B. F. Jones, J. J. Vermeire, L. Leng, L. DiFedele, L. M. Harrison, H. Xiong, Y. K. Kwong, Y. Chen, R. Bucala, E. Lolis, and M. Cappello. 2007. Structural and functional characterization of a secreted hookworm Macrophage Migration Inhibitory Factor (MIF) that interacts with the human MIF receptor CD74. *The Journal of biological chemistry* 282:23447-23456.

[49] Vermeire, J. J., Y. Cho, E. Lolis, R. Bucala, and M. Cappello. 2008. Orthologs of macrophage migration inhibitory factor from parasitic nematodes. *Trends in parasitology* 24:355-363.

[50] Yu, H. S., S. K. Park, K. H. Lee, S. J. Lee, S. H. Choi, M. S. Ock, and H. J. Jeong. 2007. Anisakis simplex: analysis of expressed sequence tags (ESTs) of third-stage larva. *Experimental parasitology* 117:51-56.

[51] Umetsu, D. T., J. J. McIntire, O. Akbari, C. Macaubas, and R. H. DeKruyff. 2002. Asthma: an epidemic of dysregulated immunity. *Nature immunology* 3:715-720.

[52] Lisbonne, M., S. Diem, A. de Castro Keller, J. Lefort, L. M. Araujo, P. Hachem, J. M. Fourneau, S. Sidobre, M. Kronenberg, M. Taniguchi, P. Van Endert, M. Dy, P. Askenase, M. Russo, B. B. Vargaftig, A. Herbelin, and M. C. Leite-de-Moraes. 2003. Cutting edge: invariant V alpha 14 NKT cells are required for allergen-induced airway inflammation and hyperreactivity in an experimental asthma model. *J Immunol* 171:1637-1641.

[53] Araujo, L. M., J. Lefort, M. A. Nahori, S. Diem, R. Zhu, M. Dy, M. C. Leite-de-Moraes, J. F. Bach, B. B. Vargaftig, and A. Herbelin. 2004. Exacerbated Th2-mediated airway inflammation and hyperresponsiveness in autoimmune diabetes-prone NOD mice: a critical role for CD1d-dependent NKT cells. *European journal of immunology* 34:327-335.

[54] Kornas, S., M. Skalska, B. Nowosad, and J. Gawor. 2007. [The communities of cyathostomes (Cyathostominae) in year-old and two-year-old Pure Blood Arabian mares]. *Wiadomosci parazytologiczne* 53:325-329.

[55] Belkaid, Y., and B. T. Rouse. 2005. Natural regulatory T cells in infectious disease. *Nature immunology* 6:353-360.

[56] Anthony, R. M., L. I. Rutitzky, J. F. Urban, Jr., M. J. Stadecker, and W. C. Gause. 2007. Protective immune mechanisms in helminth infection. *Nature reviews* 7:975-987.

[57] Pacifico, L. G., F. A. Marinho, C. T. Fonseca, M. M. Barsante, V. Pinho, P. A. J. Sales, L. S. Cardoso, M. I. Araujo, E. M. Carvalho, G. D. Cassali, M. M. Teixeira, and S. C. Oliveira. 2008. Schistosoma mansoni antigens modulate experimental allergic asthma in a murine model: a major role for CD4+CD25+Foxp3+ T cells independent of IL-10. *Infection and immunity*.

[58] Kitagaki, K., T. R. Businga, D. Racila, D. E. Elliott, J. V. Weinstock, and J. N. Kline. 2006. Intestinal helminths protect in a murine model of asthma. *J Immunol* 177:1628-1635.

[59] Park, S. K., M. K. Cho, H. K. Park, K. H. Lee, S. J. Lee, S. H. Choi, M. S. Ock, H. J. Jeong, M. H. Lee, and H. S. Yu. 2009. Macrophage migration inhibitory factor homologs of anisakis simplex suppress Th2 response in allergic airway inflammation model via CD4+CD25+Foxp3+ T cell recruitment. *J Immunol* 182:6907-6914.

[60] Akbari, O., R. H. DeKruyff, and D. T. Umetsu. 2001. Pulmonary dendritic cells producing IL-10 mediate tolerance induced by respiratory exposure to antigen. *Nature immunology* 2:725-731.

[61] Rankin, E. B., D. Yu, J. Jiang, H. Shen, E. J. Pearce, M. H. Goldschmidt, D. E. Levy, T. V. Golovkina, C. A. Hunter, and A. Thomas-Tikhonenko. 2003. An essential role of Th1 responses and interferon gamma in infection-mediated suppression of neoplastic growth. *Cancer biology & therapy* 2:687-693.

[62] Hawrylowicz, C. M., and A. O'Garra. 2005. Potential role of interleukin-10-secreting regulatory T cells in allergy and asthma. *Nature reviews* 5:271-283.

[63] Hansen, G., J. J. McIntire, V. P. Yeung, G. Berry, G. J. Thorbecke, L. Chen, R. H. DeKruyff, and D. T. Umetsu. 2000. CD4(+) T helper cells engineered to produce latent TGF-beta1 reverse allergen-induced airway hyperreactivity and inflammation. *The Journal of clinical investigation* 105:61-70.

[64] Chen, W., W. Jin, N. Hardegen, K. J. Lei, L. Li, N. Marinos, G. McGrady, and S. M. Wahl. 2003. Conversion of peripheral CD4+CD25- naive T cells to CD4+CD25+ regulatory T cells by TGF-beta induction of transcription factor Foxp3. *The Journal of experimental medicine* 198:1875-1886.

11

Cissampelos sympodialis (Menispermaceae): A Novel Phytotherapic Weapon Against Allergic Diseases?

M.R. Piuvezam, C.R. Bezerra-Santos,
P.T. Bozza, C. Bandeira-Melo, G. Vieira and H.F. Costa
Federal University of Paraiba, PB,
Oswaldo Cruz Foundation, Rio de Janeiro, RJ,
Federal University of Rio de Janeiro, RJ,
Brazil

1. Introduction

Allergic diseases affect millions of people around the world. Enhanced prevalence and the chronic characteristics of these illnesses represent an important public health problem. Most prevalent allergic diseases are classified as immediate-type reactions such as urticaria, allergic conjuctivitis, food allergy, allergic rhinitis, anaphylaxis and asthma (Sicherer & Leung, 2004; Fonacier et al., 2010; Sicherer, 2011). The immediate-type reaction terminology is applied to allergic reactions because the symptoms develop few minutes after allergen contact. The immune mechanisms responsible for the initiation of these reactions depend on the production of immunoglobulins (IgG1 and/or IgE) that activate cells such as mast cells, eosinophils and basophils. Once activated, these cells are responsible for release of inflammatory mediators, contributing to the exacerbation and maintenance of the allergic processes (Lampinen et al., 2004). Urticaria is characterized by pruritic, edematous and erythematous lesions that affect 15% to 25% of individuals during their lives. Most of the cases are acute but about 30% of patients present symptoms for more than six weeks and are considered as having chronic disease. Women are more susceptible (75%) than men and only 1% to 5% of the cases are related to IgE-dependent reaction while most of the cases are considered to be induced by physical stimuli or of idiopathic nature, including autoimmune urticaria (Antunez et al., 2006). Allergic urticaria depends on skin mast cell activation which delivers preformed mediators, mainly histamine, few minutes after allergen exposure. On the other hand activated mast cells also produce and deliver neo-formed mediators, i.e., prostaglandin D2 (PGD_2) and cisleukotrienes (*cis*LT) that stimulate inflammatory responses mediated by neutrophils, basophils, eosinophils and T lymphocytes (Funk, 2001; Harizi et al., 2008; Kambe et al., 2010). Another allergic disease of great importance in public health is allergic conjunctivitis. Allergic conjuctivities prevalence in the United States was estimated to affects about 40 million people. Allergic conjunctivitis is marked by the presence of eosinophil cells in conjunctiva mucosa (Bezerra & Santos, 2010). Food allergy, another allergic disorder, is related to the genetic susceptibility of individuals to eggs, peanuts, seafood (e.g. shrimp, lobsters, crabs, squids and mussels milk and others). Oral sensitization with shrimp tropomyosin induces in mice allergen-specific IgE, T cell response and systemic anaphylactic reactions (Capobianco et al, 2008). Food allergy has been reported in some cohort studies which describe variable rates of food allergy prevalence in the United States, Canada, the United Kindom, Singapore and the Philippines (Berin & Mayer, 2009). Approximately 1% of food allergic patients develop signs and symptoms characterized by intense diarrhea, urticaria and anaphylaxis. There are divergences about the period of exposition to food allergens and development of disease symptoms. Studies showed that allergenic food ingested during pregnancy increases the risk of higher prevalence of allergic response in infants (Sausenthaler et al., 2011). In contrary to the aforementioned, other studies suggested that earlier exposure to food allergens may promote a protective response to allergic conditions. Serologic diagnosis of patients with food allergies have demonstrated high levels of specific IgE. The pathological immune response observed in these patients depended on: (i) the presence of an adjuvant responsible for stimulating inflammatory response which is considered one necessary step to initiate lymphocyte responses, (ii) allergen doses which can induce classical or alternative mechanisms of allergic process in response to food as seen in cutaneous sensitization to food allergens and (iii) the types of mediators delivered which can lead to systemic allergic reactions such as anaphilaxis (Berin & Mayer, 2009; Sicherer & Leung, 2011). In addition, asthma, which probably may be the most important allergic disorder, affects about 300 million people in the world and causes an estimated 250,000 deaths annually. This illness is characterized by a reversible lower airway inflammation, airway hyperresponsivenss, mucus hypersecretion, leukocyte recruitment to lung tissue and airway remodeling that might cause respiratory deficits. Increased prevalence and difficulties in asthma control are responsible for the elevated costs to health systems around the world (Busse & Lemanski, 2001; Mayr et al., 2003; Bateman et al., 2008).

During asthmatic crises, patients develop an intense breathing difficulty called airway hyperreactivity (AHR). This response occurs as a consequence of the exposure of the inhaled route to the environmental allergen, thereby increasing the respiratory pause. An array of inflammatory mediators such as histamine, cisLT, PGs, cytokines, chemokines and others present in the lung tissue elicit smooth muscle cell contraction, mucus production, lung inflammation and airway remodeling. Mucus hypersecretion and bronchiole obstructions are important features of asthmatic patients. These effects of the inflammatory mediators may worsen the respiratory functions. In the last decade studies have shown the involvement of some mediators in stimulating the mucus production by cells named globlet cells. Concomitant to lung enhanced respiratory pause and lung obstruction, recruitment of inflammatory leukocytes to bronchoalveolar space initiates a cellular response that might become a destructive response to the lung tissue architecture in a chronic phase of the disease. Different leukocytes participate in the inflammatory process in the lung, i.e., neutrophils, mononuclear cells and mainly eosinophil cells (Cowden et al., 2010). Similar cellular and molecular immunological mechanisms related to asthma are described in allergic rhinitis demonstrating a strong correlation between these two allergic disorders with the same etiology. Rhinitis is an upper airway allergic inflammation and is considered co-morbidity to asthma as several studies have suggested that upper and lower airway inflammations are a unique entity. The prevalence of this disease has been increasing in many countries and an association between asthma and allergic rhinitis has been shown. Although asthma and allergic rhinitis show certain particularities, both present similar pathophysiology with IgE-dependent allergic reactions. Another severe IgE-dependent allergic reaction is the anaphylactic shock triggered by allergens such as bee venom, domiciliary dust, cockroaches, food, pollen, and/or medicines after mast cell sensitization and activation (Bateman et al., 2008). The term 'anaphylaxis' was used for the first time by Richet and Portier (1902) to describe a potentially fatal reaction that may affect different organs and systems and the process by which all the symptoms derived from pharmacologic mediators, i.e. histamine, are released by blood leukocytes as eosinophils and basophils. Mortality rate of anaphylaxis have been increasing around the world in the last decades and at least twenty people die every year in UK due to anaphylactic reactions representing one death in three million habitants a year. Although the majority of the cases of anaphylactic reactions are related to high levels of IgE and histamine, some patients do not present these serum biologic markers, suggesting in these cases an IgE-independent mechanisms (Pumphrey, 2004; Moneret-Vautrin & Mertes, 2010; Seidel et al., 2010).

2. Immune mechanisms for the initiation of allergic reactions

The allergen sensitization phase is related to multiple factors including gene polymorphisms of HLA, FcεRI-β and IL-4 family, environmental factors like vaccination for prevention of diseases, pollutants present indoors and outdoors and viral infections. IgE is a critical participant in the onset of the effector phase of allergies due to its affinity to receptors (FcεRI) present on the surface of mast cells, basophils and/or eosinophils. The cross-linking between two IgE molecules and the allergen is responsible for cellular activation and subsequent release of preformed mediators, i.e., histamine from the cytoplasmic granules as well as neo-formed mediators such as eicosanoids (leukotrienes, prostaglandins and thromboxane) (Maddox & Schwartz, 2002). These mediators increase vascular permeability, induce smooth muscle contraction causing difficulty in breathing as well as the proliferation of fibroblasts and smooth muscle cells (Kanaoka & Boyce, 2004). The IgE production by allergen-specific B cells is associated with Th2 cell profile with IL-4, IL-5 and IL-13 productions. The IL-4 and IL-13 induce in B cells the production of allegen-specific- IgE (Munitz et al., 2008) and IL-5 induces the production, activation and differentiation of bone marrow-derived eosinophil (Takatsu & Nakajima, 2008). Among the cell types mentioned above, mast cells are of fundamental importance in the first phase of allergic disease due to their wide distribution throughout the body including skin, lungs and gastrointestinal tract (Maurer & Metz, 2005). Recently, some scientific work showed that mast cells are able to migrate to the smooth muscles of the airways of asthma patients, corroborating the interaction between mediators released by mast cells and smooth muscle response in the asthmatic lung (Brightling et al., 2003).

Another important cell population in the pathophysiology of asthma is the eosinophil. This cell participates in the late phase of the inflammatory response and it was initially described as a component of defense against intestinal parasites (Gleich et al., 1993; Weller, 1997; Rothenberg, 1998). However, there are several lines of evidence that contradicts this view, and demonstrate the eosinophils as multifunctional cells involved in the initial processes and propagation of various inflammatory diseases. They are also involved in the regulation of innate and adaptive immune responses (Rothenberger & Hogan, 2006). Eosinophils can respond to different stimuli as nonspecific tissue injury, viral infections, allograft, allergens, and tumors. Additionally, these cells release cationic proteins stored in granules as eosinophil peroxidase (EPO), major basic protein (MBP), eosinophil cationic protein (ECP) and eosinophil derived neurotoxin (EDN). Eosinophils also release a range of cytokines including the Th2 profile as well as chemokines RANTES, eotaxin 1 and MIP-1α (Rothenberger & Hogan, 2006). Eosinophils participate in many pathological processes such as parasite infections, gastrointestinal disorders and allergic processes such as asthma. Several studies have revealed the presence of high levels of MBP in bronchoalveolar lavage (BAL) of asthmatic patients that induces cytotoxicity to various body tissues, especially the airway epithelium (Rothenberg, 1998). Additionally, MBP increases the reactivity of airway smooth muscle to cause dysfunction of the muscarinic M2 vagal nerve, known to contribute to the development of airway hyperreactivity, a key feature of asthma (Jacoby et al., 1993). Several studies have demonstrated that eosinophil activation in inflammatory reactions is associated with increasing number of lipid bodies (LBs) (Bozza et al., 2011). The LBs are defined as cytoplasmatic organelles rich in lipids, surrounded by a phospholipid monolayer, posses high amounts of enzymes that produce eicosanoids such as PLA2, 5-LO, 15-LO, COX, LTC$_4$ and PGE synthases and also cytokines, chemokines and several kinases related with signal transductions. However LBs are found in small quantities in non-activated cells, they are associated with a wild range of pathological conditions such as cancers, infectious and inflammatory diseases like asthma (Bozza et al., 2009). Several inflammatory mediators are able to induce the leukocyte LB formation as platelet activator factor (PAF) (De Assis et al., 2003). In eosinophils other stimuli such as prostaglandin D2 (PGD$_2$) (Mesquita-Santos et al., 2006), IL-5 (Bozza et al., 1998), RANTES and eotaxin also induced the LB formation (Vieira-de-Abreu et al., 2005). In addition, in the allergic inflammation, the new LBs are observed and this process is mediated mainly by a *cross-talk* between eotaxin/RANTES via chemokine receptors (CCR3) with MAPK, PI3K and tyrosine kinases activation and PGD2 via an unknown receptor. The main site of *cis*LT generation in eosinophils is the LBs in the pulmonary allergic inflammation (Bozza et al., 2009). Moreover, the regulation of allergic reactions is carried out by T cells called Th1 cells (Teixeira et al., 2005), which secret cytokines such as IL-2 and INF-γ, and by the Th17 cells that produce IL-17. Both profiles can reduce the eosinophil onset in the lung and the bronchial hyperreactivity (Schnyder-Candrian, et al. 2006) (Figure 1).

3. Conventional treatment of allergic diseases

A wide variety of medicines are used to treat allergic diseases. The β2-adrenergic agonist therapy is widely used as first choice for addressing the crisis of asthma (O'Byrne, 2009). Phenoterol and salbutamol are members of this group and are largely used to reverse bronchoconstriction by binding directly to β2-receptors of lung smooth muscle cells and inducing breathing relieve due to bronchodilatation. *In vitro* studies showed these drugs are responsible for increasing the levels of cAMP described as a regulatory second messenger of intracellular calcium-dependent mechanisms. Calcium is one of several molecules responsible for the smooth muscle contraction during acute phase of asthma crises (Mahn et al., 2010). Of note, side effects are observed in patients under β2-agonists therapy, mainly cardiac frequency increases in response to activation of cardiac β1-receptors. Potent anti-inflammatory steroid therapy is also used to control asthma manifestations. These medicines are indicated to block lung inflammation mediated by inflammatory leukocytes such as neutrophils, eosinophils, basophils and lymphocytes that contribute to exacerbation of inflammatory response (Jarjour et al., 2006). As consequence of inflammation, lung tissue might present a cell phenotype change, referred to as 'remodeling' which impairs the physiological lung function causing respiratory deficiency and death in some of asthmatic patients.

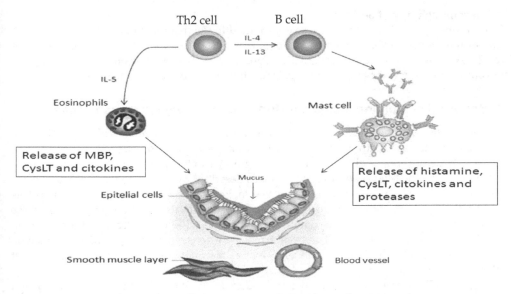

Fig. 1. Mechanism of immediate allergic reactions. Immediate allergic reactions are orchestrated by Th2 lymphocytes and its major cytokines (IL-4, IL-5 and IL-13) responsible for inducing B cell activation and IgE secretion. Mast cell sensitization depends on IgE cross-linking and binding with FcεRI, subsequent cellular activation, histamine and leukotrienes releases that are crucial to bronchospasm induction. Concomitantly, eosinophils migrate to bronchoalveolar cavity by an IL-5 (and others) dependent mechanism. Lung damage and airway remodeling are caused by cationic proteins delivered by eosinophils and matrix extracellular protein deposition.

Steroidal anti-inflammatory drugs are able to control these pathologic responses in airways by inhibition of lymphocyte functions and mainly inducing apoptosis in eosinophils, which is considered the major component of lung tissue damage. Steroids also can induce a variety of side effects like endocrine alterations, cardiovascular disturbances, psychotic crises and cancers (Belvisi, 2004). Combinations of β2-agonists and steroids are commonly used to control asthma. Another class of antiasthmatic drug that was developed about 10 years ago, the antileukotrienes (Montelukast® and derivatives). These drugs present both bronchodilator and anti-inflammatory properties. cisLT are known pro-inflammatory mediators and they induce vascular permeability, lung smooth muscle cell contraction/bronchospasm and leukocyte activation and chemotaxis (Funk, 2001). Previous studies reported cis-LT as the major bronchoconstrictor mediators in an asthmatic lung, causing sustained smooth muscle contraction. The anti-leukotriene drugs block leukotriene receptors in lung tissue, reversing bronchospasm in asthmatic patients. Additionally, leukotriene modifiers like zileutron act by blocking the 5-lipooxygenase enzyme (5-LO), thus inhibiting the leukotriene generation. Therefore, anti-leukotriene therapies strongly impair airway inflammatory response and ameliorate respiratory function (Terashima, et al. 2002; Angelova-Fischer & Tsankov, 2005). Antagonists of the enzyme phosphodiesterase, aminophylline and theophylline as well as muscarinic blockers also occupy space in the therapeutic arsenal.

3.1 Immunotherapy of asthma

Immunotherapy with anti-IgE has also contributed to the treatment of asthma patients who do not have a good response to conventional therapies (Lazaar & Panettieri, 2004; Foster et al., 2011). Despite anti-IgE therapy, which represents a major breakthrough in the treatment of asthma, the high cost of this therapy remains the major obstacle.

4. Botanical and pharmacological study with *Cissampelos sympodialis*

In northeastern Brazil, diseases such as asthma, influenza, bronchitis and rheumatism are traditionally treated with infusions of the root bark of *Cissampelos sympodialis* Eichl (Menispemaceae), popularly known in the region as milona, abuteira or orelha de onça (Correa, 1984). The Menispermaceae family was described by AL Jussieu (1789). This term is an allusion to the morphology of the seed that looks like the fourth form of the moon. This species belongs to the order Ranunculales, subdivided by Diels (1910) into eight tribes, three subtribes, 72 genera and approximately 400 species. These species are found on all continents, especially in tropical and subtropical regions. In Brazil, the Menispermaceae family is represented by 12 genera and 106 species distributed mostly in the Amazon forest (Barroso, 2004).

The genus *Cissampelos* belongs to the tribe Cocculeae, and subtribe Cissampelinae and comprises 19 species of which nine occur in Brazil (Rhodes, 1975). This genus is one of the few among the angiosperms that shows diversity and uniformity. The diversity can be seen in vegetative habitat and leaves. The uniformity is found in the sexual expression of simple flowers, pistils and small flowers. In the state of Paraiba the genus *Cissampelos* is represented by three species: *Cissampelos ovalifolia* DC, *Cissampelos glaberrima* St. Hill and *Cissampelos sympodialis* Eichl. These species are found in different types of habitat, soil and vegetation, occurring mainly in rainforests on the Atlantic coast and hills (Barbosa-Filho et al., 1997). The species *Cissampelos sympodialis* is endemic in Brazil and is found in the Northeast and Southeast, from Ceara to Minas Gerais states. This species often occurs in open areas as shrubs in sandy soil and can be distinguished mainly by the shape of the deltoid leaves (Barbosa-Filho et al., 1997). The roots of *Cissampelos sympodialis* are widely used by Indian tribes and in folk medicine to treat various diseases such as diarrhea, diseases of the genitourinary tract and especially in respiratory tract diseases such as asthma (Corrêa, 1984). Both alcoholic fraction of roots (AFR) and of leaves (AFL) and some of the chemical components (bisbenzylisoquinolinic type alkaloids) isolated from these extracts have been studied. These alkaloids have been shown to have paralytic effect, cytotoxic activity (Kupchan et al., 1965), to stimulate the central nervous system (Sur & Pradhan, 1964), to prevent hypersecretion of reactive products from neutrophils and macrophages (Castranova et al., 1991), to inhibit the inflammatory cytokine production by peripheral blood mononuclear cells (Onai et al. , 1995) and bronchodilator activity (Thomas et al., 1995). Thomas et al (1995) showed that the AFR had a relaxing effect on smooth muscle of trachea and increased the cyclic adenosine monophosphate (cAMP) levels from alveolar leukocytes in guinea pigs in a manner similar to aminophylline which antagonizes bronchial muscle contractions. Similarly, studies of AFL showed inhibition of histamine and ovalbumin (OVA)-induced bronchospasm in guinea pigs (Thomas et al., 1997a), synthesis of phosphodiesterase (PDE) IV and V in the lungs of mice and induced increased levels of cAMP in guinea pig trachea muscle cells (Thomas et al. 1997b). Also AFL had an antidepressant effect probably associated with the phosphodiesterases inhibition in rat brain

(Almeida et al., 1998), inhibited human neutrophils degranulation (Thomas et al., 1999) and induced contraction of vascular smooth muscle (Freitas et al., 2000).

5. Phytochemical study of *Cissampelos sympodialis*

Chemical studies of *Cissampelos sympodialis* led to the isolation of different alkaloids (Barbosa-Filho et al., 1997) such as bisbenzylisoquinolinic (warifteine, methilwarifteine, roraimine and simpodialine); morfinic (milonin); aporfinic (laurifolin) and oxoaporfinic (liriodenine) which have allowed for a more accurate immunopharmacological studies (Freitas et al., 1996, De Lira et al., 2002) (Table 1). Analysis of quality control of *Cissampelos sympodialis* extracts by thermogravimetry test showed that both AFL and AFR present alkaloids as major compounds and also both extracts showed the same kinetic behavior of bisbenzylisoquinolinic alkaloids (Aragão et al., 2002). Among these alkaloids warifteine showed spasmolytic activity by modifying various regulatory processes involving intracellular calcium channels and cAMP levels, which are essential for muscle contraction (Somlyo & Somlyo, 1994; Freitas et al., 1996). Therefore the purpose of our scientific study has been to develop a herbal medicine from the leaf extract of *Cissampelos sympodialis* to treat asthma as an alternative therapy.

6. Current stage of knowledge of *Cissampelos sympodialis*

6.1 Immunological study of *Cissampelos sympodialis*
Since the relaxant effect of *Cissampelos sympodialis* extracts (roots and leaves) on bronchial smooth muscle cells (Thomas et al. 1995), inhibition of phosphodiesterases (PDE) IV and V in the lung with increased levels of cAMP in muscle cells of the trachea (Thomas et al. 1997b), biological effects that corroborate with the anti-asthmatic activity of the plant were demonstrated, we began the immunological studies. Our research group, with laboratory complex located in the Laboratory of Pharmaceutical Technology (LTF), Federal University of Paraíba (UFPB), and in collaboration with Federal University of Rio de Janeiro and the Oswaldo Cruz Foundation/Rio, Brazil, has systematically studied the immunomodulatory effect of *Cissampelos sympodialis* since 1997. *In vivo* and *in vitro* tests have been conducted to understand the mechanisms of action of AFL as well as the isolated alkaloid warifteine in experimental models of allergy and inflammation.

6.2 Toxicological study of *Cissampelos sympodialis*
Several parameters can be analyzed to demonstrate the toxic potential of a plant (extracts or compounds) such as loss of weight, death, anorexia, and change of behavior. Therefore toxicological studies showed that the use of AFL in acute treatment was considered nontoxic with no deaths among rats after administration at dose of 5 g/kg orally (po) or of 2 g/kg intraperitoneally (ip) (Diniz et al., 2004). However AFL chronic treatment caused an anorexic effect in female rats and behavioral changes (Almeida et al., 2005).
The alkaloids warifteine and milonine isolated from *C. sympodialis* showed cytotoxicity in fibroblast cell line (V79) derived from hamster and in hepatocytes of Wistar rats (Melo et al., 2003). Given the mixed results of acute and chronic treatments in rats, our research group began studying the effect of chronic oral treatment (more than 15 days) with AFL into inbred BALB/c mice. We observed that this treatment induced weight gain throughout the treatment, suggesting lack of toxicity in these experimental animals (Bezerra-Santos et al., 2004).

Structure	Compound name	References
	Warifteine	Barbosa et al., 1997
	Methilwarifteine	Barbosa et al., 1997
	Milonine	Barbosa et al., 1997
	Laurifoline	Alencar, 1994
	Roraimine	De Lira et al., 2002
	Simpodialine β-N-oxide	Alencar, 1994
	Liriodenine	De Lira et al., 2001

Table 1. Alkaloids of *Cissampelos sympodialis* Eichl.

6.3 Anti-inflammatory activity of *Cissampelos sympodialis*

The inflammatory process is a complex program of intracellular signal transduction and transcription events driven by multiple pro-inflammatory mediators and cytokines (Sherwood & Toliver-Kinsky, 2004). The acute inflammation is characterized by exudation of protein-rich fluid, edema, vasodilation and cell migration, primarily of neutrophils, into the site of injury (Sherwood & Toliver-Kinsky, 2004). Investigations on the anti-inflammatory activity of AFL were performed in experimental models of acute inflammation using phlogistic agents in Swiss mice or rats. Prophylactic treatments (before the phlogistic administration) demonstrated an AFL inhibitory effect on the ear edema formation induced by either TPA (12-O-tetradecanoyl phorbol-13-acetate) or capsaicin in Swiss mice (Batista-Lima et al., 2001). The experimental model of edema induced by TPA involves the activation of phospholipase A2 and production of prostaglandins and leukotrienes while the edema induced by capsaicin involves the release of substance P, histamine and eicosanoids such as serotonin and prostaglandins. These mediators are produced and released mainly by inflammatory cells such as mast cells, basophils, eosinophils and macrophages (Funk, 2001). Based on the anti-inflammatory effect of AFL, we inferred that the plant acts on the inflammatory cells by modulating the production of mediators. Corroborating this hypothesis was the observation that prophylactic treatment of experimental animals (rats) with AFL also showed inhibition of neutrophil migration into the intraperitoneal cavity induced by carrageenan (Batista-Lima et al., 2001). The migration of neutrophils into the peritoneal cavity of rats induced by carrageenan is dependent on the release of eicosanoids and chemotactic agents such as leukotriene B4 and/or IL-8, respectively, produced by mast cells and/or resident macrophages (Lefebvre et al., 2010, Nakagome & Nagata, 2011). Taken together the results support the hypothesis that AFL treatment is modulating cytokines as well as antiinflammatory mediator effects.

7. Immunomodulatory activity of *Cissampelos sympodialis*

7.1 Effect of *Cissampelos sympodialis* on IL-10 and NO production

Although eicosanoids and chemotactic agents produced by inflammatory cells are responsible for triggering the inflammatory process, these cells are also responsible for producing cytokines which control inflammation. IL-10 produced by mononuclear cells has been described as a potent regulatory molecule in the inflammatory process (Moore et al., 2001). Surprisingly, *in vitro* studies showed, for the first time, that the inhibitory effect of AFL on the proliferative response of BALB/c mice spleen cells stimulated with the mitogen concanavalin A was associated with the production of IL-4 and IL-10 by these cells (Piuvezam et al., 1999). Macrophages are cells that produce IL-10 and from this perspective, we investigated the effect of AFL on murine resident and elicited (sodium thioglycollate) macrophages. The experimental model used for this purpose was the infection of macrophages with trypomastigote form of *Trypanosoma cruzi*. The AFL treatment induced an increase in the release of trypomastigote forms by the cells with increase in IL-10 production. This phenomenon was shown in both types of macrophages (resident or elicited). The AFL was also able to increase the production of IL-10 even in the absence of the parasite. In addition, AFL inhibited the NO synthesis induced by interferon-gamma (IFN-γ) and lipopolysaccharide (Ding, et al., 1988; Alexandre-Moreira et al., 2003). Therefore these results confirm the effect of AFL in modulating the microbicidal activity of macrophages by increasing the IL-10 production as well as inhibition of NO synthesis.

7.2 Effect of *Cissampelos sympodialis* on the immunoglobulin production

B cells are responsible for the production of immunoglobulins (Ig) after antigen recognition and activation (Snapper & Paul, 1987; Wong & Koh, 2000). Asthma reaction is an immediate-type reaction mediated mainly by IgE (Busse & Lemanski, 2001; Mayr, et al., 2003). The release of mediators associated with the inflammatory cells to the reaction site induces the clinical symptoms of asthma (Maddox & Schwartz, 2002) such as bronchocontraction, mucus production and the strangling sensation (Funk, 2001). Based on the asthma symptoms and the fact that Brazilian folk medicine has systematically used *Cissampelos sympodialis* to prevent asthma symptoms, several studies have been conducted using the experimental model of asthma to demonstrate the AFL effect. The strain of inbred BALB/c mice is hypersensitive to ovalbumin (OVA) with the production of OVA-specific IgE, pulmonary hyperactivity and mucus production after sensitization and challenge with OVA. The chronic oral treatment (15 days before OVA sensitization) with AFL inhibited the total OVA-specific IgE production and increased the production of IFN-γ by spleen cells of these mice (Bezerra-Santos et al., 2004). Alexandre-Moreira and co-workers (2003) demonstrated that AFL inhibited activated B cell function through an increase in intracellular cAMP levels. Several studies have identified cAMP as an antagonist of B cell proliferation induced by mitogens (Cohen & Rothstein, 1989). Also it was demonstrated that cAMP is a second messenger that plays an important role in the regulation of B cell apoptosis (Myklebust et al., 1999). In general, an increase in cAMP levels is associated with anti-inflammatory and immunosuppressive effects (Cohen & Rothstein, 1989; Wong & Koh, 2000; Torgersen et al., 2002). Finally, the finding that AFL inhibited immunoglobulin secretion suggests a therapeutic use for the *Cissampelos sympodialis* extract in conditions associated with up regulation of B cell function and enhanced immunoglobulin secretion such as allergic diseases as well as autoimmune disease.

7.3 Activity of *Cissampelos sympodialis* in anaphylactic shock reaction

Anaphylaxis is a severe allergic reaction and is often fatal. It is mediated by IgE antibodies, mast cells and their mediators such as histamine. Medicines, insect bites and certain foods can trigger anaphylactic shock in genetically predisposed individuals (Teo et al., 2009; Dybendal et al., 2003). To have a better understanding of the effect of AFL treatment in allergic reactions, we evaluated the therapeutic potential of the acute treatment (five days before sensitization) in experimental model of anaphylactic shock using ovalbumin (OVA) challenge. The results demonstrated that AFL treatment was able to inhibit up to 70% death of OVA-sensitized mice after 1 hour of the OVA challenge. However, the same treatment was not able to inhibit the anaphylactic shock induced by compound 48/80. These data show that the effect of the extract is dependent on mechanisms involving IgE production (Bezerra-Santos et al., 2005).

7.4 Eosinophil lipid body inhibition by *Cissampelos sympodialis*

LBs are specialized organelles in the synthesis and storage of arachidonic acid derivatives such as prostaglandins and leukotrienes, and are present in the cytoplasm of various leukocytes and activated eosinophils (Bozza & Viola, 2010). A single treatment with AFL inhibited the formation of lipid bodies in eosinophils from mice sensitized and challenged with OVA. These results suggest that the extract is capable of modulating the synthesis of inflammatory mediators important in the chemotaxis of inflammatory cells to the lungs during asthma attacks, as well as contraction mediators that cause bronchospasm.

8. Warifteine, a bisbenzylisoquinoline alkaloid from *Cissampelos sympodialis*

Warifteine is a major bisbenzylisoquinolinic alkaloid found in AFR as well as AFL. The isolated compound is an amorphous yellow crystal and the chemical name is (R)-2,8,13,13a,14,15,16,25-Octahydro- 18,30- dimethoxy-14 -methyl -4,6:9,12:21,24 -trietheno-3H pyrido (3',2':14,15) (1,11) dioxacycloeicosino (2,3,4- ij) isoquinoline-5,19-diol with molecular weight of 592.68084 g/mol. Warifteine is insoluble in polar solvents but in acidic conditions becomes a water-soluble salt, allowing its *in vivo* and *in vitro* analysis without addition of other toxic solvents. Warifteine becomes an important compound marker for the extract standardization of the plant as well as a candidate for a phytomedicine (Cerqueira-Lima et al., 2010).

8.1 Warifteine inhibits the histamine release

Allergic reactions trigger organic changes according to body region affected as atopic dermatitis (skin), hay fever or rhinitis (upper respiratory tract), asthma (lower respiratory tract), food allergy (digestive tract), anaphylactic shock (systemic reaction) (Cavalher-Machado et al., 2004; Sicherer & Leung, 2011). All of these conditions are consequence of sensitized mast cell degranulation which releases several mediators (histamine, CisLT or prostaglandins) that cause smooth muscle contraction. Histamine is also of fundamental importance in triggering the allergic symptoms such as swelling (Baroody & Naclerio, 2000), itching (Davidson & Giesler, 2010), bronchospasm (Larsen, 2001) and anaphylactic shock (Valent et al., 2011). Warifteine effect in mast cell degranulation was then investigated. Initial findings came from *in vitro* assays which showed that warifteine was able to relax smooth muscle independently of endothelium, i.e., it did not only control the tone muscle in vessels but also relaxed the bronchioles muscles (Freitas et al., 1996). Warifteine then becomes an important tool in attempting to prevent or reverse the respiratory distress occurring during asthmatic attacks (Priel et al., 1994). To evaluate the alkaloid activity on mast cell degranulation we used several experimental models. At first OVA-sensitized mice were orally treated with warifteine then OVA-challenged in their paws. An inhibition of edema formation was observed (Costa et al., 2008). Passively IgE anti-DNP/BSA-sensitized-paw of rats were treated with warifteine and challenged with DNP/BSA and the results demonstrated that the treatment inhibited the hyperalgesia reaction, showing modulation among mast cells, vessels and nerves. Mimicking a local allergic reaction like a bee sting, the intra dermal administration of the secretagogue compound 48/80 in mice induces mast cell degranulation with histamine release and consequently induction of scratching behavior (Inagaki et al., 2002). We demonstrated that warifteine treatment inhibited the itching, indicating a direct effect in mast cell degranulation (Costa et al., 2008). Mast cells from dorsal subcutaneous tissue and peritonea from OVA sensitized rats were cultured with warifteine and after OVA challenge the histamine release was measured. The warifteine inhibited significantly the histamine release from tissue and peritoneal mast cells in a similar manner to sodium cromoglycate (CGS) (Costa et al., 2008). These data indicate that warifteine is inhibiting the mast cell degranulation and histamine release.

8.2 Warifteine inhibits the B cell functions

Several models have been employed for analyzing B cell response *in vitro*. Anti-IgM antibodies (Ab) have been used as a model for studying signals induced by binding to B cell surface Ig (Mond et al., 1995) and also T-independent type 2 antigens (TI-2), which activate B cells through a broad cross-linking of their Toll-like receptors (TLR) (Vos et al., 2000; Peng, 2005). Warifteine was then analyzed on B cells. It was observed that warifteine inhibited both B cell proliferation and Ig secretion induced by TLR ligands (LPS, Pam3Cys and CpG oligodeoxynucleotide) or anti-IgM Ab. These effects were not due to a toxicity since warifteine neither induced alteration in propidium iodide labeling of fresh spleen B cells or modified XTT metabolization by the B cell line A20. Also the inhibitory effect of B cell activated with TLR activators or anti-IgM Ab did not modify the total protein phosphorylation pattern, however it attenuated the rise in intracellular calcium levels, the phosphorylation of mitogen-activated protein kinase (MAPK) ERK and the intracellular levels of transcription factor NFκB. Warifteine also increased the cAMP level. *In vivo* study showed that pre-treatment with warifteine inhibited the anti-TNP-ficoll titles in BALB/c mice immunized with TI-2 antigen TNP-ficoll (Rocha et al., 2010). Taken together, the data showed that the alkaloid present in the AFL of *Cissampelos sympodialis* is one of the compounds responsible for the B cell modulatory effect.

8.3 Warifteine inhibits the eosinophil activity

A characteristic feature of asthma is a chronic inflammation with degeneration of bronchial epithelium in an eosinophil-dependent mechanism. Eosinophils release cationic proteins, chemotactic agents (eotaxin) and eicosanoids (*cis*-LT) (Ono et al., 2008). The treatments with warifteine or AFL inhibited eosinophil migration into the pleural and bronchoalveolar cavities of OVA sensitized BALB/c mice. Both warifteine and AFL were also capable of inhibiting the secretion of *cis*-LT and eotaxin, suggesting a role for AFL and its alkaloid in controlling the inflammatory process, thus corroborating the belief of an alternative treatment for diseases associated with eosinophil activity.

9. Cellular and molecular therapeutic targets for *Cissampelos sympodialis*

Studies performed for 15 years have contributed to the unraveling of part of the immunopharmacological mechanisms involved in *Cissampelos sympodialis* and warifteine effects. Figure 2 presents different cellular and molecular therapeutic targets for the plant extract and its alkaloid.

10. Relevance of the proposal for new herbal medicine

Some allergic diseases of major public health concerns are classified as immediate-type hypersensitivity, atopic dermatitis, food allergy, rhinitis, allergic asthma and anaphylactic shock. The incidence of allergic asthma is increasing at an alarming rate in developing countries like Brazil where around 35% of the population experience allergic diseases including asthma (Brazilian Association of Allergy and Immunopathology. 2007). Asthma is considered a public health problem. A significant variety of medicines such as bronchodilators and potent anti-inflammatory drugs that mitigate the crisis is used to treat asthma but with undesirable side effects. Our research group, with multidisciplinary profile, has been studying in a systematic way, the plant extracts of *Cissampelos sympodialis* and its components on

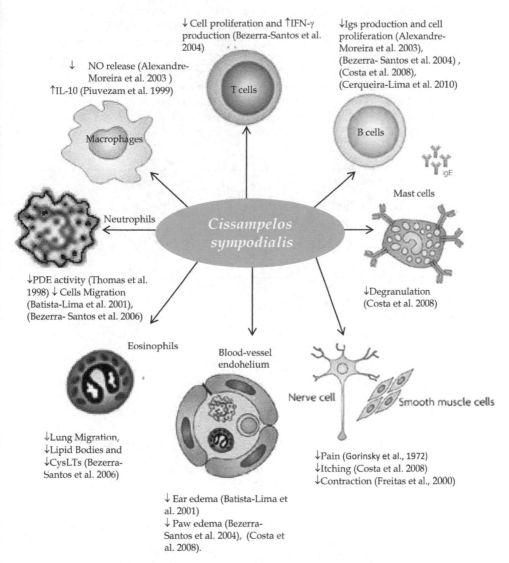

Fig. 2. Therapeutic targets for *Cissampelos sympodialis*. *In vitro* and *in vivo* studies showed that *C. sympodialis* induces IL-10 production by macrophages and IFN-γ production by splenocytes from OVA-sensitized mice. Oral treatment with AFL and warifteine inhibited OVA-specific IgE serum titer and mononuclear cell proliferation. Also both AFL as well as warifteine inhibited neutrophil and eosinophil migration and activation (PDE activity, leukotriene generation and lipid body formation) to the pleura and bronchoalveolar cavity induced by flogistic stimulus or allergens. Additionally, warifteine inhibited histamine delivery by mast cell and attenuated hyperalgesic reaction in rats.

experimental models of inflammation and allergy. The accumulated data showed that the extracts and its major alkaloid, warifteine, present potent anti-inflammatory effects, prolong the time of onset of anaphylactic shock reaction with reduction in allergen-specific IgE production, inhibit the inflammatory cell recruitment to the airways, relax airway smooth muscle in guinea pigs as well as modulate the production and release of inflammatory mediators such as histamine and cytokines. In addition, the great similarity in chemical structure among the alkaloids warifteine and milonine of *Cissampelos sympodialis* with drugs traditionally used in therapy: tubocurarine (potent muscle relaxant) and codeine (analgesic, antitussive and narcotic) respectively, (Figure 3), justified the popular use of the plant to treat respiratory diseases and the effort to produce an herbal medicine from this Brazilian plant.

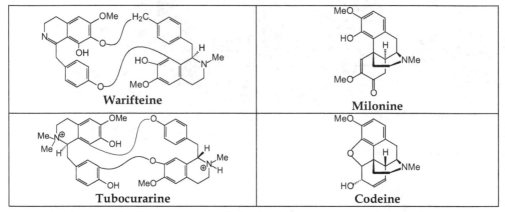

Fig. 3. Warifteine and tubocurarine are alkaloids that have the same chemical skeleton and belong to the class of bisbenzylisoquinoline. Milonine and codeine are alkaloids that have the same chemical skeleton and belong to the class of Morphinans.

11. Why *Cissampelos sympodialis* has potential as a herbal medicine?

1. *Cissampelos sympodialis* is used in folk medicine and by Indian tribes, in Northeast Brazil, for the treatment of disorders of airways such as asthma and rhinitis.
2. The preclinical data showed low or no toxicity on oral administration of the extract depending on the animal model used.
3. Studies of mechanisms of action of the extract have demonstrated efficacy in reduction of pathophysiological characteristics of allergic diseases associated with chronic inflammations such as asthma.
4. The leaf extract of the plant presents milonine, which is a morphinic alkaloid with a codeine-like chemical structure. Codeine is a classic drug with antitussive and analgesic properties.
5. Warifteine, one of the major alkaloids of the plant, presented similar effect of the extract in reducing asthma pathological profile.
6. Chemical structure of warifteine is similar to the tubocurarine chemical structure. Tubocurarine is a classic drug with muscle relaxant property.
7. Warifteine can be used as a molecular marker for the standardization of herbal medicine.

12. Acknowledgment

We thank Prof. Dr. José Maria Barbosa-Filho for the chemical expertise and for supplying the alkaloids for the immunomodulatory studies. The authors are indebted to the technical personnel of the UFPB/UFRJ/CNPq and FIOCRUZ foundation for the collaboration in the initial experiments.

13. References

Alexandre-Moreira, M.S.; Freire-De-Lima, C.G.; Trindade, M.N.; Castro-Faria-Neto, H.C.; Piuvezam, M.R. & Pecanha, L.M. (2003). *Cissampelos sympodialis* Eichl (Menispermaceae) leaf extract induces interleukin-10-dependent inhibition of Trypanosoma cruzi killing by macrophages. *Brazilian Journal of Medical and Biological Research* , VOL. 36, pp. 199-205, 0100-879X

Alencar, J. L. (1994). Isolamento e estudos das atividades relaxantes em musculatura lisa e esquelética de novos alcalóides de *Cissampelos sympodialis* Eichl.. Master's thesis (Graduate Program in Natural and Synthetic Bioactive Products) – Laboratório de Tecnologia Farmacêutica, Federal University of Paraiba, Brazil.

Almeida, R.N.; Melo-Diniz, M.F.; Medeiros, I.A.; Quintans-Junior, L.J.; Navarro, D.S.; Falcao, A.C.; Duarte, J.C. & Barbosa-Filho, J.M. (2005). Anorectic and behavioural effects of chronic *Cissampelos sympodialis* treatment in female and male rats. *Phytotherapy Research*, VOL. 19, pp. 121-124, 0951-418X

Almeida, R.N.; Navarro, D.S.; De Assis, T.S.; De Medeiros, I.A. & Thomas, G. (1998). Antidepressant effect of an ethanolic extract of the leaves of *Cissampelos sympodiulis* in rats and mice. *Journal of ethnopharmacology*, VOL. 63, pp. 247-252, 0378-8741

Angelova-Fischer, I. & Tsankov, N. (2005) Successful treatment of severe atopic dermatitis with cysteinyl leukotriene receptor antagonist montelukast. *Acta Dermatovenerologica Alpina, Panonica et Adriatica,* VOL. 14, pp. 115-119, 1581-2979

Antunez, C.; Blanca-Lopez N.; Torres, M.J.; Mayorga, C.; Perez-Inestrosa, E.; Montañez, M.I.; Fernandez, T. & Blanca, M. (2006). Immediate allergic reactions to cephalosporins: Evaluation of cross-reactivity with a panel of penicillins and cephalosporins. *Journal of Allergy and Clinical Immunology*, Vol. 117, pp. 404-410, 0091-6749

Aragão, C.F.S.; Souza, F.S.; Barros, A.C.S.; Veras, J.W.E.; Barbosa-Filho, J.M. & Macedo, R.O. (2002). Aplicação da Termogravimetria (TG) no controle de qualidade da milona (*Cissampelos sympodialis* Eichl.) Menispermaceae. *Brazilian Journal of Pharmacognosy*, VOL. 12, pp. 60-61, 0102-695X

Barbosa-Filho, J.M.; Agra, M.F. & Thomas, G. Botanical, chemical and pharmacological investigation on *Cissampelos sympodialis* species from Paraíba (Brazil). (1997). *Ciência e Cultura*, VOL. 49, pp. 386-394, 0009-6725

Baroody, F.M. & Naclerio, R.M. (2000). Antiallergic effects of H1-receptor antagonists. *Allergy*, VOL. 55, pp.17-27, 0105-4538.

Barroso, G.M. (2004). *Sistemática de angiospermas do Brasil*, UFV, ISBN 85-7269-127-8, Minas Gerais, Brasil

Bateman, E. D.; Hurd S. S.; Barnes P. J.; Bousquet, J.; Drazen J. M.; Fitzgerald, M.; Gibson P. ; Ohta K.; O'byrne P.; Pedersen S. E.; Pizzichini E.; Sullivan, S. D.; Wenzel, S. E. & Zar, H. J. (2008). Global strategy for asthma management and prevention: GINA executive summary. *European Respiratory Journal* VOL. 31, pp. 143-178, 0903-

1936Batista-Lima, K.V.; Ribeiro, R.A.; Balestieri, F.M.P.; Thomas, G. & Piuvezam, M.R. (2001). Anti-inflammatory activity of *Cissampelos sympodialis* Eichl. (Menispermaceae) leaf extract. *Acta Farmaceutica Bonaerense*, VOL. 20, pp. 275-279, 0326-2383.

Berin, M.C. & Mayer, L. (2009). Immunophysiology of experimental food allergy. *Mucosal Immunology*, VOL. 2, pp. 24-32, 1933-0219

Bezerra, H.L. & Santos, G.I.V. Tracoma em pacientes com conjuntivite alérgica. (2010). *Arquivos Brasileiros de Oftalmologia*, VOL. 73, pp. 235-239, 0004-2749

Bezerra-Santos, C.R.; Balestieri, F.M.; Rossi-Bergmann, B.; Pecanha, L.M. & Piuvezam, M.R. (2004). *Cissampelos sympodialis* Eichl. (Menispermaceae): oral treatment decreases IgE levels and induces a Th1-skewed cytokine production in ovalbumin-sensitized mice. *Journal of Ethnopharmacology*, VOL. 95, pp. 191-197, 0378-8741

Bezerra-Santos, C.R.; Peçanha, L.M.T. & Piuvezam, M.R. (2005) *Cissampelos sympodialis* Eichl. (Menispermaceae) inhibits anaphylactic shock reaction in murine allergic model. *Brazilian Journal of Pharmacognosy*, VOL. 15, pp. 287-291, 0102-695X

Bezerra-Santos, C.R.; Vieira-De-Abreu, A.; Barbosa-Filho, J.M.; Piuvezam, M.R. & Bozza, P.T. (2006). Anti-Allergic properties of *Cissampelos sympodialis* and its isolated alkaloid warifteine. *International Immunopharmacology*, VOL. 6, pp. 1152-1160, 1567-5769.

Belvisi, M.G. (2004). Regulation of inflammatory cell function by corticosteroids. *Proceedings of the American Thoracic Society*, VOL. 1, pp. 207-214, 1546-3222

Brazilian Association of Allergy and Immunopathology (2007) General Information, 10/02/2007, Available from: http://www.sbai.org.br/duvidas. htm.

Brightling, C.E.; Symon, F.A.; Holgate, S.T.; Wardlaw, A.J.; Pavord, I.D. & Bradding, P. (2003). Interleukin-4 and -13 expression is co-localized to mast cells within the airway smooth muscle in asthma. *Clinical and Experimental Allergy* , VOL. 33, pp. 1711-1716, 0954-7894.

Bozza, P.T.; Bakker-Abreu, I.; Navarro-Xavier, R.A. & Bandeira-Melo, C. (2011). Lipid body function in eicosanoid synthesis: An update. *Prostaglandins, Leukotrienes and Essential Fatty Acids*, doi:10.1016/j.plefa.2011.04.020, 0952-3278

Bozza P. T., Magalhães K. G. & Weller, P. F. (2009). Leukocyte lipid bodies – Biogenesis and functions in inflammation. *Biochimica et Biophysica Acta*. VOL. 1791, pp. 540–551, 1388-1981

Bozza, P.T. & Viola, J.P.B. (2010). Lipid droplets in inflammation and cancer. *Prostaglandins, Leukotrienes and Essential Fatty Acids*, VOL. 82, pp. 243–250, 0952-3278

Bozza, P.T.; Yu, W.; Cassara, J. & Weller, P.F. (1998). Pathways for eosinophil lipid body induction: differing signal transduction in cells from normal and hypereosinophilic subjects. *Journal of Leukocyte Biology*, VOL. 64, pp.563-569, 0741-5400

Busse, W.W. & Lemanske, R.F.(2001). Asthma. *The New England Journal of Medicine*, VOL. 344, pp. 350-362, 0028-4793.Capobianco, F.; Butteroni, C.; Barletta, B.; Corinti, S.; Afferni, C.; Tinghino, R.; Boirivant, M. & Di Felice, G. (2008). Oral sensitization with shrimp tropomyosin induces in mice allergen-specific IgE, T cell response and systemic anaphylactic reactions. *International Immunology*, VOL. 20, pp. 1077-1086, 0953-8178

Castranova, V.; Kang, J.H.; Ma, J.K.; Mo, C.G.; Malanga, C.J.; Moore, M.D.; Schwegler-Berry, D. & Ma, J.Y. (1991). Effets of bisbenzylisoquinoline alkaloids on alveolar macrophages: Correlation between binding, affinity, inhibitory pontency, and antifibrotic potential. *Toxicology and Applied Pharmacology*, VOL. 108, pp. 242-252, 0041-008X

Cavalher-Machado, S.C.; De Lima, W.T.; Damazo, A.S.; De Frias Carvalho, V.; Martins, M.A.; Silva, P.M. & Sannomiya, P. (2004). Down-regulation of mast cell activation and airway reactivity in diabetic rats: role of insulin. *The European Respiratory Journal*, VOL. 24, pp. 552-558, 0903-1936

Cerqueira-Lima, A.T.; Alcântara-Neves, N.M.; de Carvalho, L.C.; Costa, R.S.; Barbosa-Filho, J.M.; Piuvezam, M.; Momtchilo, R.; Barboza, R.; de Jesus Oliveira, E.; Marinho, A. & Figueiredo, C.A. (2010). Effects of *Cissampelos sympodialis* Eichl. and its alkaloid, warifteine, in an experimental model of respiratory allergy to Blomia tropicalis. *Current Drug Targets*, VOL. 11, pp. 1458-1467, 1389-4501

Cohen, D.P. & Rothstein, T.L. (1989). Adenosine 3',5'-cyclic monophosphate modulates the mitogenic response of murine B lymphocytes. *Cellular Immunology*, VOL. 121,pp. 113-119, 0008-8749

Corrêa, M.P. (1984). *Dicionário de Plantas Úteis do Brasil e das Exóticas Cultivadas* (1). Instituto Brasileiro de Defesa Florestal, Rio de Janeiro, Brasil.

Costa H.F.; Bezerra-Santos, C.R.; Barbosa-Filho, J.M.; Martins, M.A. & Piuvezam M.R. (2008). Warifteine, a bisbenzylisoquinoline alkaloid, decreases immediate allergic and thermal hyperalgesic reactions in sensitized animals, *International Immunopharmacology* VOL.8, pp. 519-525, 1567-5769.

Cowden, J.M.; Riley, J.P.; Ma J.Y.; Thurmond R.L. & Dunford P.J. (2010). Histamine H4 receptor antagonism diminishes existing airway inflammation and dysfunction via modulation of Th2 cytokines. *Respiratory Research*, VOL. 11, pp. 1-12, 1465-9921

Davidson, S. & Giesler, G.J. (2010). The multiple pathways for itch and their interactions with pain. *Trends in Neurosciences*, VOL.33, pp.550-558, 0166-2236

De Assis, E.F.; Silva, A.R.; Caiado, L.F.; Marathe, G.K.; Zimmerman, G.A.; Prescott, S.M.; Mcintyre, T.M.; Bozza, P.T. & De Castro-Faria-Neto, H.C. (2003). Synergism between platelet-activating factor-like phospholipids and peroxisome proliferator-activated receptor gamma agonists generated during low density lipoprotein oxidation that induces lipid body formation in leukocytes. *The Journal of Immunology*, VOL. 171, pp.2090-2098, 0022-1767

De Lira, G.A.; De Andrade, L.M.; Florencio, K.C.; Da Silva, M.S.; Barbosa-Filho, J.M. & Leitao Da-Cunha, E.V. (2002). Roraimine: a bisbenzylisoquinoline alkaloid from *Cissampelos sympodialis* roots. *Fitoterapia*, VOL. 73, pp. 356-358, 0367-326X

Dybendal, T.; Guttormsen, A.B.; Elsayed, S.; Askeland, B.; Harboe, T. & Florvaag, E. (2003). Screening for mast cell tryptase and serum IgE antibodies in 18 patients with anaphylactic shock during general anaesthesia. *International Archives of Allergy and Immunology*, VOL. 47, pp. 1211-1218, 1018-2438

Ding, A.H.; Nathan, C.F. & Stuehr, D.J. (1988). Release of reactive nitrogen intermediates and reactive oxygen intermediates from mouse peritoneal macrophages. Comparison of activating cytokines and evidence for independent production. *The Journal of Immunology*, VOL. 141, pp. 2407-2412, 0022-1767

Diniz, M.F.F.M.; Melo, A.F.M.; Santos, H.B.; Silva, V.B. & Medeiros, I.A. (2004). Pre-clinical toxicological acute assays with the leaves of *Cissampelos sympodialis* Eichl in mice. *Revista Brasileira de Ciências da Saúde*, VOL. 8, pp. 135-142, 1415-2177

Freitas, M.R.; Cortes, S.F.; Thomas, G. & Barbosa Filho, J.M. (1996). Modification of Ca2+ metabolism in the rabbit aorta as a mechanism of spasmolytic action of warifteine, a bisbenzylisoquinoline alkaloid isolated from the leaves of *Cissampelos sympodialis* Eichl. (Menispermaceae). *The Journal of Pharmacy and Pharmacology*, VOL. 48, pp. 332-336, 0022-3573

Freitas, M.R.; Lemos, V.S.; Queiroga, C.E.; Thomas, G.; Medeiros, I.A. & Cortes, S.F. (2000). Mechanisms of the contractile effect of the hydroalcoholic extract of *Cissampelos sympodialis* Eichl. in the rat aorta. *Phytomedicine*, VOL. 7, pp. 63-67, 0944-7113.

Fonacier, L. S.; Dreskin S.C. & Leung D.Y.M. (2010). Allergic skin diseases. *Journal of Allergy and Clinical Immunology*, VOL. 125, pp.138-149, 1528-4050

Foster, B.; Foroughi, S.; Yin, Y.; Prussin, C. (2011). Effect of anti-IgE therapy on food allergen specific T cell responses in eosinophil associated gastrointestinal disorders. *Clinical and Molecular Allergy*. VOL. 9, pp.1-8.

Funk, C.D. Prostaglandins and Leukotrienes: Advances in Eicosanoid Biology. (2001). *Science,*VOL. 294, pp. 1871- 1875, 0036-8075

Gleich, G.J.; Adolphson C.R. & Leiferman, K.M. (1993). The biology of the eosinophilic leukocyte. *Annual Review of Medicine*, VOL.44, pp.85–101, 0066-4219

Gorinsky, C.; Luscombe, D.K. & Nicholls, P.J. (1972). Neuromuscular blocking and local anaesthetic activities of warifteine hydrochloride, an alkaloid isolated from Cissampelos ovalifolia D.C. *The journal of Pharmacy Pharmacology*. VOL. 24, pp.147-148, 0022-3573

Harizi, H.; Corcuff, J.B. & Gualde, N. (2008). Arachidonic-acid-derived eicosanoids: roles in biology and immunopathology. *Trends in Molecular Medicine* VOL. 14, pp. 461-469, 1471-4914

Inagaki, N.; Igeta, K.; Kim, J.F.; Nagao, M.; Shiraishi, N.; Nakamura, N. & Nagai, H. (2002). Involvement of unique mechanisms in the induction of scratching behavior in BALB/c mice by compound 48/80. *European Journal of Pharmacology*, VOL. 448, pp. 175- 183, 0014-2999

Jacoby, D.B.; Gleich, G.J. & Fryer, A.D. (1993). Human eosinophil major basic protein is an endogenous allosteric antagonist at the inhibitory muscarinic M2 receptor. The *Journal of Clinical Investigation*, VOL. 91, pp. 1314-1318, 0021-9738.

Jarjour N.N.; Wilson S.J., Koenig S.M.; Laviolette, M.; Moore W. C.; Davis, W.B.; Doherty, D.E.; Hamid, Q.; Israel, E.; Kavuru M.S.; Ramsdell, J.W.; Tashkin, D. P.; Reilly, D.S.; Yancey S.W.; Edwards, L.D.; Stauffer, J.L.; Dorinsky, P. M. & Djukanovic, R. (2006). Control of airway inflammation maintained at a lower steroid dose with 100/50 mg of fluticasone propionate/salmeterol. *Journal of Allergy and Clinical Immunology,* VOL. 118, pp. 44-52, 0091-6749.

Kambe, N.; Nakamura, Y.; Saito, M. & Nishikomori, R. (2010). The Inflammasome, an Innate Immunity Guardian, Participates in Skin Urticarial Reactions and Contact Hypersensitivity. *Allergology International*, VOL. 59, pp. 105-113, 1323-8930

Kanaoka, Y. & Boyce, J.A. Cysteinyl leukotrienes and their receptors: cellular distribution and function in immune and inflammatory responses. (2004). *The Journal of Immunology*, VOL. 173, pp. 1503-1510, 0022-1767

Kupchan, S.M.; Patel, A.C. & Fujita, E. (1965). Tumor inhibitors. VI. Cissampareine, new cytotoxic alkaloid from *Cissampelos pareira*. Cytotoxicity of bisbenzylisoquinoline alkaloids. *Journal of Pharmaceutical Sciences*, VOL. 54, pp. 580-583, 0022-3549

Lampinen, M.; Carlson, M.; Hakansson, L.D. & Venge, P. (2004). Cytokine-regulated accumulation of eosinophils in inflammatory disease. *Allergy*, VOL. 59, pp. 793-805, 0105-4538.

Larsen, J.S. (2001). Do antihistamines have a role in asthma therapy? *Pharmacotherapy*, VOL. 21, pp. 28-33, 0277-0008

Lazaar, A.L. & Panettieri, R.A. (2004). Pathogenesis and treatment of asthma. Recent advances. *Drug Discovery Today: Disease Mechanisms*, VOL. 1, pp. 111-116, 1740-6765.

Lefebvre, J.S.; Marleau, S.; Milot, V.; Lévesque, T.; Picard, S.; Flamand, N. & Borgeat P. (2010). Toll-like receptor ligands induce polymorphonuclear leukocyte migration: key roles for leukotriene B4 and platelet-activating factor. *The FASEB Journal*, VOL. 24, pp. 637-647, 0892-6638

Maddox, L. & Schwartz, D.A. (2002). The pathophysiology of asthma. *Annual Review of Medicine*, VOL. 53, pp. 477-498, 0066-4219

Maurer, M. & Metz, M. (2005). The status quo and quo vadis of mast cells. *Experimental Dermatololgy*, VOL. 14, pp. 923-929, 0906-6705.

Mayr, S.I.; Zuberi, R.I. & Liu, F.T. (2003). Role of immunoglobulin E and mast cells in murine models of asthma. *Brazilian Journal of Medical and Biological Research*, VOL. 36, pp. 199-205, 0100-879X

Mahn, K.; Ojo, O.O.; Chadwick, G.; Aaronson, P.I.; Ward, J.P.T. & Lee, T.H. (2010). Ca2+ homeostasis and structural and functional remodelling of airway smooth muscle in asthma. *Thorax*, VOL. 65, pp. 547-552, 0040-6376

Melo, P.S.; De Medeiros Cavalcante, H.M.; Barbosa-Filho, J.M.; De Fatima Formiga Melo Diniz, M.; De Medeiros, I.A. & Haun, M. (2003). Warifteine and milonine, alkaloids isolated from *Cissampelos sympodialis* Eichl: cytotoxicity on rat hepatocyte culture and in V79 cells. *Toxicology Letters*, VOL. 142, pp. 143-151, 0378-4274.

Mesquita-Santos, F. P.; Vieira-De-Abreu, A.; Calheiros, A. S.; Figueiredo, I. H.; Castro-Faria-Neto, H. C.; Weller, P. F.; Bozza P. T.; Diaz, B. L. & Bandeira-Melo, C. (2006). Cutting edge: prostaglandin D2 enhances leukotriene C4 synthesis by eosinophils during allergic inflammation: synergistic in vivo role of endogenous eotaxin. *Journal of Immunology*, VOL. 176, pp. 1326-1330, 0022-1767

Mond, J.J.; Vos, Q.; Lees, A. & Snapper, C.M. (1995). T cell independent antigens. *Current Opinion in Immunology*, VOL. 3, pp. 349-354, 0952-7915.

Moneret-Vautrin, D. A.; Mertes, P. M. (2010). Anaphylaxis to general anesthetics. *Chemical Immunology and Allergy*. VOL. 95, pp. 180-189.

Moore, K. W.; De Waal R. M.; Coffman R. L. & O'garra, A. (2001). Interleukin-10 and the interleukin-10 receptor. *Annual Review of Immunology*. VOL. 19, pp.683-765, 0732-0582

Munitz, A.; Brandt, E. B.; Mingler, M.; Finkelman, F.D. & Rothenberg, M.E. (2008). Distinct roles for IL-13 and IL-4 via IL-13 receptor I and the type II IL-4 receptor in asthma pathogenesis. *Proceedings of the National Academy of Sciences of the United States of America*, VOL. 105, pp. 7240-7245, 0027-8424

Myklebust, J.H.; Josefsen, D.; Blomhoff, H.K.; Levy, K.; Finn, O.; Naderi, S.; Reed, J.C. & Smeland, E.B. (1999). Activation of cAMP signaling pathway increases apoptosis in human B precursor cells and is associated with down regulation of Mcl-1 expression. *Journal of Cellular Physiology*, VOL. 180, pp. 71-80, 1097-4652

Nakagome, K. & Nagata, M. (2011). Pathogenesis of airway inflammation in bronchial asthma. *Auris Nasus Larynx*, VOL. 38, pp. 555–563, 0385-8146

O'Byrne, P.M. Allergen-induced airway inflammation and its therapeutic intervention. (2009). *Allergy, asthma & immunology research*, VOL. 1, pp.3-9, 2092-7355

Onai, N.; Tsunokawa, Y.; Suda, M.; Watanabe, N.; Nakamura, K.; Sugimoto, Y. & Kobayashi, Y. (1995). Inhibitory effects of bisbenzylisoquinoline alkaloids on induction of proinflammatory cytokines, interleukin-1 and tumor necrosis factor-alpha. *Planta Medica*, VOL. 61, pp. 497-501, 0032-0943.

Ono, E.; Taniguchi M.; Mita H.; Higashi N.; Fukutomi Y.; Tanimoto H.; Sekiya K.; Oshikata C.; Tsuburai, T.; Tsurikisawa, N.; Otomo M.; Maeda, Y.; Matsuno O.; Miyazaki E.; Kumamoto, T. & Akiyama, K. (2008). Increased urinary leukotriene E4 concentration in patients with eosinophilic pneumonia. *European Respiratory Journal*, VOL. 32, pp. 437–442, 0903-1936

Peng, S.L. Signaling in B cells via Toll-like receptors. (2005). *Current Opinion in Immunology* VOL. 17, pp. 230–236, 0952-7915

Piuvezam, M.R.; Pecanha, L.M.; Alexander, J. & Thomas, G. (1999). *Cissampelos sympodialis* Eichl. leaf extract increases the production of IL-10 by concanavalin-A-treated BALB/c spleen cells. *Journal of Ethnopharmacology*, VOL. 67, pp. 93-101, 0378-8741

Priel, B.; Heimer, D.; Rabinowitz, B. & Hendler, N. (1994). Perceptions of asthma severity: the role of negative affectivity. *The Journal of Asthma*, VOL. 31, pp. 479-484, 0277-0903

Pumphrey, R. Anaphylaxis: can we tell who is at risk of a fatal reaction? (2004). *Current Opinion in Allergy and Clinical Immunology*, VOL. 4, pp.285-290, 1528-4050

Rhodes, D.G. (1975). A revision of the genus Cissampelos. *Phytologia*, VOL. 30, pp. 415-485, 0031-9430.

Rocha, J.D.B.; Decoté-Ricardo, D.; Redner, P.; Lopes, U.G.; Barbosa-Filho J.M.; Piuvezam, M.R.; Arruda- Hinds, L. & Peçanha, L.M.T. (2010). Effect of the alkaloid warifteine purified from *Cissampelos sympodialis* on B lymphocyte function *in vitro*. *Planta Medica*, VOL. 76 (4), pp.325-330.

Rothenberg, M.E. (1998). Eosinophilia. *The New England journal of medicine*, VOL. 338, pp. 1592-1600, 0028-4793.

Rothenberg, M.E. & Hogan, S.P. (2006). The Eosinophil. *Annual Review of Immunology*, VOL. 24, pp.147-74. 0732-0582.

Sausenthaler. S.; Heinrich, J. & Koletzko, S. (2011). Early diet and the risk of allergy: what can we learn from the prospective birth cohort studies GINIplus and LISAplus? *The American Journal of Clinical Nutrition. ajcn.001180; First published online May 4, 2011.*

Seidel, S.; Voller, B.; Geusau, A. & Wöhrl, S. (2010). Severe anaphylaxis to hymenoptera stings: does the basal serum tryptase concentration really matter? *Annals of Allergy, Asthma and Immunology*. VOL. 105, pp. 185-187.

Schnyder-Candrian, S.; Togbe, D.; Couillin, I.; Mercier, Isabelle.; Brombacher, F.; Quesniaux, V.; Fossiez, F. ; Ryff, B. & Schnyder, B. (2006). Interleukin-17 is a negative regulator of established allergic asthma. The *Journal of Experimental Medicine*, VOL. 203, pp. 2715-2725, 0022-1007.

Sherwood, E. R. & Toliver-Kinsky, T. Mechanisms of the inflammatory response. (2004). *Best Practice & Research Clinical Anaesthesiology*, VOL.18, pp. 385–405, 1521-6896

Sicherer, S.H. Epidemiology of food allergy. (2011). *Journal of Allergy and Clinical Immunology*, VOL. 127, pp.594-602, 1528-4050

Sicherer, S.H. & Leung, D.Y. (2004). Advances in allergic skin disease, anaphylaxis, and hypersensitivity reactions to foods, drugs, and insect stings. *Journal of Allergy and Clinical Immunology*, VOL. 114, pp. 118-124, 0091-6749.

Sicherer, S.H. & Leung, D.Y. (2011). Advances in allergic skin disease, anaphylaxis, and hypersensitivity reactions to foods, drugs, and insects in 2010. *Journal of Allergy and Clinical Immunology*, VOL. 137, pp. 326-335, 0091-6749.

Snapper, C.M. & Paul, W.E. (1987). B cell stimulatory factor-1 (interleukin-4) prepares resting murine B cells to secrete IgG1 upon subsequent stimulation with bacterial lipopolysaccharide. *The Journal of Immunology*, VOL. 139, pp. 10-17, 0022-1767

Somlyo, A.P. & Somlyo, A.V. (1994). Smooth muscle: excitation-contraction coupling, contractile regulation, and the cross-bridge cycle. *Alcoholism: clinical and experimental research*, VOL. 18, pp. 138-143, 0145-6008

Sur, R.N. & Pradhan, S.N. (1964). Studies on Cissampelos Alkaloids. I. Action of Hayatin Derivatives on the Central Nervous System of Cats and Dogs. *Archives Internationales de Pharmacodynamie et de Therapie* , VOL. 152, pp. 106-114, 0003-9780

Takatsu K. & Nakajima H. IL-5 and eosinophilia. (2008). *Current Opinion in Immunology*, VOL.20, pp.288–294, 0952-7915

Teixeira, L.K.; Fonseca, B.P.; Barboza, B.A. & Viola, J.P. (2005). The role of interferon-gamma on immune and allergic responses. *Memórias do Instituto Oswaldo Cruz*, VOL. 100, pp. 137-144, 0074-0276

Terashima, T.; Amakawa, K.; Matsumaru, A.; Yamaguchi, K. (2002). Correlation between cysteinyl leukotriene release from leukocytes and clinical response to a leukotriene inhibitor. *Chest*, VOL. 122, pp. 1566-1570, 0012-3692

Teo, S–L.; Gerez, I.F.A. & Ang, E.Y. (2009) Food-dependent Exercise-induced Anaphylaxis – A Review of 5 Cases. *Annals of the Academy of Medicine, Singapore*. VOL. 38, pp. 905-909, ISSN

Thomas, G.; Araújo, C.C.; Duarte, J.C.; De Souza, D.P. (1997a). Bronchodilator activity of an aqueous fraction of an ethanol extract of the leaves of *Cissampelos sympodialis* Eichl. (Menispermaceae) in the guinea pig. *Phytomedicine*, VOL. 4, pp. 233-238, 0944-7113.

Thomas, G.; Araújo, C.C.; Agra, M.F. & Diniz, M.F.F. (1995). Preliminary studies on the hydroalcoholic extract of the root of *Cissampelos sympodialis* Eichl in guinea-pig tracheal strips and bronchoalveolar leukocytes. *Phytotherapy Research*, VOL. 9, pp. 473-477, 0951-418X.

Thomas, G.; Burnes, F.; Pyne, S. & Pyne, N.J. (1997b). Characterization of the extract from the leaves of *Cissampelos sympodialis* Eichl. (Menispermaceae) on spontaneous tone of isolated trachea, cyclic nucleotide phosphodiesterase activity and intracellular cAMP. *Phytotherapy research*, VOL. 11, pp. 496-499, 0951-418X.

Thomas, G.; Selak, M. & Henson, P.M. (1999). Effects of the aqueous fraction of the ethanol extract of the leaves of *Cissampelos sympodialis* Eichl. in human neutrophils. *Phytotherapy research*, VOL. 13, pp. 9-13, 0951-418X.

Torgersen, K.M.; Vang, T.; Abrahamsen, H.; Yaqub, S. & Tasken, K. (2002). Molecular mechanisms for protein kinase-A mediated modulation of immune function. *Cellular Signalling*, VOL. 14, pp. 1-9, 0898-6568

Vos, Q.; Lees, A.;Wu, Z.Q.; Snapper, C.M. & Mond, J.J. (2000) B cell activation by T cell independent type 2 antigen as an integral part of the humoral immune response to pathogenmicroorganisms. *Immunological Reviews*; VOL. 176, pp. 154–170, 0105-2896

Valent, P.; Horny, H.P.; Triggiani, M. & Arock. M. (2011). Clinical and Laboratory Parameters of Mast Cell Activation as Basis for the Formulation of Diagnostic Criteria. *International Archives of Allergy and Immunology* VOL. 156, pp. 119–127, 1018-2438

Vieira-De-Abreu, A.; Assis, E.F.; Gomes, G.S.; Castro-Faria-Neto, H.C.; Weller, P.F.; Bandeira-Melo, C. & Bozza, P.T. Allergic challenge-elicited lipid bodies compartmentalize in vivo leukotriene C4 synthesis within eosinophils. (2005). *American Journal of Respiratory Cell and Molecular Biology*, VOL. 33, pp. 254-261, 1044-1549

Weller, P.F. Human eosinophils. (1997). *Journal of Allergy and Clinical Immunology*, VOL. 100, pp.283–287, 0091-6749.

Wong, W.S.F. & Koh, D.S.K. (2000). Advances in immunopharmacology of asthma. *Biochemical Pharmacology*, VOL. 59, pp. 1323-1355, 0006-2952

12

Pharmaceutical Treatment of Asthma Symptoms in Elite Athletes – Doping or Therapy

Jimmi Elers and Vibeke Backer
Copenhagen University,
Denmark

1. Introduction

According to the World Health Organization (WHO), 300 million people suffer from asthma, a disease which is increasing in western societies, and furthermore asthma is the most common chronic disease among children, adolescents and young adults. A steady increase in the prevalence of asthma, has been seen in most countries in recent decades (Thomsen et al 2011) and the higher frequency of asthma in young people may partly explain the high frequency found in elite athletes – although both frequency of asthma symptoms and use of anti-asthmatic medication are different than expected. Moreover, the frequency of airway hyperresponsiveness (AHR) in elite athletes is higher than expected as well as the frequency of asthma-like symptoms (cough, wheeze, shortness of breath and chest tightness) which might be caused by exhaustive ventilation, but the pathogenesis is still unknown.

The frequency of asthma among the general population is around 7-10%; whereas the frequency of asthma among elite athletes is found to be higher, especially among endurance athletes (Pedersen et al 2008b). It seems as asthma is something they gain, as only one third of Olympic athletes had childhood asthma. Although asthma among the general public is a permanent phenomenon, it seems to be different in elite athletes, as asthma apparently disappeared after retiring from the sport (Fitch et al 2008).

2. Asthma among athletes

Asthma is a chronic respiratory condition classically characterised by airway inflammation and airway hyperresponsiveness (AHR) to multiple stimuli (Anderson et al 2009). AHR is defined as a pathological bronchoconstrictive response to a given stimulus . AHR to a direct stimulus (e.g. methacholine) acts through airway smooth muscles and the response is thought to be independent of airway inflammation. Whereas response to an indirect stimulus (e.g. exercise, hyperventilation, mannitol) acts through a release of inflammatory mediators, such as histamine, prostaglandins, and leukotrienes, which causes contraction of the airway smooth muscle cells. Airway inflammation in asthma is characterised by inflammatory cells, such as eosinophils, mast cells, and macrophages. The inflammation causes remodelling of the basal membrane, enlargement of the mass of smooth muscles, and disturbance of the surface area. Permanent use of controller therapy with inhaled steroids (ICS) is needed in asthma, as well as relief therapy with short-acting beta$_2$-agonists (SABA), long-acting beta$_2$-agonists (LABA) or others.

Elite athletes, with or without asthma, have asthma-like symptoms during their training season, especially cough, phlegm and shortness of breath is a dominant complain among athletes (Lund et al 2009). Furthermore, athletes are more often found with AHR to direct stimuli and less to direct stimuli than found in normal subjects thus suggesting a respiratory illness. Variation in action of the different provocative agents is related to the fact that response to an indirect challenge would reflect an ongoing inflammation better than would direct tests, and perhaps thus reflect the presence of classical asthma, whereas AHR to direct agents indicates airway smooth muscle dysfunction and, in some cases, asthma (Pedersen et al 2008a, Sue-Chu et al 2010).

The definition of asthma includes respiratory symptoms, variable airway obstruction and airway hyperresponsiveness to multiple agents. The respiratory symptoms in patients with common asthma and the elite athletes with or without asthma are similar, which leave a diagnostic problem in these cases where symptoms are the single diagnostic parameter available. Whereas, the differences between common asthma and asthma among elite athletes are predominantly related to the airway responsiveness to inhaled agents, the day-to-day variability of lung function as well as the content of the inflammatory cells which predominantly are neutrophilic cells and not eosinophilic.

3. Exercise-induced asthma and bronchoconstriction in elite athletes

Exercise-induced bronchoconstriction (EIB) is an acute, transient narrowing of the airway that occurs during and particularly after exercise. In most scientific papers, exercise-induced asthma (EIA) are defined as respiratory symptoms and a significant reduction in FEV1 after exercise, i.e. Δ FEV$_1$ $\geq$ 10%, whereas EIB is a significant reduction in FEV1 ($\geq$10%) when tested, independent of symptoms or not. In population samples, the prevalence of EIB (16%) is the same as the findings of AHR to histamine (16%), although only 6% had responsiveness to both test (Backer et al 1992). EIB is believed to be more specific to asthma, but less sensitive, as the number of false negative results is a problem when research and clinical situations settings are evaluated (Anderson & Kippelen 2005). The frequency of AHR is frequently found above 40%, which is higher than the frequency of asthma. Elite athletes claim that exercise is the most prominent trigger of asthma symptoms, as they very seldom complain of respiratory symptoms at rest or during the night.

The pathogenesis of asthma-like symptoms in elite athletes is multifactorial, and is not completely understood. However, deep, exhaustive ventilation during exercise brings atmospheric air which is cold and dry and this manoeuvre overcomes the ability of the upper airways to warm up and humidify the air reaching the smaller airways(Anderson & Kippelen 2005). This brings about airway narrowing due to osmotic and thermal evaporative water loss, and some vascular involvement. These airway differences, together with some degree of inflammation, lead to a respiratory condition described as EIB or sports asthma. This abnormal response is most often found in endurance sports, such as cross-country skiing , swimming, rowing, cycling, fast-track skating and long distance running.

The symptoms of exercise-induced bronchoconstriction range from mild impairment of performance with minor reduction in lung function after exercise to severe bronchospasm with large reduction in FEV$_1$. In athletes, however, the most common symptoms include cough, wheezing, chest tightness, dyspnoea, and fatigue. These symptoms are frequently found in healthy subjects, subjects with asthma, subjects who are not in good condition and sometimes in subjects suffering from an extrathoracal disorder such as vocal cord dysfunction (VCD).

In conclusion, the most frequent complaint among healthy and diseased athletes is respiratory symptoms during exercise. Furthermore, healthy elite athletes often have AHR with a pattern which differ from the general asthma patient. Lastly, the types of cells involved in the inflammation are different from those in normal asthmatics.

4. Diseases mimicking exercise-induced asthma

Not all that wheezes is asthma. When the diagnosis of asthma is based on respiratory symptoms alone, misdiagnosis may occur. Patients may present with respiratory distress, such as wheezy, when experiencing a low level of fitness, a psychological condition, inhalation of airborne irritants, rhinosinusitis, or gastroesophageal reflux disease. Moreover, exercise-induced symptoms can occur as periodic occurance of laryngeal obstruction (POLO) or exercise induced laryngeal obstruction (EILO) and present with asthma like symptoms. These diseases include conditions such as vocal cord dysfunction (VCD), exercise-induced paradoxical arytenoid motion (EPAM), exercise-induced laryngomalacia (EIL), exercise-induced laryngochalasia, angioedema, vocal cord tumours, and vocal cord paralysis. There seems to be a substantial overlap between EILO and EIA, at least in elite athletes. It could be of minor importance, but it could also have a major influence on the diagnostic procedure in the daily care settings of those with asthma-like symptoms. When POLO/EILO is misdiagnosed as asthma, patient are erroneously treated with anti-asthma therapy, even high doses because of "resistant disease".

These diseases are easily recognized by performing a Flow/Volume curve where a classical cutoff of the inspiratory loop is apparent. On the other hand, a specific diagnose of the actual pathology need laryngeal examination during exercise. The definitive diagnosis of laryngeal obstruction might require laryngoscopy during strenuous exercise. Heimdal et al (Heimdal et al 2006) recently published a paper describing a model for use when performing the continuous laryngoscopy exercise test (CLE). Patients with asthma should start asthma medication, and for those with satisfactory adherence who do not achieve well-controlled disease, other reasons for persistent respiratory symptoms should be explored. In such cases CLE should be performed.

5. Treatment

Treatment of elite athletes with asthma can be divided into non-pharmacological and pharmacological treatment. During the last decades the International Olympic Committee (IOC) increased their focus on the increasing use of anti-asthmatic medication by Olympic and other elite athletes. At the 1996 Olympic Games in Atlanta 3.7% of the athletes used beta2-agonists, 5.6% at the 1998 Winter Games in Nagano, and 5.7% at the Sydney Games 2000. The IOC and the World Anti Doping Agency (WADA) have had many changes in the anti-doping regulations on beta2-agonists through the years, partly due to concerns regarding ergogenic effects and partly because of health risk concerns. Due to the increased use of beta2-agonists as mentioned above the IOC introduced a criterion of demonstration of asthma by an objective measure of reversibility or bronchial airway hyperresponsiveness in order approved use of beta2-agonist. This resulted in a 27% reduction in the use of beta2-agonists in the 2004 Games in Athen.

5.1 Pharmacological treatment

Treatment of asthma and exercise-induced bronchoconstriction (EIB) in elite athletes should follow international asthma treatment guidelines like the Global Initiative for Asthma (GINA), see Figure 1 (Bateman et al 2008). The main purpose of pharmacotherapy is control of asthma symptoms, reducing airway inflammation and airway hyperresponsiveness, achieving normal lung function, and prevent exacerbations

Step1	Step2	Step3	Step4	Step5
	Asthma education	and	Environmental control	
Short-acting beta2-agonist as needed		Short-acting beta2-agonist as needed		
	Select one	Select one	Select one	Select one
	Low-dose inhaled corticosteroid	Low-dose inhaled corticosteroid + Long acting beta2-agonist	Medium or high-dose inhaled corticosteroid + Long acting beta2-agonist	Oral glucocorticosteroid
	Leukotriene modifier	Medium or high-dose inhaled corticosteroid	Leukotriene modifier	Anti-IgE treatment
		Low-dose inhaled corticosteroid + Leukotriene modifier	Theophylline	
		Low-dose inhaled corticosteroid + Theophylline		

Fig. 1. Management approach. Adapted from GINA.

5.2 Beta2-agonists

Inhaled short acting beta2-agonists (SABA), e.g. salbutamol and terbutaline, are first choice therapy for fast relief of EIB. Moreover, SABA is useful in preventing EIB if taken 15 minutes before exercise. Frequent and increased use indicates uncontrolled asthma and should result in reassessment of treatment strategies. Side effects are tremor, tachycardia, palpitations and headache, which increase in frequency and intensity with higher doses. With high systemic doses hypopotassemia and muscle convulsions can occur. Systemic use of beta2-agonists by elite athletes is entirely prohibited according to the Prohibited List, see Table 1.

Inhaled long acting beta2-agonists (LABA), e.g. salmeterol and formoterol, are used in management of uncontrolled asthma treated with inhaled corticosteroid alone. LABA is used as add-on therapy to inhaled corticosteroids, either as fixed combination or in two separate devices. LABA should never be used as monotherapy in asthma due to risk of serious adverse events with increased risk of mortality in case of exacerbation. In a review from 2005 it was concluded that combined fluticasone and salmeterol was superior to fluticasone as monotherapy in preventing EIA. Furthermore, in a randomized, double-blinded study combined budesonide/formoterol was compared with budesonide alone, asthma control was better with reduced symptoms when treated with combination of budesonide/formoterol. A new study from 2010 confirms previous findings with more efficacy when inhaled budesonide is combined with formoterol among adults and adolescents with moderate to severe asthma. These findings indicate that it is not an effect related to the specific drug, but a class effect of the combination.

I SUBSTANCES AND METHODS PROHIBITED AT ALL TIMES (IN- AND OUT-OF-COMPETITION):

S0. Non-approved substances
S1. Anabolic agents
S2. Peptide hormones, growth factors and related substances
S3. Beta2-agonists
S4. Hormone antagonists and modulators
S5. Diuretics and other masking agents
M1. Enhancement of oxygen transfer
M2. Chemical and physical manipulation
M3. Gene doping

II SUBSTANCES AND METHODS PROHIBITED IN-COMPETITION:

S0-5 and M1-3 defined above
S6. Stimulants
S7. Narcotics
S8. Cannabinoids
S9. Glucocorticosterooids

III SUBSTANCES PROHIBITED IN PARTICULAR SPORTS:

P1. Alcohol
P2. Beta-Blockers

Table 1. The 2011 Prohibited List by World Anti-Doping Agency.

It is well known that regular use of beta2-agonist could lead to development of tolerance to bronchodilation (i.e. reduced bronchodilator response during acute asthma) and bronchoprotection (i.e. reduced ability to prevent exercise-induced bronchoconstriction). Tolerance to bronchodilator develops rapidly, after only few doses, and regardless of ongoing treatment with inhaled corticosteroid. Tolerance to bronchoprotection develops after few weeks of treatment and regardless of ongoing treatment with inhaled corticosteroids. The decreased bronchoprotection might result in increased use of beta2-

agonist and higher risk of side effects. Though theoretical concerns that regular beta2-agonist treatment may lead to tolerance and failure to respond to emergency asthma treatment, there is little evidence that this is a clinical problem. However, as elite athletes exercise daily and often several times a day, use of beta2-agonists, either before exercise to prevent bronchoconstriction or during/after due to bronchoconstriction, would exceed the maximal recommend weekly use in the GINA guidelines, indicating that other treatment strategies than SABA in case of EIB are needed.

5.3 Inhaled corticosteroids

Inhaled corticosteroids (ICS) are the most used and most effective inhaled anti-inflammatory drug available. ICS improves asthma symptoms, self-reported quality of life and lung function, reduces airway inflammation and airway hyperresponsiveness and furthermore, ICS has been found to reduce number and severity of exacerbations and asthma mortality (Jeffery et al 1992, Suissa et al 2000). GINA guidelines recommend ICS when asthma is uncontrolled with non-pharmacological interventions and rescue therapy alone. Effects are observed after 7-14 days, while full effects are seen after eight weeks of treatment.

Our current knowledge about effects of ICS on exercise-induced bronchoconstriction is based on adults and children with asthma. Existing studies ranges from three weeks to two years duration of treatment, mostly conducted in a parallel design. A study with 40 adult asthmatic subjects randomized to 6 weeks treatment with placebo or 800 micrograms budesonide twice a day showed a post-exercise fall in FEV_1 of 7% in the budesonide group and to 22% in the placebo group. Similar findings are reported in asthmatic children.

5.4 Leukotriene modifiers

Leukotriene modifiers have anti-inflammatory and bronchodilatory effects. Leukotriene modifiers are administered orally and once daily for montelukast and twice daily for zileuton. Montelukast is used as add-on treatment in case of uncontrolled asthma with medium dose ICS as monotherapy(Lofdahl et al 1999). Prevention of EIA is another indication in elite athletes with asthma. Studies report a reduced post-exercise fall in FEV_1 and a reduced period of bronchoconstriction after exercise when treated with montelukast compared to placebo in non-smoking asthmatic subjects. No studies have reported development of tolerance during regular use.

5.5 Cromoglycate

In a study from 2010 treatment with sodium cromoglycate decreased the FEV_1 fall after a eucapnic voluntary hyperpnoea (EVH) challenge in elite athletes with EIB (Anderson et al 2010). This finding support that release of mast cell mediators is an important factor for the severity of EIB. However, use of cromones in asthmatic elite athletes is limited.

6. Non-pharmacological interventions

Asthmatic athletes with pollen allergy should avoid prolonged outdoor endurance exercise in areas with high pollen counts. Exercise in temperatures below minus 15 degrees Celsius should be avoided, particularly in areas with air pollution or other airway irritants.

Few studies have investigated correlation between physical warm-up and degree of EIA in asthmatic athletes and a warm-up period has been shown to induce refractoriness to

EIA without itself inducing significant bronchoconstriction. The protective effect of different types of warm-up has been compared in controlled studies, but no consensus is found. Different study protocols and designs make it difficult to compare the existing studies, but physical warm-up in some form and extent seems generally to have a protective effect on EIA, and physical warm-up should be advised for all athletes with asthma. Breathing filters may reduce EIB among those exercising in cold conditions. A study from 2000 compared response to exercise in cold air (decrease in FEV_1) in nine patients with EIA when given no treatment, given premedication with a beta2-agonist, wearing a heat-and-moisture-exchanging facemask, and given both premedication and facemask. The mean maximal change in FEV_1 was 27% with no treatment, 12% with facemask, 7% with premedication, and no change with the combination of premedication and facemask. Another study from 2006 examined effects of a heat exchanger mask, placebo mask, and premedication with a beta2-agonist. Five patients with EIA performed a treadmill exercise test while breathing cold air. It was concluded that a heat exchanger mask prevented cold exercise-induced fall in lung function as effectively as treatment with beta2 agonist before exercise in cold air.

During the last decade some research has focused on nutritional factors, especially omega-3-polyunsaturated fatty acids' influence on airway inflammation and exercise-induced bronchoconstriction. A review from 2005 concluded that omega-3-polyunsaturated fatty acid supplementation reduces the degree of exercise-induced bronchoconstriction compared with placebo in patients with EIA. The review was based on a small number of studies with limited range of clinically important outcomes. Further controlled and well-designed research is needed to establish any evidence-based recommendations.

7. Treatment or doping

As mentioned above the IOC and WADA have increased their attention on the status of beta2-agonists on the "The 2010 Prohibited List" (www.wada-ama.org). Until the end of 2009 granting of a Therapeutic Use Exemption (TUE) was necessary for use of inhaled salbutamol, terbutaline, salmeterol and formoterol. From 2010 use of inhaled salbutamol and salmeterol in therapeutic doses are allowed. From 2010 use of inhaled terbutaline and formoterol is still prohibited and requires a TUE and a reasonable explanation of why these drugs are prescribed when other equal drugs are permitted. Use of inhaled corticosteroids in therapeutic doses is permitted, except when used in a fixed combination with formoterol, which requires a TUE. Use of oral or topical antihistamines or leukotriene modifiers is permitted. Use of systemic corticosteroids is prohibited during competition. Systemic intake of beta2-agonist and clenbuterol is strictly prohibited in elite athletes. The criteria for granting a TUE, the "Prohibited List", and guidelines are available on WADA's website (www.wada-ama.org). As the anti-doping legislation and the prohibited list are continually updated, it is important to be familiar with the current regulations before prescribing asthma medication to an elite athlete with asthma. The 2011 Prohibited List is shown in Table 2. For details visit WADA´s website.

In the academic societies of sports and pulmonary medicine it is discussed whether or not beta2-agonists have any ergogenic, i.e. performance enhancing effects, and if it should be considered doping or not. According to the World Anti-Doping Agency (WADA) minimum two of three criteria must be met in order to consider a substance or method for inclusion on the Prohibited List:

1. The substance or method can be performance enhancing
2. The use of the substance or the method can endanger the athlete´s health
3. The use of the substance or method is against the spirit of sport

As it appears a substance or method can be listed without being performance enhancing. Due to health issues the IOC considers inhaled use of beta2-agonist without need unacceptable. Beta2-agonists have received much attention the last decades because of side effects, and few studies have reported and the US Food and Drug Administration have issued some concerns about beta2-agonists and side effects/serious adverse events. Regarding health issues in elite athletes using beta2-agonists the IOC is concerned about athletes using beta2-agonists without need and in supratherapeutic doses. Studies in asthmatic children have shown both significant raised and normal blood levels of myocardial stress markers after inhalation of beta2-agonists in ten times prophylactic doses. Studies with unrestrained rats have documented dose-response myocyte apoptosis after administration of the beta2-agonists formoterol and clenbuterol. Significant changes in human cardiac electrophysiological properties is seen after administration of salbutamol 5 mg as a single dose.

Several studies have investigated the ergogenic effects of inhaled and oral beta2-agonists conducted with healthy well-trained men, most studies in therapeutic doses. The extensive research on therapeutic doses of inhaled beta2-agonsits clearly rules out any ergogenic effects. Only few studies have shown ergogenic effects of inhaled salbutamol, but these are limited by enrolment of recreational subjects. It is now a common opinion that inhaled beta2-agonists in therapeutic doses has no advantageous effects in healthy athletes. However, animal and human studies, where beta2-agonists are given in systemic supra-therapeutic doses daily for few weeks, have shown evidence of improvement of muscle strength and endurance performance. Pluim et al. concluded in a systematic review and meta-analyses of randomized controlled trials on beta2-agonists and physical performance published in 2011 that there is some evidence indicating that systemic beta2-agonists may have a positive effect on physical performance in healthy subjects(Pluim et al 2011). Clenbuterol, another beta2-agonist used in veterinary medicine via prescription as a bronchodilator, cardiotonic and tocolytic agent. However used in supratherapeutic doses in animals and humans it is misused as a growth promotor with anabolic and lipolytic effects.

8. References

[1] Anderson SD, Brannan JD, Perry CP, Caillaud C, Seale JP. 2010. Sodium cromoglycate alone and in combination with montelukast on the airway response to mannitol in asthmatic subjects. *J. Asthma.* 47(4):429-33
[2] Anderson SD, Charlton B, Weiler JM, Nichols S, Spector SL, Pearlman DS. 2009. Comparison of mannitol and methacholine to predict exercise-induced bronchoconstriction and a clinical diagnosis of asthma. *Respir Res.* 10:4
[3] Anderson SD, Kippelen P. 2005. Exercise-induced bronchoconstriction: pathogenesis. *Curr. Allergy Asthma Rep.* 5(2):116-22

[4] Backer V, Ulrik CS, Hansen KK, Laursen EM, Dirksen A, Bach-Mortensen N. 1992. Atopy and bronchial responsiveness in random population sample of 527 children and adolescents. *Ann. Allergy.* 69(2):116-22

[5] Bateman ED, Hurd SS, Barnes PJ, Bousquet J, Drazen JM, FitzGerald M, Gibson P, Ohta K, O'Byrne P, Pedersen SE, Pizzichini E, Sullivan SD, Wenzel SE, Zar HJ. 2008. Global strategy for asthma management and prevention: GINA executive summary. *Eur. Respir J* 31(1):143-78

[6] Fitch KD, Sue-Chu M, Anderson SD, Boulet LP, Hancox RJ, McKenzie DC, Backer V, Rundell KW, Alonso JM, Kippelen P, Cummiskey JM, Garnier A, Ljungqvist A. 2008. Asthma and the elite athlete: summary of the International Olympic Committee's consensus conference, Lausanne, Switzerland, January 22-24, 2008. *J Allergy Clin Immunol.* 122(2):254-60, 260

[7] Heimdal JH, Roksund OD, Halvorsen T, Skadberg BT, Olofsson J. 2006. Continuous laryngoscopy exercise test: a method for visualizing laryngeal dysfunction during exercise. *Laryngoscope* 116(1):52-7

[8] Jeffery PK, Godfrey RW, Adelroth E, Nelson F, Rogers A, Johansson SA. 1992. Effects of treatment on airway inflammation and thickening of basement membrane reticular collagen in asthma. A quantitative light and electron microscopic study. *Am. Rev. Respir. Dis.* 145(4 Pt 1):890-9

[9] Lofdahl CG, Reiss TF, Leff JA, Israel E, Noonan MJ, Finn AF, Seidenberg BC, Capizzi T, Kundu S, Godard P. 1999. Randomised, placebo controlled trial of effect of a leukotriene receptor antagonist, montelukast, on tapering inhaled corticosteroids in asthmatic patients. *BMJ.* 319(7202):87-90

[10] Lund TK, Pedersen L, Anderson SD, Sverrild A, Backer V. 2009. Are asthma-like symptoms in elite athletes associated with classical features of asthma? *Br. J Sports Med.* 43(14):1131-5

[11] Pedersen L, Lund TK, Barnes PJ, Kharitonov SA, Backer V. 2008a. Airway responsiveness and inflammation in adolescent elite swimmers. *J Allergy Clin Immunol.* 122(2):322-7, 327

[12] Pedersen L, Winther S, Backer V, Anderson SD, Larsen KR. 2008b. Airway responses to eucapnic hyperpnea, exercise, and methacholine in elite swimmers. *Med. Sci. Sports Exerc.* 40(9):1567-72

[13] Pluim BM, de Hon O, Staal JB, Limpens J, Kuipers H, Overbeek SE, Zwinderman AH, Scholten RJ. 2011. beta-Agonists and physical performance: a systematic review and meta-analysis of randomized controlled trials. *Sports Med.* 41(1): 39-57

[14] Sue-Chu M, Brannan JD, Anderson SD, Chew N, Bjermer L. 2010. Airway hyperresponsiveness to methacholine, adenosine 5-monophosphate, mannitol, eucapnic voluntary hyperpnoea and field exercise challenge in elite cross-country skiers. *Br. J. Sports Med.* 44(11):827-32

[15] Suissa S, Ernst P, Benayoun S, Baltzan M, Cai B. 2000. Low-dose inhaled corticosteroids and the prevention of death from asthma. *N. Engl. J. Med.* 343(5):332-6

[16] Thomsen SF, van der SS, Kyvik KO, Skytthe A, Skadhauge LR, Backer V. 2011. Increase in the heritability of asthma from 1994 to 2003 among adolescent twins. *Respir. Med.*

Permissions

The contributors of this book come from diverse backgrounds, making this book a truly international effort. This book will bring forth new frontiers with its revolutionizing research information and detailed analysis of the nascent developments around the world.

We would like to thank Celso Pereira, PhD, MD, for lending his expertise to make the book truly unique. He has played a crucial role in the development of this book. Without his invaluable contribution this book wouldn't have been possible. He has made vital efforts to compile up to date information on the varied aspects of this subject to make this book a valuable addition to the collection of many professionals and students.

This book was conceptualized with the vision of imparting up-to-date information and advanced data in this field. To ensure the same, a matchless editorial board was set up. Every individual on the board went through rigorous rounds of assessment to prove their worth. After which they invested a large part of their time researching and compiling the most relevant data for our readers. Conferences and sessions were held from time to time between the editorial board and the contributing authors to present the data in the most comprehensible form. The editorial team has worked tirelessly to provide valuable and valid information to help people across the globe.

Every chapter published in this book has been scrutinized by our experts. Their significance has been extensively debated. The topics covered herein carry significant findings which will fuel the growth of the discipline. They may even be implemented as practical applications or may be referred to as a beginning point for another development. Chapters in this book were first published by InTech; hereby published with permission under the Creative Commons Attribution License or equivalent.

The editorial board has been involved in producing this book since its inception. They have spent rigorous hours researching and exploring the diverse topics which have resulted in the successful publishing of this book. They have passed on their knowledge of decades through this book. To expedite this challenging task, the publisher supported the team at every step. A small team of assistant editors was also appointed to further simplify the editing procedure and attain best results for the readers.

Our editorial team has been hand-picked from every corner of the world. Their multi-ethnicity adds dynamic inputs to the discussions which result in innovative outcomes. These outcomes are then further discussed with the researchers and contributors who give their valuable feedback and opinion regarding the same. The feedback is then collaborated with the researches and they are edited in a comprehensive manner to aid the understanding of the subject.

Apart from the editorial board, the designing team has also invested a significant amount of their time in understanding the subject and creating the most relevant covers. They scrutinized every image to scout for the most suitable representation of the subject and create an appropriate cover for the book.

The publishing team has been involved in this book since its early stages. They were actively engaged in every process, be it collecting the data, connecting with the contributors or procuring relevant information. The team has been an ardent support to the editorial, designing and production team. Their endless efforts to recruit the best for this project, has resulted in the accomplishment of this book. They are a veteran in the field of academics and their pool of knowledge is as vast as their experience in printing. Their expertise and guidance has proved useful at every step. Their uncompromising quality standards have made this book an exceptional effort. Their encouragement from time to time has been an inspiration for everyone.

The publisher and the editorial board hope that this book will prove to be a valuable piece of knowledge for researchers, students, practitioners and scholars across the globe.

List of Contributors

Luis Garcia-Marcos and Manuel Sanchez-Solis
University of Murcia, Spain

Lia Fernandes
Department of Psychiatry and Mental Health, Faculty of Medicine, University of Oporto, Psychiatry Service of S. João Hospital, Oporto, Portugal

Esther Hafkamp-de Groen and Hein Raat
Erasmus MC-University Medical Center Rotterdam, The Netherlands

Anne-Judith Waligora-Dupriet and Marie-José Butel
EA 4065 Département Périnatalité, Microbiologie, Médicament, Faculté des Sciences Pharmaceutiques et Biologiques, Université Paris Descartes, Sorbonne Paris Cité, France

Akio Matsuda and Kyoko Futamura
Department of Allergy and Immunology, National Research Institute for Child Health and Development, Tokyo, Japan

Clayton MacDonald and Marianna Kulka
Institute for Nutriscience and Health, National Research Council, Canada

Celso Pereira, Graça Loureiro, Beatriz Tavares and Filomena Botelho
Immunoallergology Department, Coimbra University Hospital, Portugal

Elaine A. Cruz and Michelle F. Muzitano
Faculdade de Farmacia, Macae Campus, Universidade Federal do Rio de Janeiro, Brazil

Sonia S. Costa
Nucleo de Pesquisa de Produtos Naturais, Universidade Federal do Rio de Janeiro, Brazil

Bartira Rossi-Bergmann
Instituto de Biofísica Carlos Chagas Filho, Universidade Federal do Rio de Janeiro, Brazil

C.A. Araujo
Department of Immunology, St Jude Children's Research Hospital, Memphis, TN, USA

M.F. Macedo-Soares
Laboratory of Immunopathology, Butantan Institute, Sao Paulo, SP, Brazil

Hak Sun Yu
Department of Parasitology, School of Medicine, Pusan National University, Yangsan-si, South Korea

M.R. Piuvezam, C.R. Bezerra-Santos, P.T. Bozza, C. Bandeira-Melo, G. Vieira and H.F. Costa
Federal University of Paraiba, PB, Oswaldo Cruz Foundation, Rio de Janeiro, RJ, Federal University of Rio de Janeiro, RJ, Brazil

Jimmi Elers and Vibeke Backer
Copenhagen University, Denmark

Printed in the USA
CPSIA information can be obtained
at www.ICGtesting.com
JSHW011435221024
72173JS00004B/814